Pediatric Neuroendocrinology

This book has been printed with financial support from Pfizer Italia

Endocrine Development

Vol. 17

Series Editor

P.-E. Mullis Bern

Workshop, May 17–19, 2009 Villasimius (Cagliari), Italy

Pediatric Neuroendocrinology

Volume Editors

Sandro Loche Cagliari
Marco Cappa Rome
Lucia Ghizzoni Turin
Mohamad Maghnie Genova
Martin O. Savage London

37 figures and 18 tables, 2010

KARGER Basel · Freiburg · Paris · London · New York · Bangalore · Bangkok · Shanghai · Singapore · Tokyo · Sydney

Sandro Loche
Regional Hospital for
Microcytaemia
Cagliari, Italy

Marco Cappa
Department of Pediatrics
Pediatric Hospital Bambino Gesù
Rome, Italy

Lucia Ghizzoni
Division of Endocrinology and
Metabolism
Department of Internal Medicine
University of Turin, Turin, Italy

Mohamad Maghnie
Department of Pediatrics
IRCCS G. Gaslini
University of Genova
Genova, Italy

Martin O. Savage
Department of Endocrinology
John Vane Science Centre
London, UK

Library of Congress Cataloging-in-Publication Data

Pediatric neuroendocrinology / volume editors, Sandro Loche ... [et al.].
p. ; cm. -- (Endocrine development, ISSN 1421-7082 ; v. 17)
Workshop, May 17-19, 2009, Villasimius (Cagliari), Italy.
Includes bibliographical references and indexes.
ISBN 978-3-8055-9032-1 (hardcover : alk. paper)
1. Pediatric neuroendocrinology--Congresses. I. Loche, Sandro. II.
Series: Endocrine development, v. 17. 1421-7082 ;
[DNLM: 1. Puberty--physiology--Congresses. 2. Growth
Hormone--physiology--Congresses. 3. Pituitary-Adrenal
System--physiology--Congresses. W1 EN3635 v. 17 2010 / WS 450 P371 2010]
RJ418.P436 2010
618.92'8--dc22

2009036721

Bibliographic Indices. This publication is listed in bibliographic services, including Current Contents®

Disclaimer. The statements, opinions and data contained in this publication are solely those of the individual authors and contributors and not of the publisher and the editor(s). The appearance of advertisements in the book is not a warranty, endorsement, or approval of the products or services advertised or of their effectiveness, quality or safety. The publisher and the editor(s) disclaim responsibility for any injury to persons or property resulting from any ideas, methods, instructions or products referred to in the content or advertisements.

Drug Dosage. The authors and the publisher have exerted every effort to ensure that drug selection and dosage set forth in this text are in accord with current recommendations and practice at the time of publication. However, in view of ongoing research, changes in government regulations, and the constant flow of information relating to drug therapy and drug reactions, the reader is urged to check the package insert for each drug for any change in indications and dosage and for added warnings and precautions. This is particularly important when the recommended agent is a new and/or infrequently employed drug.

www.karger.com
Printed in Switzerland on acid-free and non-aging paper (ISO 9706) by Reinhardt Druck, Basel
ISSN 1421–7082
ISBN 978–3–8055–9302–1
e-ISBN 978–3–8055–9303–8

Contents

Preface

Pediatric neuroendocrinology is an important field of clinical and scientific interest, which has rarely been addressed as a single entity. Consequently, this is a particularly welcomed volume. In this issue of *Endocrine Development*, an eclectic group of high-quality clinicians and scientists has been assembled to provide focussed updates of their particular fields of interest. The scope of pediatric neuroendocrinology and its potential disturbances is wide and has direct relevance to both pediatric and adult endocrinology, as major pediatric pathology is likely to have implications in adult life.

The principle hypothalamic-pituitary axes with discussion of the neurobiology and its disturbances in a range of topics including neurogenesis, sleep and its abnormalities, sexual differentiation, onset of puberty, and stress are all covered here. The physiology and pathophysiology of ghrelin, leptin and kisspeptin are described as well as the pharmacological effects of modulating the hypothalamo-pituitary-adrenal axis. Contributions with a more clinical orientation include those on disease entities such as abnormal puberty, central adrenal insufficiency, pituitary tumors and Cushing's disease. Advances in investigations such as neuroimaging and the molecular characteristics of pituitary adenomas are provided by the leaders of their respective fields. Finally, two chapters on the extremes of disordered energy balance, namely hypothalamic obesity and anorexia nervosa, highlight the endocrine disturbances in and the therapeutic options for these serious conditions.

This volume covers a wide range of topics in pediatric neuroendocrinology and informs the reader of the latest scientific developments as well as the diagnostic and molecular techniques and therapeutic options available today. We believe that the volume will benefit scientists and clinicians involved in the care of children with neuroendocrine disorders.

S. Loche, M. Cappa, L. Ghizzoni, M. Maghnie, M.O. Savage

Loche S, Cappa M, Ghizzoni L, Maghnie M, Savage MO (eds): Pediatric Neuroendocrinology.
Endocr Dev. Basel, Karger, 2010, vol 17, pp 1–10

The Transcriptome and the Hypothalamo-Neurohypophyseal System

Charles Colin Thomas Hindmarch · David Murphy

Henry Wellcome Laboratories for Integrative Neuroscience and Endocrinology, University of Bristol, Bristol, UK

Abstract

The hypothalamo-neurohypophyseal system (HNS) is a highly specialised region of the brain that is comprised of the magnocellular neurons of the paraventricular (PVN) and supraoptic (SON) nuclei, the axons of which project to the neural lobe of the pituitary. The PVN and the SON are involved in a broad spectrum of activities including, but not restricted to, osmotic regulation, cardiovascular control, parturition and lactation, energy homeostasis and the stress response resulting in a function-related plasticity of these tissues, allowing them the modulation necessary to reply to the physiological demands in an appropriate manner. We hypothesise that the HNS response to physiological stimulation is underpinned by changes in gene transcription. Affymetrix microarrays with 31,099 probes representing the total rat genome, were interrogated with RNA targets from SON, PVN and the neuro-intermediate lobe dissected from naïve rats as well as those responding to physiological and pathological cues. The data generated are comprehensive catalogues of genes that are expressed in each tissue, as well as lists of genes that are differentially regulated following changes in the physiological state of the animal.

The brain is often described as the most complex 'thing' in the universe. That this most complicated 'thing' is the result of a process typified by its simplicity whereby graduated changes in operation provide a substrate for selection pressure is remarkable enough. Even more remarkable is that the complexity of the brain and the animal as a whole is dependant on the information encoded by just 25,000 genes, a number that does not differ significantly between the rat and the human. The plasticity of the genome to respond to changes in the internal and external environment is mediated by the expression of each individual gene, in each cell, in concert. Collectively these transcript expressions may be defined as the transcriptome; the total transcript expression of the genome.

Work in our laboratories has sought to comprehensively catalogue the transcriptome of hypothalamic structures that are involved in osmoregulation. To this end, microarray gene chips have been employed to measure the simultaneous expression levels of the whole genome. Gene chip data rely on the ratio between the hybridisation of labelled target mRNA from a normal and a treated biological unit to multiple probes representing a specific transcript. This ratio is related to the level of mRNA expression between the two units with the signal from each unit being representative of the relative amount of a particular transcript in each condition (fig. 1). The desired end point of the microarray study is not necessarily to determine which genes are being expressed in a particular paradigm (though this is an obvious benefit), but to gain a perspective on the relative expression of each gene simultaneously in response to the paradigm. The hypothesis assumed by microarray experiments is that the biological environment is under transcriptomic control and that co-expression of different gene populations cooperatively maintain the stability of the biological environment.

Osmoregulation

Osmotic stability is aggressively defended in mammalian organisms [1] that must maintain a wet internal environment in a dry external environment; fluids lost through excretion, perspiration or expiration must be replaced quickly. Osmoregulation is a highly conserved mechanism that provides a means by which an organism can maintain a constant prescribed level of water and salts within the intra- and extracellular fluid. The path of least resistance here is a behavioural adaptation to replacing water by actively seeking out water. However, since water is not always readily available, this mechanism is complemented by a physiological approach to limit the amount of water lost in times of osmotic stress. The main mechanism involves the brain peptide hormone vasopressin (Avp) which acts on the kidney to conserve water.

Detection of Hyperosmolality

Dehydration effectively increases the relative concentration of sodium and other electrolytes in the extracellular fluid with the result that water is drawn from cells. Although all cells are subject to this cellular dehydration, certain cells are particularly responsive to it and are able to communicate the change in osmolality to the brain. The subfornical organ (SFO) is a circumventricular organ that is capable of detecting changes in osmotic status, is unprotected by the blood-brain barrier (BBB) and is well connected with the hypothalamus. In contrast with regions protected by the BBB, the SFO is well vascularised with highly fenestrated capillaries allowing effective diffusion of peripheral signals that the SFO can 'taste'. Direct connections between the SFO and the vasopressinergic magnocellular neurons of the supraoptic (SON) and paraventricular (PVN) nuclei have been demonstrated [2]. Moreover, these connections are functionally active and responsive to changes in osmolality since intravenous injection of NaCl in the rat regulates the immediate early gene c-fos mRNA and Fos protein in the SFO, the PVN and the SON.

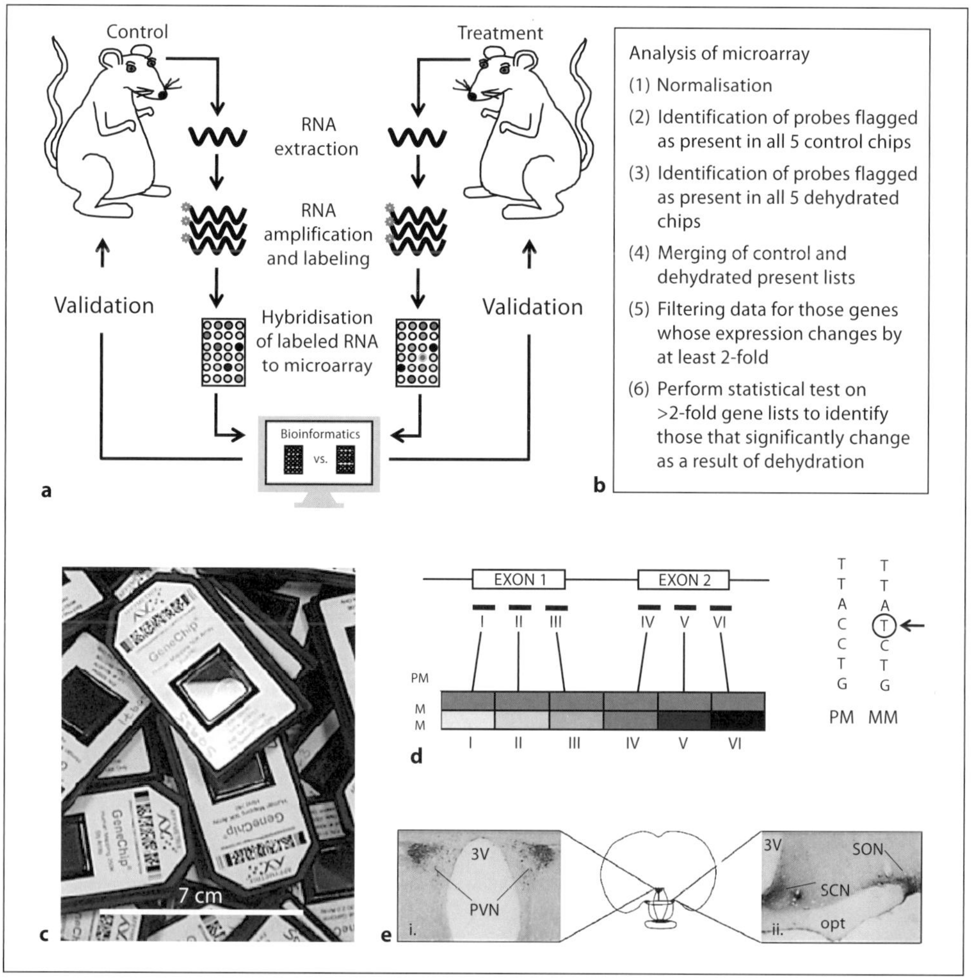

Fig. 1. **a** Typical microarray workflow, where mRNA extracted from tissue dissected from either a control or a treated animal is amplified, labelled and hybridised to a gene chip. Each chip, control or treated, results in signal intensities for each of the genes that are represented on the array. By comparing the signals of control and treated datasets, a signal ratio is generated that can be used for fold-change filtering and statistical testing. Identification of gene targets using bioinformatical approaches are validated using molecular and physiological approaches. **b** A generalised microarray experiment analysis [15]. **c** The Affymetrix GeneChip® Rat Genome 230 2.0 microarray is comprised to 31,099 probesets, representing 30,000 transcripts from over 28,000 rat genes. **d** Each gene is represented by 1 or more probesets. The signal intensity of the probeset is the function of multiple probes that are a perfect match (PM) to the RNA sequence. Each PM sequence is complemented by an mismatch (MM) probe, an identical sequence with a single nucleotide-difference. This MM can be used for signal correction. **e** Immunohistochemistry Dab staining using an anti-vasopressin (Avp) antibody. Avp immunoreactivity can be seen in the (i) lateral magnocellular portion of the paraventricular nucleus (PVN) seated at the top of the 3rd ventricle (3V), and (ii) the supraoptic nucleus (SON) which is at the boundary of the optic tract (opt) and the suprachiasmatic nucleus (SCN) where vasopressingergic neurons are also present.

This Fos expression can be abolished in the PVN and SON but not the SFO when the connection between the SFO and the hypothalamus is severed [3]. Also, destruction of the SFO results in the partial abolishment of osmotically induced Avp release [4]. For total abolishment, however, destruction of the entire lamina terminalis is required [5].

The Hypothalamo-Neurohypopyseal System

The hypothalamo-neurohypophyseal system (HNS) is a highly specialised region of the brain that is comprised of the magnocellular neurons of the PVN and the SON that project their nuclei to the posterior lobe of the pituitary (PP). The PVN and the SON are involved in a broad spectrum of activities including, but not restricted to, osmotic regulation, cardiovascular control, parturition and lactation, energy homeostasis and the stress response [6–10] resulting in a function-related plasticity of these tissues and allowing them the modulation necessary to reply to the physiological demands in an appropriate manner. Seated in a position immediately lateral to the boundary of the optic tract (fig. 1), the SON is a relatively homogeneous population of large (10–40 μm cell body diameter) and densely packed magnocellular neurons, the axons from which proceed to the neural lobe of the pituitary where they terminate [11]. The main known role of the magnocellular neurons is confined to the appropriate synthesis and secretion of two closely related hormones; vasopressin (Avp) and oxytocin (Oxt) that are involved in osmoregulation and reproductive duties, respectively. While the SON is a relatively homogeneous population of MCNs that terminate in a single hypophyseal location, the PVN is a rather more complicated structure. Situated slightly caudal to the SON, the PVN is located on either side of the third ventricle and may be split into eight discrete subdivisions of either large magnocellular or smaller (10–15 μm cell body diameter) parvocellular neurons (fig. 1). The parvocellular neurons project in a more diverse manner than that of the magnocellular neurons, terminating in numerous central sites and therefore being involved in a wide range of biological functions. For example in response to stress, the parvocellular regulation of corticotropin-releasing factor (CRF) and vasopressin together with their subsequent release into the anterior pituitary portal blood system results in adrenal release of glucocorticoids via adrenocorticotropin hormone stimulation [7]. Also, through parvocellular projections to sympathetic preganglionic motor neurons of the rostrol ventrolateral medulla (RVLM) and the intermediolateral cell column, PVN is able to directly influence sympathetic nerve traffic [9].

Function-Related Plasticity

Upon activation, the neuronal populations of the SON and PVN undergo a dramatic event called function related plasticity, defined by Hatton as the power that fluctuating physiological conditions have to reversibly alter the structural relationships among the various cell types as well as the functional pathways over which information is transmitted [12]. In line with this definition various stimuli including: dehydration, decreases in blood pressure, late stages of pregnancy, parturition and lactation, induce morphological, electrical and biosynthetic changes in the SON and PVN that are fully reversible upon removal of the stimulus [12]. These morphological changes are accompanied by biochemical events such as a strong activation of the cyclic adenosine monophosphate (cAMP) pathway in both SON and PVN [13] and transcriptional events that extend beyond simple Avp and Oxt genesis [14].

A Comprehensive Description of the HNS Transcriptome

That the SON and PVN undergo morphological and biosynthetic changes as a result of appropriate stimulation implies that function-related plasticity is necessary to create a favourable environment for the proportional and appropriate delivery of the hormone payload. We hypothesise that the elegant plasticity of the hypothalamus in response to dehydration is under the direct control of gene transcription and have therefore catalogued gene expression within the male rat SON, PVN and neurointermediate lobe of the pituitary (NIL). For each tissue we generated a list of genes that are statistically considered to be present in each of the 5 independent experimental chips in the control or dehydrated state [15]. These lists were then combined so that a single list of genes considered present in either the control or dehydrated animal could be used as a basis for further filtering and statistical analysis. In total, 183 genes were significantly ($p < 0.05$) regulated by greater than 2-fold in the SON. Of these 183 transcripts, the literature confirmed that 13% of them have already been described in the SON and 6% of the 183 are specifically regulated as a result of osmotic cues. It is also interesting to note that 17 of the transcripts identified as being significantly regulated in the SON as a consequence of the hyperosmolality in this study appear to be regulated in an opposite direction by hypo-osmolality induced by pharmacological manipulation with Avp [16]. When the PVN data were subjected to the same fold change threshold and statistical testing as the SON, it appears that only 12 genes are regulated. Given the common function of the SON and PVN it is perhaps surprising that such a great disparity in the number of regulated genes exists, until one remembers that in contrast to the SON, the PVN is a heterogeneous population of neurons involved in multiple biological functions that extend beyond osmoregulation. It is likely that a combination of noise generated from parvocellular neurons involved in, for example, the stress response, together with the stringent statistical cut-offs we have applied to our data has resulted in the lower number of regulated genes noticed in this tissue; a 1.5-fold cut-off results in a greater number of significantly regulated genes. To further investigate the phenotypic differences that exist between the SON and PVN, we compared the transcriptome data from the two tissues to identify which population of mRNAs in the PVN might be specifically parvo- or magnocellular in nature. The data were arranged so that those genes that have an expression level of greater than 5-fold in either tissue under either euhydrated or dehydrated states were revealed. In the control state, several genes known to be confined to parvocellular regions were revealed including corticotropin-releasing hormone [17].

When the list of genes regulated by greater than 2-fold following dehydration were compared between the SON and PVN, 7 of the 12 PVN genes are commonly regulated in the SON, presumably confirming their magnocellular credentials. One of these genes, gonadotropin-inducible ovarian transcription factor 1 (Giot-1), provided an ideal candidate for validation. Transcription factors are mature proteins capable of binding to the promoter sequence of a specific gene, thus regulating its transcription. The importance of transcription factors to our hypothesis that transcriptional events underpin hypothalamic plasticity is immediately clear. With this in mind, the SON data were statistically analysed without a fold-change cut-off being applied. This resulted in 2,453 transcripts of which 38 were identified as mRNAs that encode known transcription factors [18]. Using the subjective criteria of novelty and abundance, 5 transcription factors; Giot-1, Giot-2β, cAMP-responsive element-binding protein 3-like 1 (Creb3l1), CCAAT/enhancer-binding protein-β (Cebpb) and activating transcription factor 4 (Atf4) were selected for validation. Using in situ hybridisation histochemistry, the regulation of all 5 transcription factors was confirmed in the SON following dehydration. In the PVN, Giot-1 Creb3l1 and Atf4 were all significantly regulated following dehydration whereas Giot2 and Cebpb only just failed to reach significance. Presumably these transcription factors are expressed following chronic (72-hour) dehydration so that either a proportional response to the continued osmotic stress is maintained or a recovery may be initiated upon rehydration. Additionally, we confirmed that the upstream signalling pathways that regulate the Giot-1 transcript in the HNS are cAMP dependent. The activity of the Giot-1 proximal promotor has already been demonstrated to be induced by cAMP intracellular pathways through a cAMP-responsive element (CRE) site [19]. We have demonstrated that unilateral injection of an adenoviral construct encoding PKIα, a specific inhibitor of protein kinase A, significantly reduced the upregulation of Giot-1 noticed in the dehydrated PVN [18]. Interestingly, the Giot-1 promotor has also been shown to be the target of the orphan nuclear receptor (Nr4a1) [20] transcription factor, that is also upregulated following dehydration in the SON [15].

Although Nr4a1 is upregulated in the SON following dehydration, our data shows that this mRNA is downregulated in the NIL. Further comparison of the SON and the NIL data reveals that there are 26 genes that are significantly regulated by greater than 1.5-fold in opposite directions as a result of dehydration (10 up in SON/down in NIL and 16 down in SON/up in NIL). It has been hypothesised that some transcripts that increase in abundance in the NIL as a consequence of dehydration are in fact transported from the magnocellular cell bodies, down the axons to nerve terminals in the posterior pituitary. One such transcript encodes Avp [21] also identified here as being up-regulated by 2.5-fold in the NIL. The 16 transcripts identified, represent candidates for further study of anterograde axonal transport between the SON and the NIL. These data also identified 10 transcripts that are downregulated in the NIL but upregulated in the SON one of which, c-fos, has been suggested to be stored in the axons of the HNS and transported in a retrograde fashion in response to osmotic stimulation [22]. Whether the other 9 transcripts are subject to retrograde transport or just differently regulated in each tissue is not clear, but it is interesting to note that all three members of the orphan nuclear receptor subfamily (Nr4a1–3) are downregulated in the NIL, and Nr4a1 and Nr4a3 are both upregulated in the SON. Also interesting is the downregulation of pro-hormone convertases type 1 and 2 (Pcks 1 and 2) in the NIL and a corresponding upregulation in the SON following dehydration. The role of these proprotein convertases is to mediate post-translational modification of regulatory neuropeptides including provasopressin proinsulin, proglucagon, prosomatostatin, proCrf and Vgf. The expression of both PC1 and PC2 transcript has been observed in the magnocellular neurons of both the SON and PVN where both PCs are found in both Avp and Oxt neurons, while PC2 has also been observed in the parvocellular region of the PVN [23]. Interestingly, the same study showed that only PC2 mRNA was localised in Crf neurons suggesting specificity in processing.

The HNS Transcriptome Is Highly Strain Dependent

Physiologists are adept at breeding particular traits into rodents that make them candidates for particular biological investigations. For example, marked differences in the hypothalamo-pituitary-adrenal axis (HPA) in different strains of rat exist [24] and the HPA of the inbred Wistar-Kyoto (WKY) rat strain, is particularly responsive to stress [25]. Outbred Sprague-Dawley (SD) and outbred Wistar rats differ in posterior pituitary weight and vasopressin gene product content, and whilst reserpine administration, which depletes catecholamine vesicles and inhibits vasopressin release, has no effect on PP Avp content in SD rats, it elicited a fall in Wistar animals [26]. Strain-dependent differences in sodium appetite and intake, and behavioural responses to salt excess, have also been reported [27, 28].

The wealth of transcriptome information that we have collected from various strains has afforded us the opportunity to re-mine old data with new questions. Data collected from 'control' SD, 'control' Wistar and 'control' Wistar-Kyoto (WKY) rats, each involved in a different experimental paradigm has been mined specifically to answer questions about the strain specific nature of transcriptome expression; the results are surprising. When data were arranged so that those genes whose expression is greater than 2-fold in either the SD-SON or SD-NIL or the WKY-SON or

WKY-NIL were revealed, the expression of a large number of genes seems to be strain specific. In the SD-SON, 1,099 genes are enriched compared to the WKY-SON. Also, there are 374 genes that are enriched in the WKY-SON compared to the SD [29]. The same pattern of enrichment is noticed in the NIL too where 558 genes are SD specific and 309 genes WKY specific. The PVN data benefit from a third strain of rat, the Wistar. Interestingly, there are fewer enriched genes between the Wistar and the WKY-PVN than between SD-PVN, presumably reflecting the closer genetic relationship between these two strains.

In the light of this highly strain-dependent transcriptome expression we are left with an interesting issue to resolve. Given the apparent strain-dependent transcriptome expression noticed in the HNS, how is the highly conserved phenotype of osmoregulation achieved? Transcriptome-wide data are not currently available to satisfactorily answer this question; however, because dehydration results in an increase in vasopressin transcription, synthesis and discharge from the HNS in all strains of rats, we can hypothesise that the transcriptome expression between strains is more similar following dehydration than it is under 'control' conditions. The extension of this hypothesis is that the environmental conditions act as a phenotypic switch that aligns gene expression to a common purpose. The fitness of different strains to respond to such a switch will therefore be governed by the extent to which the strain-common or strain-unique genes are expressed. By analogy, the mixing of different primary gene colours will result in a strain-dependent spectrum of phenotypes that act as a substrate for selection pressure by the switch.

Conclusion

The analysis of transcriptome-wide data commonly results in lists of genes expressed in a particular tissue under different conditions with an emphasis placed on how the expression of each gene is changed beyond a prescribed cut-off. Interpretation of such data with a one-gene-at-a-time approach not only undermines the sentiment behind the approach but also ignores an important facet of the biological complexity that the researcher hopes to describe using that data. A disparity exists between the number of genes expressed by the human or rat genomes and the number of biological tasks they are required to achieve, a problem only resolved when one considers that the expression of any individual gene is part of a larger transcriptome-wide network of gene expressions rather than a discrete event. Work in our laboratory now seeks to describe the HNS transcriptome using this hypothesis, examining the relationships between all of the individual gene expressions to identify the role that the individual units of transcription play in the larger physiological response to osmotic stress.

References

1 Antunes-Rodrigues J, de Castro M, Elias LL, Valenca MM, McCann SM: Neuroendocrine control of body fluid metabolism. Physiol Rev 2004;84:169–208.

2 Weiss ML, Hatton GI: Collateral input to the paraventricular and supraoptic nuclei in rat. I. Afferents from the subfornical organ and the anteroventral third ventricle region. Brain Res Bull 1990;24:231–238.

3 Starbuck EM, Fitts DA: Subfornical organ disconnection and Fos-like immunoreactivity in hypothalamic nuclei after intragastric hypertonic saline. Brain Res 2002;951:202–208.

4 Mangiapane ML, Thrasher TN, Keil LC, Simpson JB, Ganong WF: Role for the subfornical organ in vasopressin release. Brain Res Bull 1984;13:43–47.

5 McKinley MJ, Gerstberger R, Mathai ML, Oldfield BJ, Schmid H: The lamina terminalis and its role in fluid and electrolyte homeostasis. J Clin Neurosci 1999;6:289–301.

6 Sabatier NLG: Vasopressin and Fluid Balance: Running Hard to Stand Still. Amsterdam, Elsevier, 2006.

7 Scott LV, Dinan TG: Vasopressin and the regulation of hypothalamic-pituitary-adrenal axis function: implications for the pathophysiology of depression. Life Sci 1998;62:1985–1998.

8 Tung YC, Ma M, Piper S, Coll A, O'Rahilly S, Yeo GS: Novel leptin-regulated genes revealed by transcriptional profiling of the hypothalamic paraventricular nucleus. J Neurosci 2008;28:12419–12426.

9 Badoer E: Hypothalamic paraventricular nucleus and cardiovascular regulation. Clin Exp Pharmacol Physiol 2001;28:95–99.

10 Higuchi T, Okere CO: Role of the supraoptic nucleus in regulation of parturition and milk ejection revisited. Microsc Res Tech 2002;56:113–121.

11 Alonso G, Assenmacher I: Radioautographic studies on the neurohypophysial projections of the supraoptic and paraventricular nuclei in the rat. Cell Tissue Res 1981;219:525–534.

12 Hatton GI: Function-related plasticity in hypothalamus. Annu Rev Neurosci 1997;20:375–397.

13 Carter DA, Murphy D: Cyclic nucleotide dynamics in the rat hypothalamus during osmotic stimulation: in vivo and in vitro studies. Brain Res 1989; 487:350–356.

14 Lightman SL, Young WS 3rd: Vasopressin, oxytocin, dynorphin, enkephalin and corticotrophin-releasing factor mRNA stimulation in the rat. J Physiol 1987;394:23–39.

15 Hindmarch C, Yao S, Beighton G, Paton J, Murphy D: A comprehensive description of the transcriptome of the hypothalamoneurohypophyseal system in euhydrated and dehydrated rats. Proc Natl Acad Sci USA 2006;103:1609–1614.

16 Yue C, Mutsuga N, Verbalis J, Gainer H: Microarray analysis of gene expression in the supraoptic nucleus of normoosmotic and hypoosmotic rats. Cell Mol Neurobiol 2006;26:959–978.

17 Sawchenko PE, Swanson LW: Localization, colocalization, and plasticity of corticotropin-releasing factor immunoreactivity in rat brain. Fed Proc 1985; 44:221–227.

18 Qiu J, Yao S, Hindmarch C, Antunes V, Paton J, Murphy D: Transcription factor expression in the hypothalamo-neurohypophyseal system of the dehydrated rat: upregulation of gonadotrophin inducible transcription factor 1 mRNA is mediated by cAMP-dependent protein kinase A. J Neurosci 2007;27: 2196–2203.

19 Yazawa T, Mizutani T, Yamada K, et al: Involvement of cyclic adenosine 5′-monophosphate response element-binding protein, steroidogenic factor 1, and Dax-1 in the regulation of gonadotropin-inducible ovarian transcription factor 1 gene expression by follicle stimulating hormone in ovarian granulosa cells. Endocrinology 2003;144:1920–1930.

20 Song KH, Park YY, Kee HJ, et al: Orphan nuclear receptor Nur77 induces zinc finger protein GIOT-1 gene expression, and GIOT-1 acts as a novel corepressor of orphan nuclear receptor SF-1 via recruitment of HDAC2. J Biol Chem 2006;281:15605–15614.

21 Murphy D, Levy A, Lightman S, Carter D: Vasopressin RNA in the neural lobe of the pituitary: dramatic accumulation in response to salt loading. Proc Natl Acad Sci USA 1989;86:9002–9005.

22 Skutella T, Probst JC, Jirikowski GF: c-fos mRNA is present in axons of the hypothalamo-neurohypophysial system of the rat. Cell Mol Biol (Noisy-legrand) 1995;41:793–798.

23 Dong W, Seidel B, Marcinkiewicz M, Chretien M, Seidah NG, Day R: Cellular localization of the prohormone convertases in the hypothalamic paraventricular and supraoptic nuclei: selective regulation of PC1 in corticotrophin-releasing hormone parvocellular neurons mediated by glucocorticoids. J Neurosci 1997;17:563–575.

24 Harbuz MS, Jessop DS, Lightman SL, Chowdrey HS: The effects of restraint or hypertonic saline stress on corticotrophin-releasing factor, arginine vasopressin, and proenkephalin A mRNAs in the CFY, Sprague-Dawley and Wistar strains of rat. Brain Res 1994;667:6–12.

25 Malkesman O, Maayan R, Weizman A, Weller A: Aggressive behavior and HPA axis hormones after social isolation in adult rats of two different genetic animal models for depression. Behav Brain Res 2006;175:408–414.

26 Edwards BA: Variability in neurosecretory material and responses to reserpine of the pituitary neural lobe in five strains of rat. Acta Endocrinol (Copenh) 1980;93:402–406.
27 Leshem M, Kavushansky A, Devys JM, Thornton S: Enhancement revisited: the effects of multiple depletions on sodium intake in rats vary with strain, substrain, and gender. Physiol Behav 2004;82:571–580.
28 Drueke TB, Muntzel M: Heterogeneity of blood pressure responses to salt restriction and salt appetite in rats. Klin Wochenschr 1991;69(suppl 25):73–78.
29 Hindmarch C, Yao S, Hesketh S, et al: The transcriptome of the rat hypothalamic-neurohypopyseal system is highly strain-dependent. J Neuroendocrinol 2007;19:1009–1012.

Charles Colin Thomas Hindmarch
Henry Wellcome Laboratories for Integrative Neuroscience and Endocrinology
University of Bristol
Bristol BS1 3NY (UK)
Tel. +44 117 3313072, E-Mail c.hindmarch@bristol.ac.uk

Loche S, Cappa M, Ghizzoni L, Maghnie M, Savage MO (eds): Pediatric Neuroendocrinology.
Endocr Dev. Basel, Karger, 2010, vol 17, pp 11–21

Role of Sleep and Sleep Loss in Hormonal Release and Metabolism

Rachel Leproult · Eve Van Cauter

Department of Medicine, University of Chicago, Chicago, Ill., USA

Abstract

Compared to a few decades ago, adults, as well as children, sleep less. Sleeping as little as possible is often seen as an admirable behavior in contemporary society. However, sleep plays a major role in neuroendocrine function and glucose metabolism. Evidence that the curtailment of sleep duration may have adverse health effects has emerged in the past 10 years. Accumulating evidence from both epidemiologic studies and well-controlled laboratory studies indicates that chronic partial sleep loss may increase the risk of obesity and weight gain. The present chapter reviews epidemiologic studies in adults and children and laboratory studies in young adults indicating that sleep restriction results in metabolic and endocrine alterations, including decreased glucose tolerance, decreased insulin sensitivity, increased evening concentrations of cortisol, increased levels of ghrelin, decreased levels of leptin and increased hunger and appetite. Altogether, the evidence points to a possible role of decreased sleep duration in the current epidemic of obesity. Bedtime extension in short sleepers should be explored as a novel behavioral intervention that may prevent weight gain or facilitate weight loss. Avoiding sleep deprivation may help to prevent the development of obesity, particularly in children.

Hormones that Influence Glucose Regulation and Appetite Control Are Influenced by Sleep

The temporal organization of the release of the counterregulatory hormones growth hormone (GH) and cortisol as well as the release of hormones that play a major role in appetite regulation, such as leptin and ghrelin, is partly dependent on sleep timing, duration and quality. Glucose tolerance and insulin secretion are also markedly modulated by the sleep-wake cycle [1]. Sleep propensity and sleep architecture are in turn controlled by the interaction of two time-keeping mechanisms in the central nervous system, circadian rhythmicity (i.e. intrinsic effects of biological time, irrespective of the sleep or wake state) and sleep-wake homeostasis (i.e. a measure of the duration of prior wakefulness, irrespective of time of day).

Circadian rhythmicity is an endogenous oscillation with a near 24-hour period generated in the suprachiasmatic nuclei of the hypothalamus. The ability of the SCN nuclei to generate a circadian signal is not dependent on cell-to-cell interaction and synchronization. Instead, single SCN cells in culture can generate circadian neural signals [2]. The generation and maintenance of circadian oscillations in SCN neurons involve a series of clock genes (including at least *per1, per 2, per3, cry1, cry2, tim, clock, B-mal1, CKIε/δ*), often referred to as 'canonical', which interact in a complex feedback loop of transcription/translation [3, 4]. Circadian timing is transmitted to other areas of the brain and to the periphery via direct neuronal connections with other parts of the hypothalamus, via the control of sympathetic nervous activity and via hormonal signals, including melatonin. The molecular and neuronal mechanisms that measure the duration of prior wakefulness and are thus responsible for the homeostatic control of sleep have not been fully elucidated. Human sleep is comprised of rapid-eye-movement (REM) sleep and non-REM sleep. Deep non-REM sleep is characterized by 'slow waves' in the electroencephalogram (EEG), which reflect a mode of synchronous firing of thalamo-cortical neurons. The intensity of non-REM sleep may be quantified by slow wave activity (SWA; EEG spectral power in the 0.5–4 Hz frequency range). Slow waves of larger amplitude and greater regularity are reflected in higher SWA and in deeper sleep. Because SWA decreases in the course of the sleep period, is higher after sleep deprivation (i.e. extended wakefulness) and lower when the waking period has been interrupted by a long nap (i.e. shorter wakefulness), SWA is considered as the major marker of homeostatic sleep pressure. Converging evidence implicates adenosine, an inhibitory neurotransmitter, in sleep homeostasis in mammals [5]. Prolonged wakefulness results in increased levels of extracellular adenosine, which partly derive from ATP degradation, and adenosine levels decrease during sleep [6]. The adenosine receptor antagonist, caffeine, inhibits SWA [7]. It has been proposed that the restoration of brain energy during SWS involves the replenishment of glycogen stores [8]. The results of experiments testing this hypothesis have been mixed. A recent and well-supported hypothesis regarding sleep homeostasis is that the level of SWA in early sleep is a function of the strength of cortical synapses developed during wakefulness and that the decline in SWA across the sleep period reflects the downscaling of these synapses [9].

The major mechanisms by which the modulatory effects of circadian rhythmicity and sleep-wake homeostasis are exerted on peripheral physiological systems include the modulation of hypothalamic activating and inhibiting factors controlling the release of pituitary hormones and the modulation of sympathetic and parasympathetic nervous activity.

The relative contributions of the circadian signal versus homeostatic sleep pressure vary from endocrine axis to endocrine axis. It has been well-documented that GH is a hormone essentially controlled by sleep-wake homeostasis. Indeed, in men, the most reproducible pulse of GH occurs shortly after sleep onset, during slow wave sleep (SWS, stages 3 and 4) when SWA is high. In both young and older men, there is a 'dose-response' relationship between SWS and nocturnal GH release. When the sleep period is displaced, the major GH pulse is also shifted and nocturnal GH release during sleep deprivation is minimal or frankly absent. This impact of sleep pressure on GH is particularly clear in men but can also be detected in women.

The 24-hour profile of cortisol is characterized by an early morning maximum, declining levels throughout the daytime, a period of minimal levels in the evening and first part of the night, also called the quiescent period, and an abrupt circadian rise during the later part of the night. Manipulations of the sleep-wake cycle only minimally affect the wave shape of the cortisol profile. Sleep onset is associated with a short-term inhibition of cortisol secretion that may not be detectable when sleep is initiated in the morning, i.e. at the peak of corticotropic activity. Awakenings (final as well as during the sleep period) consistently induce a pulse in cortisol secretion. The cortisol rhythm is therefore primarily controlled by circadian rhythmicity. Modest effects of sleep deprivation are clearly present as will be shown below.

The 24-hour profiles of two hormones that play a major role in appetite regulation, leptin, a satiety hormone secreted by the adipocytes, and ghrelin, a hunger hormone released primarily from stomach cells, are also influenced by sleep. The human leptin profile is mainly dependent on meal intake and therefore shows a morning minimum and increasing levels throughout the daytime culminating in a nocturnal maximum. Under continuous enteral nutrition, a condition of constant caloric intake, a sleep-related elevation of leptin is observed, irrespective of the timing of sleep. Ghrelin levels decrease rapidly after meal ingestion and then increase in anticipation of the following meal. Both leptin and ghrelin concentrations are higher during nocturnal sleep than during wakefulness. Despite the absence of food intake, ghrelin levels decrease during the second part of the night suggesting an inhibitory effect of sleep per se. At the same time, leptin is elevated, maybe to inhibit hunger during the overnight fast.

The brain is almost entirely dependent on glucose for energy and is the major site of glucose disposal. Thus, it is not surprising that major changes in brain activity, such as those associated with sleep-wake and wake-sleep transitions, impact glucose tolerance. Cerebral glucose utilization represents 50% of total body glucose disposal during fasting conditions and 20–30% postprandially. During sleep, despite prolonged fasting, glucose levels remain stable or fall only minimally, contrasting with a clear decrease during fasting in the waking state. Thus, mechanisms operative during sleep must intervene to prevent glucose levels from falling during the overnight fast. Experimental protocols involving intravenous glucose infusion at a constant rate or continuous enteral nutrition during sleep have shown that glucose tolerance deteriorates as the evening progresses, reaches a minimum around mid sleep and then improves to return to morning levels [10, 11]. During the first part of the night, decreased glucose tolerance is due to decreased glucose utilization both by peripheral tissues (resulting from muscle relaxation and rapid hyperglycemic effects of sleep-

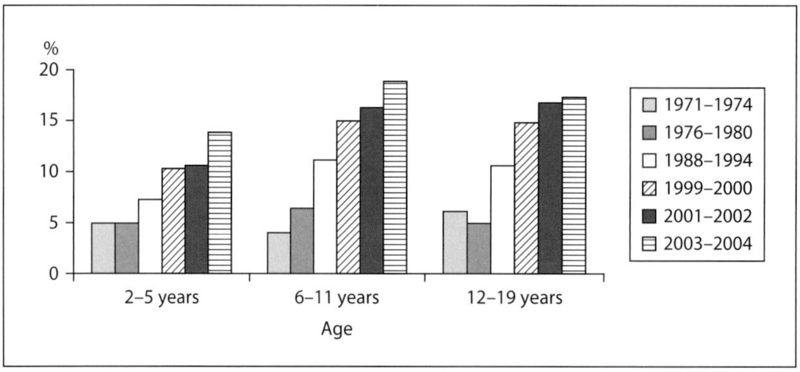

Fig. 1. Prevalence of overweight (>95th percentile) among American children and adolescents ages 2 to 19 years old from 1971 to 2004.

onset GH secretion) and by the brain, as demonstrated by PET imaging studies that showed a 30–40% reduction in glucose uptake during SWS relative to waking or REM sleep. During the second part of the night, these effects subside as light non-REM sleep and REM sleep are dominant, awakenings are more likely to occur, GH is no longer secreted and insulin sensitivity increases.

These important modulatory effects of sleep on hormonal levels and glucose regulation suggest that sleep loss may have adverse effects on endocrine function and metabolism. It is only during the past decade that a substantial body of evidence has emerged to support this hypothesis. Indeed, earlier work had only involved conditions of total sleep deprivation which are necessarily short term and therefore of dubious long-term clinical implication. The more recent focus on the highly prevalent condition of chronic partial sleep deprivation resulted in a major re-evaluation of the importance of sleep for health, and particularly for the risks of obesity and diabetes. In the two sections below, we first summarize the evidence from epidemiologic studies and then the evidence from laboratory studies.

Obesity and Sleep Loss: Epidemiologic Evidence

The increasing prevalence of obesity in both children and adults is affecting all industrialized countries. Figure 1 shows the change in the prevalence of overweight among American children per age category (2–5, 6–11 and 12–19 years) from 1971 to 2004 [12]. The prevalence of overweight went from about 5% in 1971 to about 15% in 2004 in each age category.

Increases in food intake and decreases in physical activity are the two most obvious reasons for the alarming increase in prevalence of obesity but experts agree that other factors must also be involved. Among those, reductions in sleep duration has

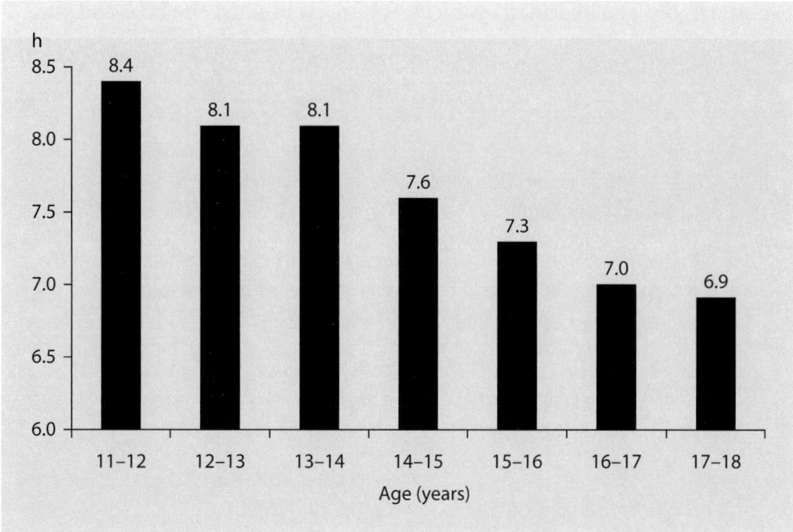

Fig. 2. Self-reported sleep duration in American adolescents in 2004.

been proposed to be one of the most likely contributing factors [13]. Over the past few decades, nightly sleep duration (by self-report) has decreased in a mirror image with the increase in the prevalence of obesity. In 2008, the poll conducted by the National Sleep Foundation [14] revealed that American adults sleep on average 6 h 40 min during weekdays and 7 h 25 min during the weekend. In contrast, in 1960, the average sleep duration was 8.5 h [15]. Thus, over less than 50 years, a reduction of sleep duration by 1.5–2 h seems to have occurred. Short sleep durations seems to be also typical in American adolescents. Well-documented laboratory studies have shown that, when given a 10-hour opportunity to sleep for several days, children between 10 and 17 years of age sleep for about 9 h, indicating that sleep need is not less than 9 h [16]. In stark contrast with this physiologic sleep need are the sleep durations self-reported by American children between 11 and 18 years old in 2006 [17]. Even in the youngest children, the amount of sleep is less than 9 hours and drops to 7 h or less in 16- to 18-year-olds (fig. 2).

Is there an association between the prevalence of obesity and the prevalence of short sleep duration? Cross-sectional studies have examined associations between sleep duration and BMI in both children and adults and prospective studies have tested the hypothesis that short sleep duration at baseline predicted weight gain or the incidence of obesity over the follow-up period. All studies controlled for a variety of potential confounders. In adults, as of May 2009, a total of 29 cross-sectional studies and 6 prospective studies originating from a wide variety of industrialized countries have been published. Thirty of these 35 studies had positive findings. Obesity risk generally increased for sleep durations under 6 h. There have been 20 cross-sectional

Table 1. Prospective studies of sleep (reported by the parents) and obesity risk in boys and girls.

Reference	Number of subjects and years of follow-up	Results	Country of origin
Lumeng et al. [18], 2007	n = 785 aged 9–10 years (3rd grade) and 11–12 years (6th grade)	short sleep duration in 3rd grade is associated with overweight in 6th grade	USA
Agras et al. [19], 2004	n = 150 sleep reported at 3-5 years weight measured at 9.5 years	less sleep time in childhood is a risk factor for childhood overweight	USA
Reilly et al. [20], 2005	n = 7,758 sleep reported at 38 months obesity measured at 7 years	short sleep duration (<10.5 h) at age 3 years is associated with a risk of obesity	UK
Taveras et al. [21], 2008	n = 915 sleep reported at 6 months, 1 year and 2 years BMI z score measured at 3 years	short sleep duration (<12 h/day) during infancy is associated with a higher BMI z score at 3 years	USA
Touchette et al. [22], 2008	n = 1,138 sleep duration reported yearly from 2.5 to 6 years BMI measured at 2.5 and 6 years	persistent short sleepers (<10 h) increases risk of overweight and obesity in later childhood	Canada
Sugimori et al. [23], 2004	n = 8,170 sleep and BMI measured at ages 3 and 6 years	short sleep duration (≤9 h) is associated with a risk of obesity in boys, not in girls	Japan
Snell et al. [24], 2007	n = 2,281 aged 3–12 years at baseline and 5 years later	less sleep is associated with higher BMI, 5 years later	USA

studies in children and all had positive findings. Prospective studies are particularly important because they provide an indication regarding the direction of causality. Also, an overweight child is at higher risk of becoming an overweight or obese adult. Table 1 summarizes the 7 prospective epidemiologic studies so far that have examined sleep duration and obesity risk in boys and girls. All 7 studies showed a significant association between short sleep duration at baseline and weight gain or incidence of overweight or obesity over the follow-up period.

In conclusion, the epidemiologic data consistently support a link between short sleep and obesity risk. Negative studies were mostly focusing on older adult populations. Of note, two cross-sectional studies used objectively recorded sleep, rather than self-report, and also found a significant association between short sleep and higher BMI. A major limitation of nearly all these studies is that there was no assessment of sleep quality or sleep disorders and therefore it is generally not known if short sleep was the result of bedtime restriction in a healthy sleeper or of the inability to achieve more sleep in an individual suffering from a sleep disorder.

Epidemiologic studies in adults have also shown associations between short sleep and diabetes risk [25]. Studies are needed to determine if the increased prevalence of type 2 diabetes in children and young adults is also partly predicted by short sleep.

Obesity, Diabetes and Sleep Loss: Evidence from Laboratory Studies

There has been no laboratory study so far that has examined the impact of experimental recurrent sleep restriction on hormones and metabolism in children. The existing laboratory studies were all conducted in young to middle-aged adults.

The first well-controlled laboratory study that tested the hypothesis that partial sleep deprivation could affect the metabolic and endocrine function was published 10 years ago [26]. Young lean subjects were studied (1) after building a state of sleep debt by restricting bedtime to 4 h for 6 nights, (2) after full recovery, obtained by extending the bedtime period to 12 h for 7 nights, and (3) under normal condition of 8 h in bed. This latter 8-hour bedtime condition was performed 1 year after the two other sleep conditions. Figure 3 shows the 24-hour profiles of leptin, cortisol, GH and HOMA (homeostatic model assessment, an integrated measure of glucose and insulin, that is the product of glucose concentration (mmol/l) by insulin concentration (mIU/l) divided by 22.5) under the 3 bedtime conditions. Caloric intake was the same in the 3 conditions, i.e. 3 identical carbohydrate-rich meals. Posture and physical activity were also controlled as continuous bed rest was enforced during blood sampling. Clearly, overall leptin levels, evening cortisol levels, and the HOMA response to breakfast varied in a dose-response relationship with sleep duration. Shorter sleep duration was associated with greater disturbances in these hormonal and metabolic variables. Leptin levels were lowest when the subjects were in a state of sleep debt, signaling the brain an unnecessary need for extra caloric intake. Evening cortisol levels were highest when the subjects were in a state of sleep debt. A state of sleep debt therefore appears to delay the normal return to low levels of corticotropic activity. HOMA levels post-breakfast were the highest in a state of sleep debt indicating a decrease in glucose tolerance and/or a decrease in insulin sensitivity. The 24-hour GH profiles in the 8- and 12-hour bedtime conditions were qualitatively similar, with a trend for lower post-sleep peak values in the extended bedtime that is consistent with a reduced homeostatic drive for sleep with the decreased duration of the wake period. In the state of sleep debt, a GH pulse prior to sleep onset was observed, in addition to the normal post-sleep onset GH pulse. The elevation of GH concentrations during waking could have an adverse impact on glucose metabolism.

A subsequent study [27] examined appetite regulation after 2 nights of 4 h in bed and after 2 nights of 10 h in bed, in a randomized cross-over design. This study confirmed the decrease in leptin levels seen in the previous study, with a 18% decrease of

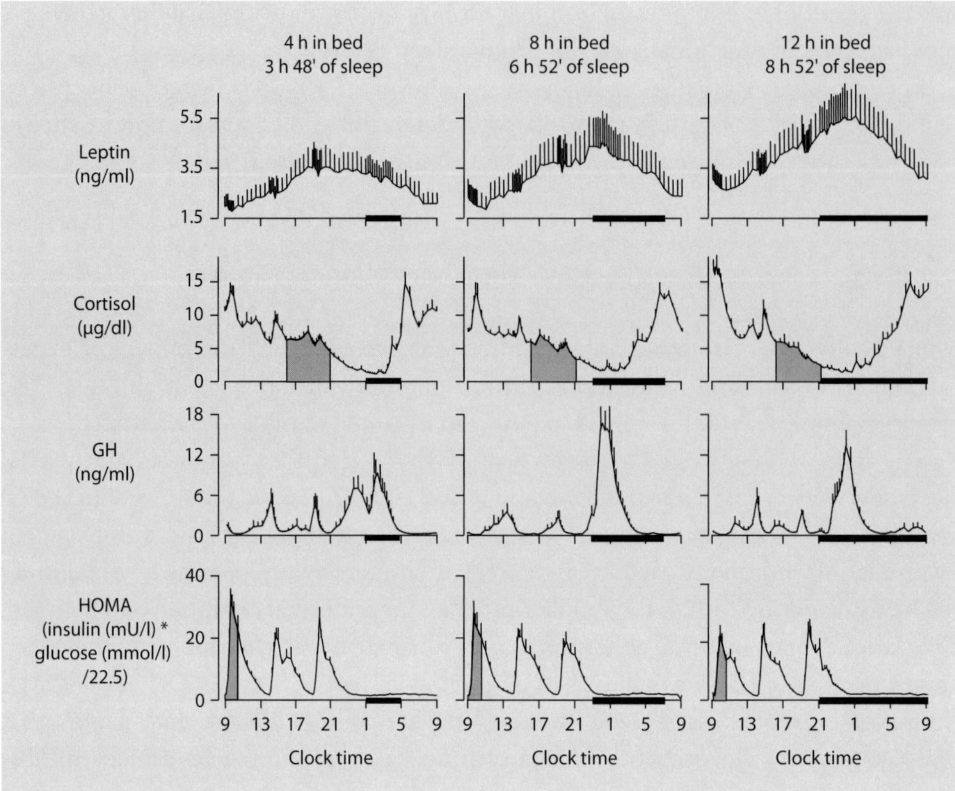

Fig. 3. Relationship between sleep duration and leptin, cortisol, GH and HOMA.

leptin levels after the short nights relative to the long nights. Furthermore, ghrelin was assayed and showed a 28% increase after the 2 nights of 4 h in bed. Questionnaires on hunger and appetite were completed and indicated a 24% increase in hunger and a 23% increase in global appetite after the 4-hour nights versus the 10-hour nights. Appetite for high carbohydrate nutrients was the most affected with a 32% increase. Importantly, the subjective report of increased hunger was correlated with the increase in ghrelin to leptin ratio (i.e. hunger factor/satiety factor). These observations suggest that in real life, when food is available everywhere and all the time, sleep deprived people may consume excessive amounts of calories, particularly from carbohydrates. A recent study tested this hypothesis using a randomized cross-over design with either extension or restriction of the usual bedtime period by 1.5 h for 2 weeks in the laboratory [28]. The subjects were middle-aged overweighed individuals who were exposed to unlimited amounts of palatable food presented in 3 meals per day and snacks were continuously available. The volunteers consumed excessive amounts of calories from meals under both sleep conditions but consumed more calories from snacks when sleep was restricted rather than extended.

Table 2. Alterations in glucose metabolism after sleep loss: 2 laboratory studies

	p	% change from well-rested condition
5 nights of 4-hour bedtimes (n = 11)		
Glucose tolerance ($\% \cdot min^{-1}$)	≤0.003	−43 ± 12
Acute insulin response to glucose ($\mu U \cdot ml^{-1} \cdot min$)	≤0.03	−27 ± 10
Glucose effectiveness	≤0.05	−25 ± 19
Insulin sensitivity, $10^4 min^{-1} (\mu U/ml)^{-1}$	≤0.04	−24 ± 9
Disposition index	0.004	−50 ± 6
3 nights of slow-wave sleep suppression (n = 9)		
Glucose tolerance, $\% \cdot min^{-1}$	≤0.03	−23 ± 9
Acute insulin response to glucose, $\mu U \cdot ml^{-1} \cdot min$	≤0.73	+11 ± 11
Glucose effectiveness	≤0.19	−15 ± 10
Insulin sensitivity, $10^4 min^{-1} (\mu U/ml)^{-1}$	≤0.009	−25 ± 8
Disposition index	≤0.02	−20 ± 7

Several studies have also shown that recurrent partial sleep restriction or experimentally reduced sleep quality results in decreased insulin resistance, another risk factor for weight gain and obesity. Remarkably, the decrease in insulin sensitivity was not associated with a compensatory increase in insulin release, and therefore diabetes risk was elevated.

The upper part of table 2 presents a re-analysis of the data from intravenous glucose tolerance testing (ivGTT) performed in the initial 'sleep debt study' [26] after 5 days of bedtime restriction to 4 h per night and when the subjects were fully rested at the end of the recovery period. Glucose tolerance was decreased by more than 40% when the subjects were in the state of sleep debt. This may be partly due to a decrease in brain glucose utilization as Sg (glucose effectiveness) which quantifies non-insulin-dependent glucose disposal, was significantly reduced. Insulin-dependent glucose disposal was also decreased since the glucose disposition index was markedly lower. Consistent findings have been observed in several follow-up studies [29, 30].

Recently, a study showed that reduced sleep quality, without change in sleep duration, can also have adverse effects on glucose metabolism [31]. Slow-wave sleep was suppressed by delivering acoustic stimuli that replaced deep sleep SWS by shallow NREM sleep (stage 2) for 3 consecutive nights, mimicking the impact of four to five decades of aging. The lower part of table 2 shows the results of an ivGTT performed at baseline and after 3 nights of SWS suppression. The findings are qualitatively similar to those seen after 5 nights of bedtime curtailment but of lesser magnitude as would be expected since the intervention was of shorter duration.

Conclusions

Rapidly accumulating evidence suggests that sleep disturbances, including insufficient sleep due to bedtime curtailment and poor sleep quality, may represent novel risk factors for obesity and type 2 diabetes. While laboratory studies have been conducted in adults only, a large number of epidemiologic studies in pediatric populations have demonstrated associations between short sleep and adiposity that are often stronger than those seen in adult populations. Sleep curtailment appears to be an increasingly prevalent behavior in children and, in the United States, adolescents may well be the most sleep-deprived age group with a difference between self-reported sleep and estimated sleep need of more than 2 h daily. There is a paucity of knowledge regarding how insufficient sleep and sleep disorders may affect pubertal development and growth, despite the fact that it has been known for several decades that the release of sex steroids and GH is markedly dependent on sleep during the pubertal transition. An increasing number of children are obese and may suffer from obstructive sleep apnea. The impact of this sleep disorder, which is known to promote insulin resistance and reduced testosterone in adults, on neuroendocrine release and metabolic function in children is in urgent need of rigorous study.

Acknowledgements

Part of the work described in this article was supported by US National Institute of Health grants P01 AG-11412, R01 HL-075079, P60 DK-20595, R01 DK-0716960, R01 HL-075025 and M01 RR000055 and by US Department of Defense award W81XWH-07-2-0071.

References

1 Van Cauter E, Copinschi G: Endocrine and other biological rhythms; in DeGroot L, Jameson J (eds): Endocrinology. Philadelphia, Saunders, 2006, pp 235–256.
2 Welsh DK, et al: Individual neurons dissociated from rat suprachiasmatic nucleus express independently phased circadian firing rhythms. Neuron 1995;14:697–706.
3 Lowrey PL, Takahashi JS: Mammalian circadian biology: elucidating genome-wide levels of temporal organization. Annu Rev Genomics Hum Genet 2004;5:407–441.
4 Vitaterna M, Pinto L, Turek F: Molecular genetic basis for mammalian circadian rhythms; in Kryger MH, Dement WC (eds): Principles and Practices of Sleep Medicine, ed 4. New York, Saunders, 2005, pp 363–374.
5 Landolt HP: Sleep homeostasis: a role for adenosine in humans? Biochem Pharmacol 2008;75:2070–2079.
6 Porkka-Heiskanen T, et al: Adenosine: A mediator of the sleep-inducing effects of prolonged wakefulness. Science 1997;276:1255–1258.
7 Retey JV, et al: A functional genetic variation of adenosine deaminase affects the duration and intensity of deep sleep in humans. Proc Natl Acad Sci USA 2005;102:15676–15681.
8 Benington JH, Heller HC: Restoration of brain energy metabolism as the function of sleep. Prog Neurobiol 1995;45:347–360.
9 Tononi G, Cirelli C: Sleep function and synaptic homeostasis. Sleep Med Rev 2006;10:49–62.
10 Van Cauter E, et al: Modulation of glucose regulation and insulin secretion by circadian rhythmicity and sleep. J Clin Invest 1991;88:934–942.
11 Simon C, et al: Slow oscillations of plasma glucose and insulin secretion rate are amplified during sleep in humans under continuous enteral nutrition. Sleep 1994;17:333–338.

12 Centers for Disease Control and Prevention. Prevalence of Overweight Among Children and Adolescents: United States, 2003–2004 [online]. 2007 [cited April 12, 2008]; Available from: http://www.cdc.gov/nchs/products/pubs/pubd/hestats/overweight/overwght_child_03.htm.
13 Keith SW, et al: Putative contributors to the secular increase in obesity: exploring the roads less traveled. Int J Obes (Lond) 2006;30:1585–1594.
14 National Sleep Foundation: Sleep in America Poll. Washington, 2008.
15 Kripke D, et al: Short and long sleep and sleeping pills. Is increased mortality associated? Arch Gen Psychiatry 1979;36:103–116.
16 Carskadon MA, Acebo C: Regulation of sleepiness in adolescents: update, insights, and speculation. Sleep 2002;25:606–614.
17 National Sleep Foundation: Sleep in America Poll. Washington, 2006.
18 Lumeng JC, et al: Shorter sleep duration is associated with increased risk for being overweight at ages 9 to 12 years. Pediatrics 2007;120:1020–1029.
19 Agras WS, et al: Risk factors for childhood overweight: a prospective study from birth to 9.5 years. J Pediatr 2004;145:20–25.
20 Reilly J, et al: Early life risk factors for obesity in childhood: cohort study. Br Med J 2005;330:1357.
21 Taveras EM, et al: Short sleep duration in infancy and risk of childhood overweight. Arch Pediatr Adolesc Med 2008;162:305–311.
22 Touchette E, et al: Associations between sleep duration patterns and overweight/obesity at age 6. Sleep 2008;31:1507–1514.
23 Sugimori H, et al: Analysis of factors that influence body mass index from ages 3 to 6 years: a study based on the Toyama cohort study. Pediatr Int 2004;46:302–310.
24 Snell EK, Adam EK, Duncan GJ: Sleep and the body mass index and overweight status of children and adolescents. Child Dev 2007;78:309–323.
25 Knutson KL, Van Cauter E: Associations between sleep loss and increased risk of obesity and diabetes. Ann NY Acad Sci 2008;1129:287–304.
26 Spiegel K, Leproult R, Van Cauter E: Impact of sleep debt on metabolic and endocrine function. Lancet 1999;354:1435–1439.
27 Spiegel K, et al: Sleep curtailment in healthy young men is associated with decreased leptin levels, elevated ghrelin levels and increased hunger and appetite. Ann Intern Med 2004;141:846–850.
28 Nedeltcheva AV, Kilkus JM, Imperial J, Kasza K, Schoeller DA, Penev PD: Sleep curtailment is accompanied by increased intake of calories from snacks. Am J Clin Nutr 2009;89:126–133.
29 Spiegel K, et al: Sleep loss: a novel risk factor for insulin resistance and Type 2 diabetes. J Appl Physiol 2005;99:2008–2019.
30 Buxton O, et al: Sleep restriction for one week reduces insulin sensitivity measured using the euglycemic hyperinsulinemic clamp technique. Sleep 2008;31:A107.
31 Tasali E, et al: Slow-wave sleep and the risk of type 2 diabetes in humans. Proc Natl Acad Sci USA 2008; 105:1044–1049.

Eve Van Cauter, PhD
Department of Medicine, MC1027
5841 S. Maryland Avenue
Chicago, IL 60637 (USA)
Tel. +1 773 702 0169, Fax +1 773 702 7686, E-Mail evcauter@medicine.bsd.uchicago.edu

Loche S, Cappa M, Ghizzoni L, Maghnie M, Savage MO (eds): Pediatric Neuroendocrinology.
Endocr Dev. Basel, Karger, 2010, vol 17, pp 22–35

Sexual Hormones and the Brain: An Essential Alliance for Sexual Identity and Sexual Orientation

Alicia Garcia-Falgueras · Dick F. Swaab

Netherlands Institute for Neuroscience, an Institute of the Royal Netherlands Academy of Arts and Sciences, Amsterdam, The Netherlands

Abstract

The fetal brain develops during the intrauterine period in the male direction through a direct action of testosterone on the developing nerve cells, or in the female direction through the absence of this hormone surge. In this way, our gender identity (the conviction of belonging to the male or female gender) and sexual orientation are programmed or organized into our brain structures when we are still in the womb. However, since sexual differentiation of the genitals takes place in the first two months of pregnancy and sexual differentiation of the brain starts in the second half of pregnancy, these two processes can be influenced independently, which may result in extreme cases in transsexuality. This also means that in the event of ambiguous sex at birth, the degree of masculinization of the genitals may not reflect the degree of masculinization of the brain. There is no indication that social environment after birth has an effect on gender identity or sexual orientation.

Sex Differences in Cognition and Aggression: Little Effect of the Social Environment

Boys and girls behave in different ways and one of the stereotypical behavioral differences between them, that has often been said to be forced upon them by upbringing and social environment, is their behavior in play. Boys prefer to play with cars and balls, whereas girls prefer dolls. This sex difference in toy preference is present very early in life (3–8 months of age) [1]. The idea that it is not society that forces these choices upon children but a sex difference in the early development of their brains and behavior is also supported by monkey behavioral studies. Alexander and Hines [2], who offered dolls, toy cars and balls to green Vervet monkeys found the female monkeys consistently chose the dolls and examined these ano-genitally, whereas the male monkeys were more interested in playing with the toy cars and with the ball. 'Neutral' toys, such as a picture book and a toy dog, did not show sex differences in either humans or monkeys. A similar result was reported in rhesus monkeys, showing that toy preference can develop without explicit gender socialization [3–5]. Testosterone levels during pregnancy plays a role in this, because girls who are exposed to high levels of testosterone in the womb in the case of congenital adrenal hyperplasia (CAH), tend to choose boys as playmates, play preferentially with boys' toys, are generally wilder, present less interest in infants than other girls and are called tomboys [6, 7]. In addition they have some male-typical direction personality features [7]. It thus seems that these sex differences are originated early on in our evolution, before the hominids, and that they are imprinted during intrauterine development under the influence of testosterone [8] and its receptor [9]. It should be noted that children's toy preferences are not necessary predicting an adult gender identity disorder [10].

A similar conclusion can be inferred from the sex differences in spontaneous drawings. Japanese research shows that subject matter, choice of color and composition of drawings by boys and girls show clear sex differences, influenced by the hormones to which the child's brain was exposed in the womb. Girls tend to draw human figures, mainly girls and women, flowers and butterflies. Boys, however, prefer to draw more technical objects, weapons and fighting, and means of transport, such as cars, trains and airplanes, in birds-eye view compositions. Drawings by girls exposed to too high testosterone levels in the womb due to CAH begin to show male characteristics some 5–6 years later, even when treated immediately after birth [11]. Apparently, exposure to higher levels of male hormones has important and lasting effects on behavior and artistic pattern expression. Aggressive behavior in men has been related as well with prenatal testosterone levels [12], although those levels can be variable postnatally depending on the time of the day, seasonal changes and other tonic circadian rhythms [13] such as an aggressive stimuli in men [12] and sexual behavior in both sexes [14].

Organizational and Activational Effects of Sex Hormones

The fetal testicles and ovaries develop in the sixth week of pregnancy. This occurs under the influence of a cascade of genes, starting with the sex-determining gene on the Y chromosome (*SRY*). The production of testosterone and the peripheral conversion of testosterone into dihydrotestosterone between weeks 6 and 12 of pregnancy are essential for the formation of a boy's penis, prostate and scrotum. Instead, the development of the female sexual organs in the womb is based primarily on the absence of androgens [15].

Once the differentiation of the sexual organs into male or female is settled, the next thing that is differentiated is the brain, under the influence, mainly, of sex hormones such as testosterone, estrogen and progesterone on the developing brain cells and under the presence of different genes as well [15]. The changes brought about in this stage are permanent. Later, during puberty, the brain circuits that were organized in the womb are activated by sex hormones. There are at present many additional candidate genes for a role in sexual differentiation of the brain without the involvement of hormones, since it has been found that 50 genes are expressed at different levels in the brains of male and female mouse fetuses, even before the hormones come into play [16]. Thus, sexual differentiation of the brain is not caused by hormones alone, even though they are very important for gender identity and sexual orientation.

There are two critical periods in human development where testosterone levels are known to be higher in boys: the first surge occurs during mid-pregnancy, when testosterone levels peak in the fetal serum between weeks 12 and 18 of pregnancy and in weeks 34–41 of pregnancy the testosterone levels of boys are ten times higher than those of girls [15]. The second surge takes place in the first 3 months after birth. At the end of pregnancy, when the α-fetoprotein level declines, the fetus is more exposed to estrogens from the placenta, this exposure inhibiting the hypothalamus-hypophysial-gonadal axis of the developing child. The testosterone level in boys at this time is as high as it will be in adulthood, although a large part of the hormone circulates bound. Also at this time the testosterone level is higher in boys than in girls. During these two periods, therefore, girls do not show high levels of testosterone. These fetal and neonatal peaks of testosterone, together with the functional steroid receptor activity, are thought to fix the development of structures and circuits in the brain for the rest of a boy's life (producing 'programming' or 'organizing' effects). Later, the rising hormone levels that occur during puberty 'activate' circuits and behavioral patterns that were built during development, in a masculinized and de-feminized direction for male brains or in a feminized and de-masculinized direction for female brains.

As sexual differentiation of the genitals takes places much earlier in development (i.e. in the first 2 months of pregnancy) than sexual differentiation of the brain, which starts in the second half of pregnancy and becomes overt upon reaching adulthood, these two processes may be influenced independently of each other. In rare cases, this may result in transsexuality, i.e. people with male sexual organs who feel female or vice versa. It also means that in the event of an ambiguous sex at birth, the degree of masculinization of the genitals may not always reflect the degree of masculinization of the brain [15, 17]. In addition, gender identity may be determined by prenatal hormonal influences, even though the prenatal hormonal milieu might be inadequate for full genital differentiation [15].

The brain structure differences that result from the interaction between hormones, genes and developing brain cells are thought to be the basis of sex differences in a wide spectrum of behaviors, such as gender role (behaving as a man or a woman in society), gender identity (the conviction of belonging to the male or female gender), sexual orientation (heterosexuality, homosexuality or bisexuality), and sex differences regarding cognition, aggressive behavior and language organization. Factors that interfere with the interactions between hormones and the developing brain systems during development in the womb may permanently influence later behavior.

Programmed Gender Identity Is Irreversible

The irreversibility of programmed gender identity is clearly illustrated by the sad story of the John-Joan-John case (i.e. the case of David Reimer). In the 1960s and 1970s, in the context of the Behaviorism, it was postulated that a child is born as a *tabula rasa* and is subsequently forced in the male or female direction by society's conventions. Although it is true that, by the age of 2–3 years, children during preschool year are able to correctly label themselves and others according to gender [18], there is no evidence that external or social events might modify these processes. However, J. Money argued that: 'Gender identity is sufficiently incompletely differentiated at birth as to permit successful assignment of a genetic male as a girl. Gender identity then differentiates in keeping with the experiences of rearing' [19]. This view had devastating results in the John-Joan-John case (Colapinto). Money maintained that gender imprinting does not start until the age of 1 year, and that its development is well advanced by the age of 3–4 years [20]. This was, indeed, the basis for the decision to make a girl out of an 8-month-old boy who lost his penis due to a mistake during minor surgery (i.e. an operation to correct phimosis). The testicles of this child were removed before he reached the age of 17 months in order to facilitate feminization. The child was dressed in girl's clothes, received psychological counseling and was given estrogens in puberty. According to Money, this child developed as a normal female. However, Milton Diamond later made it clear that this had not been the case at all. In adulthood, this child changed back to male, married, and adopted several children [21]. Unfortunately, John had a troubled life and committed suicide in 2004. This story illustrates the enormous programming influence of the intrauterine period on gender. Other cases have been described in the literature due to enzymatic disorders or to cloacal exstrophy that support the existence of early permanent programming of brain sex by biological factors and androgen exposure, rather than by social environment and learning [for revision, see 15, 17].

Neurobiological Factors of Sexual Differentiation of the Brain

In humans, the main mechanism responsible of sexual identity and orientation involves a direct effect of testosterone on the developing brain. Complete androgen insensitivity syndrome is caused by different mutations in the gene for the androgen receptor (AR). Despite their genetic (XY) masculinity, affected individuals with complete androgen insensitivity develop as phenotypical women and experience 'heterosexual' sexual orientation, fantasies and experiences, without gender problems [22]. Partial androgen insensitivity (different locus mutations in the AR) can, however, lead to dissatisfaction with the assigned female sex [23].

On the other hand, when a male fetus has a 5α-reductase-2 or 17β-hydroxysteroid dehydrogenase-3 deficiency preventing peripheral testosterone from being transformed into dihydrotestosterone, a 'girl' with a large clitoris is born. These children are generally raised as girls. However, when testosterone production increases in these XY children during puberty, this 'clitoris' grows to penis size, the testicles descend, and the child's build begins to masculinize and become muscular. Despite the fact that these children are initially raised as girls, the majority (60%) change into heterosexual males [15, 17], apparently due to the organizing effect of testosterone on early brain development and the activational testosterone production in puberty. Boys who are born with a cloacal exstrophy – i.e. with bladder exstrophy and a partly or wholly absent penis – are usually changed into girls immediately after birth. A survey showed that in adulthood only 65% of these children who were changed into girls continued to live as girls, and when individuals with gender dysphoria were excluded the figure dropped to 47% [24, 25]. From these examples it appears that the direct action of testosterone on the developing brain in boys and the lack of such action on the developing brain in girls are crucial factors in the development of male and female gender identity and sexual orientation, although other sexually dimorphic functions still need to be investigated.

Sex Differences in the Human Brain

A sex difference in brain weight is already present in children from the age of 2 years and sex differences can thus be expected throughout the brain from early in development onwards. In the adult human brain structural sex differences can be found from the macroscopic level down to the ultramicroscopic level. Functionally, too, a large number of sex differences in different brain regions have recently been described. Although a greater intrasex phenotype variability in males have been found for cognitive abilities, sexual differentiation of the human brain is also expressed in behavioral differences [17, 26].

When observed by our group, the structural difference in the intermediate nucleus of the human hypothalamus (InM) [27] was at first termed 'the sexually dimorphic nucleus of the preoptic area (SDN-POA)' [28]. We found this nucleus to be 2.5 times larger in men than in women and to contain 2.2 times as many cells [28]. The sex difference develops only after the age of 5 years and disappears temporarily after the age of 50 years [28–30]. Allen et al. [31] described four interstitial nuclei of the anterior hypothalamus (INAH1–4) and found, in men compared to women, a larger volume of the INAH3 and INAH2 subdivisions (respectively 2.8 and 2 times greater).

We recently localized and delineated the uncinate nucleus (Un). We found a sex differences in volume and neuron number in the INAH3 subdivision [32] (fig. 1), confirming previously reported data [33–35].

Other sex differences that could be related to sex differences in cognitive abilities have been found in the human anterior commissure, the interthalamic adhesion and in the corpora mamillaria [36].

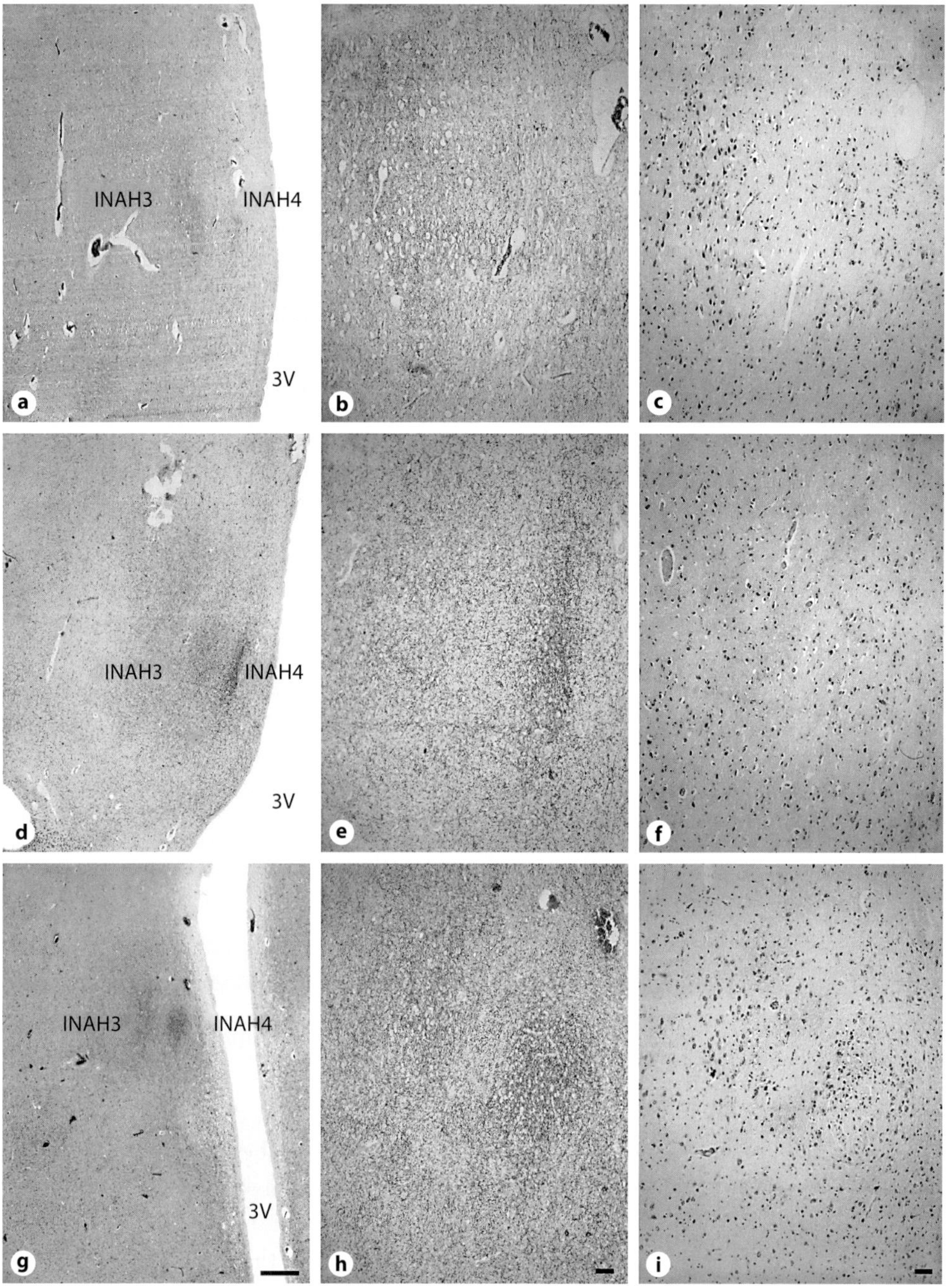

Fig. 1. Representative photomicrographs of the uncinate nucleus in man, woman and transsexual person through consecutive sections (**a–c** subject NBB # 00131; male 25 years old; **d–f** subject NBB # 01011; female 46 years old; **g–i** subject NBB # 84037; transsexual male-to-female 44 years old). **a**, **d, g** Low magnification power of the immunocytochemical stainings of Neuropeptide-Y (NPY). INAH3 and 4: interstitial nucleus of the anterior hypothalamus 3 and 4, 3V: third ventricle. Scale bar = 500 μm. **b, e, h** Details of the innervation by NPY fibers. **c, f, i** Details of the thionin consecutive staining sections. Scale bar = 63 μm. Note that the male group shows a larger number of cells in INAH3 subdivision than the transsexual and female subjetcs (**c, f. i**). From Garcia-Falgueras and Swaab [32] fig. 8, with permission.

Transsexuality

Transsexuality is the most extreme gender-identity disorder (GID) and consists of the unshakable conviction of belonging to the opposite sex, leading to a request for sex-reassignment surgery and hormonal treatment [37]. There is a vast array of factors that may lead to gender problems [for refs, see 17]. Twin and family research has shown that genetic factors play a part. Rare chromosomal abnormalities may lead to transsexuality, and it was recently found that polymorphisms of the genes for ERα and ERβ, AR repeat length polymorphism, and polymorphisms in the aromatase or CYP17 gene also produced an increased risk. Abnormal hormone levels during early development may play a role, as girls with congenital adrenal hyperplasia (CAH), who has been exposed to extreme levels of testosterone in utero, have an increased chance becoming transsexual. Although the likelihood of transsexuality developing in such cases is 300–1,000 higher than normal, the risk for transsexuality in CAH is still only 1–3%, whereas the probability of serious gender problems is 5.2%. The consensus is, therefore, that girls with CAH should be raised as girls, even when they are masculinized. Epileptic women who were given phenobarbital or diphantoin during pregnancy also have an increased risk of giving birth to a transsexual child. Both these substances change the metabolism of the sex hormones and can act on the sexual differentiation of the child's brain. There are no indications that postnatal social factors could be responsible for the occurrence of transsexuality.

Only in 23% of cases does a childhood gender problem lead to transsexuality in adulthood. With regard to sexual orientation, the most likely outcome of childhood gender identity disorder is homosexuality or bisexuality.

Transsexuality and the Brain

The theory on the origins of transsexuality is based on the fact that the differentiation of sexual organs takes place during the first couple of months of pregnancy, before the sexual differentiation of the brain. As these two processes have different timetables, it is possible, in principle, that they take different routes under the influence of different factors. If this is the case, one might expect to find, in transsexuals, female structures in a male brain and vice versa, and indeed, we did find such reversals in the central nucleus of the BSTc and in the INAH3, two brain structures that, in rats, are involved in many aspects of sexual behavior.

In men the BSTc volume was twice as large as in women and contained twice as many somatostatin neurons [38, 39]. The same was true for the INAH3, which was found to be 1.9 times larger in men than in women and to contain 2.3 as many neurons [32] (fig. 1, 2). It is remarkable that, even although a significant difference was present in total brain between man and woman ($p < 0.001$) no sex differences structural or functional were found in the INAH4 subdivision of the uncinate nucleus [32].

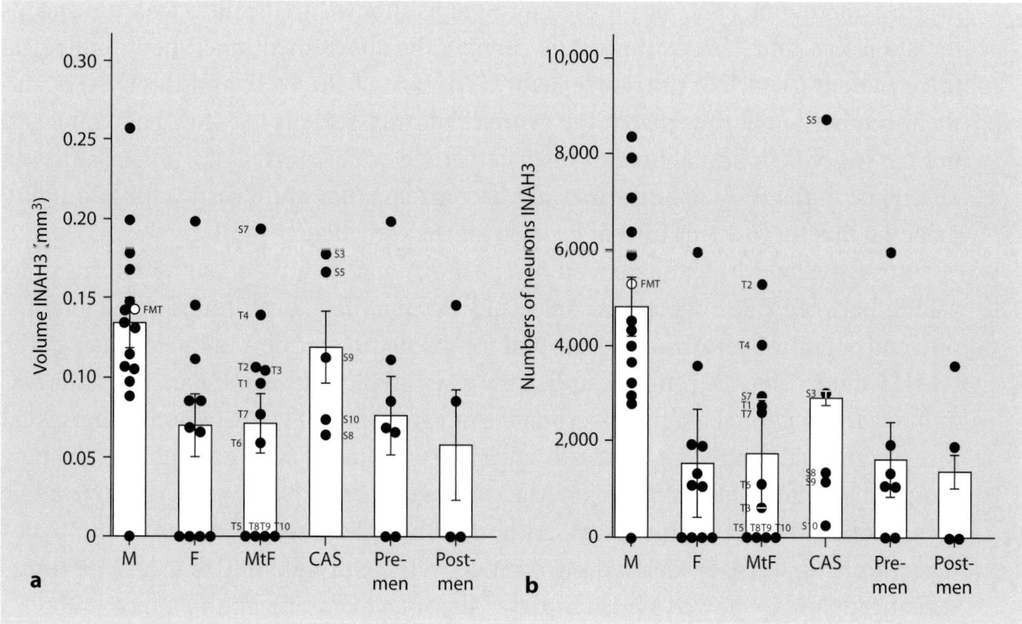

Fig. 2. **a** INAH3 volume in thionin staining in different groups, according to their gender identity and hormonal changes in adulthood. (M) control male group, (F) control female group, (MtF) male to female transsexual group, (CAS) castrated male group, (PreM) premenopausal women, (PostM) postmenopausal women. Bars represent means and standard errors of the mean (SEM). MtF and F groups were statistically different compared to the M group ($p < 0.018$ and $p < 0.013$, respectively). Hormonal changes in adulthood (CAS vs. M and PreM vs. PostM groups) showed no differences in INAH3 volume. Note that the volume of the female-to-male transsexual subject (FTM, in the male group, 51 years old) is in the male range, while the gender dysphoric male-to-female subject, who was not treated in any way (S7, in the MtF group, 84 years old), showed a male value for INAH3 volume. **b** Distribution of the INAH3 number of neurons among different groups. Bars represent means and standard errors of the mean (SEM). Statistically significant differences were found between men (M) and women (F) ($p < 0.029$) and between men (M) and male-to-female transsexual groups ($p < 0.002$). The FMT subject, in the male group, had a masculine INAH3 number of neurons and S7 subject, in the MtF group, had a similar number of neurons to the other transsexuals examined. From Garcia-Falgueras and Swaab [32] fig. 5 and 6, with permission.

In relation to sexual orientation, no difference was found in the size or number of neurons in the BSTc area, while for the INAH3 the volume has previously been found to be related to sexual orientation, being larger in heterosexual than in homosexual men [33]. In the MtF transsexuals group we found a completely female BSTc and INAH3. Until now we have only been able to obtain material from one female to male (FtM) transsexual, and his BSTc and INAH3 indeed turned out to have all the male characteristics. We were able to exclude the possibility that the reversal of sex differences in the BSTc and INAH3 were caused by changing hormone levels in adulthood, by including and comparing the results with a group of men that were gonadectomized because of prostate carcinoma [32], and it therefore seems that we are dealing with a developmental effect. Our observations thus support the above-mentioned neurobiological theory about the origin of transsexuality. The size of the BSTc and the INAH3 and their number of neurons match the gender that transsexuals feel they belong to, and not the sex of their sexual organs, birth certificate or passport. Unfortunately, the sex difference in the BSTc volume does not become apparent until early adulthood [40], meaning that this nucleus cannot be used for the early diagnosis of transsexualism.

In transsexual MtF patients who receive hormonal treatment, some intermediate values, between those typical for men and women, have been found for lateralization and cognitive performance [41] and for the neuropeptide Y stained values in the INAH3 subdivision [32] (fig. 1), indicating a sex atypical development. The same was found with functional magnetic resonance imaging (fMRI) study in non-homosexual MtF transsexual people (i.e. erotically attracted to women), who were not treated hormonally: a number of brain areas in the transsexual hypothalamus were activated by pheromones in a sex-atypical way. Although the functional reactions in the hypothalamus to an estrogen-derived pheromone were predominantly female, MtF transsexual people also showed some characteristics of a male activation pattern [42].

Sexual Orientation

Sexual orientation in humans is also determined during early development, under the influence of our genetic background and factors that influence the interactions between the sex hormones and the developing brain [for references see 17]. The apparent impossibility of getting someone to change their sexual orientation [43] is a major argument against the importance of the social environment in the emergence of homosexuality, as well as against the idea that homosexuality is a lifestyle choice.

The presence of a genetic component of over 50% in the development of sexual orientation is apparent from family and twin studies. However, exactly which genes play a role is not yet clear. A number of genetic studies have suggested maternal transmission, indicating X-linked inheritance. The X-chromosome has accumulated genes involved in sex, reproduction and cognition. A meta-analysis of four linkage studies suggested that Xq28 plays an important role in male homosexuality. However, 16 years after the initial findings the exact genes involved have not yet been identified. A different technique also indicated a role for the X-chromosome in male sexual orientation. Women with gay sons appeared to have an extreme skewing of X-inactivation as compared to mothers without gay sons. Although this unusual methylation pattern supports a possible role of the X-chromosome in male homosexuality, its mechanism of action is far from clear. Given the complexity of the development of sexual orientation, it is likely to involve many genes. A genome-wide linkage screening indeed identified several chromosomal regions and candidate genes for further exploration.

Abnormal hormone levels originating from the child itself during intrauterine development may influence sexual orientation, as is apparent from the large percentage of bisexual and homosexual girls with CAH. Between 1939 and 1960 some two million pregnant women in the US and Europe were prescribed diethylstilbestrol (DES) in order to prevent miscarriage. DES is an estrogen-like substance that actually turned out not to prevent miscarriage; furthermore, it also found, in small dosages, not only to give a slightly elevated risk of cervical cancer but also to increase the chance of bisexuality or homosexuality in girls.

The chance that a boy will be homosexual increases with the number of older brothers he has. This phenomenon is known as the fraternal birth order effect and is putatively explained by an immunological response by the mother to a product of the Y chromosome of her sons. The chance of such an immune response to male factors would increase with every pregnancy resulting in the birth of a son. Prenatal exposure to nicotine, amphetamine, or thyroid-gland hormones increases the chances of giving birth to lesbian daughters. A stressed pregnant woman has a greater chance of giving birth to a homosexual son. An interesting hypothesis is that the changes in androgen concentration during pregnancy as a result of environmental stress factors may influence the fetal central nervous system as an adaptive adjustment to the environment [44].

Although it has often been postulated that postnatal development is also important for the direction of sexual orientation, there is no solid proof for this. On the contrary, children who were born after artificial insemination with donor sperm and who were raised by a lesbian couple are heterosexually oriented [45]. There is also no proof for the idea that homosexuality is the result of a deficient upbringing, or that it is a 'lifestyle choice' or an effect of social learning [43]. It is curious, therefore, that some children are still forbidden to play with homosexual friends, an unthinkable attitude left over from the idea that homosexuality is 'contagious' or can be learned.

Sexual Orientation and the Brain

Several structural and functional differences in the brain have been described in relation to sexual orientation [for a review, see 17]. We found the first difference in the SCN, or brain clock, which turned out to be twice as large in homosexual compared with heterosexual men [46, 47].

In 1991, LeVay [47] reported that homosexual men, just like heterosexual women, have a smaller volume of the frontal part of the hypothalamus (INAH3). In 1992, Allen and Gorski reported that the anterior commissure of homosexual men is larger than that of heterosexual men. This structure, which is larger in women than in men, takes care of left-right connections within the temporal cortex, and is thus involved in sex differences in cognitive abilities and language. As shown by Savic and Lindström [48], this difference in size may possibly be related to the sex-atypical hemispheric asymmetries observed in homosexual men and homosexual women [47, 48]. No differences were found in the BSTc volume or number of somatostatin neurons in homosexual compared to heterosexual men [38, 39].

Functional scanning has recently also shown differences in the hypothalamus in relation to sexual orientation: the hypothalamus of homosexual men turned out not to be as responsive to a classic antidepressant (fluoxetine) as that of heterosexual men, which suggests a different kind of activity of the serotonergic system [49].

There are some human studies that point to the presence of unconsciousness personal communication through pheromones. Savic and Lindström [48] used pheromone compounds derived from progesterone and excreted in perspiration in concentrations that are 10 times higher in men than in women and probed pheromones influence sexual behavior and stimulate activation in the hypothalamus of heterosexual women and homosexual men in the same way, but the one used in this study not elicit a PET response in the hypothalamus of heterosexual men. Apparently, heterosexual men are not stimulated by a male scent, which suggests that pheromones contribute to determining our behavior in relation to our sexual orientation [48]. In a follow-up study, lesbian women, as compared to heterosexual women, reacted in a sex-atypical, almost reciprocal way to pheromones. These observations, too, show that there are hypothalamic circuits that function in a way that depends on our sexual orientation.

Savic's previous studies raised the question of whether certain sexually dimorphic features in the brain, which are unlikely to be directly involved in reproduction, may differ between homosexual and heterosexual individuals. They showed hemispheric asymmetry, using volumetric MRI, and functional connectivity of the amygdala, using PET measurements of cerebral blood flow [47, 48]. Dichotic listening performance has also been found to show a greater right ear advantage in heterosexual men as compared to heterosexual women, while lesbian women were somewhat masculinized in their functional cerebral asymmetry [50].

These studies show sex-atypical cerebral asymmetry and functional connections in homosexual subjects that cannot be primarily linked to reproduction, and suggest a linkage between sexual orientation and neurobiological entities.

Conclusions

The human fetal brain develops in the male direction through a direct action of testosterone and in the female direction through the absence of such an action. During the intrauterine period, gender identity (the conviction of belonging to the male or female gender), sexual orientation, cognition, aggression and other behaviors are programmed in the brain in a sexually differentiated way. Sexual differentiation of the genitals takes place in the first 2 months of pregnancy, whereas sexual differentiation of the brain starts in the second half of pregnancy. This means that in the event of an ambiguous sex at birth, the degree of masculinization of the genitals may not reflect the degree of masculinization of the brain.

Our observations on reversed sex differences in the brains of transsexual people support the idea that transsexuality is based on an opposite sexual differentiation of (1) sexual organs during the first couple of months of pregnancy, and (2) the brain in the second half of pregnancy. There is no proof that the social environment after birth has an effect on the development of gender or sexual orientation and hormonal changes during puberty do not seem to be responsible of the adult sexual identity and orientation, while the possible effects on sexual differentiation of the brain by endocrine disrupters in the environment and in medicines given to the pregnant mother should be investigated.

The differences observed in the INAH3 in relation to sexual orientation and gender identity and this structure's possible connection with the BSTc suggest that these two nuclei and the two earlier described nuclei that were found to be related to gender and sexual orientation, i.e. the SDN-POA (= intermediate nucleus = INAH1 and 2) and SCN, are all part of a complex network involved in various aspects of sexual behavior. Neurobiological research on sexual orientation and gender identity in humans is only just gathering momentum, but the evidence shows that humans have a vast array of brain differences. There is a need for further multidisciplinary research on the putative influence of testosterone in development, e.g. in individuals with complete androgen-insensitivity syndrome.

Acknowledgements

We thank Bart Fisser, Jasper Anik, Rawien Balesar, Arja A. Sluiter, Joop Van Heerikhuize and Ton Puts for their technical help, Jenneke Kruisbrink for her literature resource help and Mrs. Terry Reed and Dr. Michel Hofman for their critical comments. Brain material was provided by the Netherlands Brain Bank (coordinator Dr. Inge Huitinga). Financial support was obtained from the grant project number 930424 (postdoctoral fellowship, The Netherlands Institute for Neuroscience).

References

1 Alexander GM, Wilcox T, Woods R: Sex differences in infants' visual interest in toys. Arch Sex Behav 2009;38:427–433.

2 Alexander GM, Hines M: Sex differences in response to children's toys in nonhuman primates (*Cercopithecus aethiops sabaeus*). Evolution and Human Behavior 2002;23:467–479.

3 Hassett JM, Siebert ER, Wallen K: Sex differences in rhesus monkey toy preferences parallel those of children. Horm Behav 2008;54:359–364.

4 Williams CL, Pleil KE: Toy story: why do monkey and human males prefer trucks? Comment on 'Sex differences in rhesus monkey toy preferences parallel those of children' by Hassett, Siebert and Wallen. Horm Behav 2008;54:355–358.

5 Wallen K, Hassett JM: Sexual differentiation of behaviour in monkeys: role of prenatal hormones. J Neuroendocrinol 2009;21:421–426.

6 Nordenström A, Servin A, Bohlin G, et al: Sex-typed toy play behavior correlates with the degree of prenatal androgen exposure assessed by CYP21 genotype in girls with congenital adrenal hyperplasia. J Clin Endocrinol Metabol 2002;87:5119–5124.
7 Mathews GA, Fane BA, Conway GS, Brook CG, Hines M: Personality and congenital adrenal hyperplasia: possible effects of prenatal androgen exposure. Horm Behav 2009;55:285–291.
8 Hines M, Alexander GM: Monkeys, girls, boys and toys: a confirmation Letter regarding 'Sex differences in toy preferences: striking parallels between monkeys and humans'. Horm Behav 2008;54:478–479.
9 Wilson JD: Androgens, androgen receptors, and male gender role behavior. Horm Behav 2001;40: 358–366.
10 Wallien MS, Cohen-Kettenis PT: Psychosexual outcome of gender-dysphoric children. J Am Acad Child Adolesc Psychiatry 2008;47:1413–1423.
11 Iijima M, Arisaka O, Minamoto F: Sex differences in children's free drawings: a study on girls with congenital adrenal hyperplasia. Horm Behav 2001; 40:90–104.
12 Mazur A, Booth A: Testosterone and dominance in men. Behav Brain Sci 1998;21:353–363.
13 Dabbs JM Jr: Salivary testosterone measurements: reliability across hours, days, and weeks. Physiol Behav 1990;48:83–86.
14 Dabbs JM Jr, Mohammed S: Male and female salivary testosterone concentrations before and after sexual activity. Physiol Behav 1992;52:195–197.
15 Swaab DF: The human hypothalamus: basic and clinical aspects. II. Neuropathology of the hypothalamus and adjacent brain structures; in Aminoff MJ, Boller F, Swaab DF (eds): Handbook of Clinical Neurology. Amsterdam, Elsevier, 2004, p 596.
16 Dewing P, Shi T, Horvath S, Vilain E: Sexually dimorphic gene expression in mouse brain precedes gonadal differentiation. Brain Res 2003;118:82–90.
17 Swaab DF, Garcia-Falgueras A: Sexual differentiation of the human brain in relation to gender identity and sexual orientation. Funct Neurol 2009;24: 17–28.
18 Zucker KJ, Cohen-Kettenis PT: Gender identity disorder in children and adolescents; in Rowland DL, Incrocci L (eds): Handbook of Sexual and Gender Identity Disorders. Wiley, New York, 2008.
19 Money J: Ablatio penis: normal male infant sex-reassigned as a girl. Arch Sex Behavr 1975;4:65–71.
20 Money J, Erhardt AA: Man and Woman, Boy and Girl: The Differentiation and Dimorphism of Gender Identity from Conception to Maturity. Johns Hopkins University Press, Baltimore, 1972.
21 Diamond M, Sigmundson K: Sex reassignment at birth. Long-term review and clinical implications. Arch Pediatr Adolesc Med 1997;151:298–304.
22 Wisniewski AB, Migeon CJ, Meyer-Bahlburg HFL, et al: Complete androgen insensitivity syndrome: longterm medical, surgical, and psychosexual outcome. J Clin Endocrinol Metab 2000;85:2664–2669.
23 Katsumata N, Horikawa R, Tanaka T: Novel missense mutation in the P-box of androgen receptor in a patient with androgen insensitivity syndrome. Endocr J 2008;55:225–228.
24 Reiner WG, Gearhart JP: Discordant sexual identity in some genetic males with cloacal exstrophy assigned to female sex at birth. N Engl J Med 2004;350: 333–341.
25 Meyer-Bahlburg HFL: Gender identity outcome in female-raised 46,XY persons with penile agenesis, cloacal exstrophy of the bladder, or penile ablation. Arch Sex Behav 2005;34:423–438.
26 Lehre AC, Lehre KP, Laake P, Danbolt NC: Greater intrasex phenotype variability in males than in females is a fundamental aspect of the gender differences in humans. Dev Psychobiol 2009;51:198–206.
27 Koutcherov Y, Paxinos G, Mai JK: Organization of the human medial preoptic nucleus. J Comp Neurol 2007;503:392–406.
28 Swaab DF, Fliers E: A sexually dimorphic nucleus in the human brain. Science 1985;228:1112–1115.
29 Hofman MA, Swaab DF: The sexually dimorphic nucleus of the preoptic area in the human brain: a comparative morphometric study. J Anat 1989;164: 55–72.
30 Swaab DF, Gooren LJ, Hofman MA: The human hypothalamus in relation to gender and sexual orientation. Prog Brain Res 1992;93:205–219.
31 Allen LS, Hines M, Shryne JE, Gorski RA: Two sexually dimorphic cell groups in the human brain. J Neurosci 1989;9:497–506.
32 Garcia-Falgueras A, Swaab DF: A sex difference in the hypothalamic uncinate nucleus: relationship to gender identity. Brain 2008;131:3132–3146.
33 LeVay S: A difference in hypothalamic structure between heterosexual and homosexual men. Science 1991;253:1034–1037.
34 Byne W, Lasco MS, Kemether E, et al: The interstitial nuclei of the human anterior hypothalamus: an investigation of sexual variation in volume and cell size, number and density. Brain Res 2000;856:254–258.
35 Byne W, Tobet S, Mattiace LA, et al: The interstitial nuclei of the human anterior hypothalamus: an investigation of variation with sex, sexual orientation, and HIV status. Horm Behav 2001;40:86–92.

36 Swaab DF: The human hypothalamus: basic and clinical aspects. I. Nuclei of the hypothalamus; in Aminoff MJ, Boller F, Swaab DF (eds): Handbook of Clinical Neurology. Amsterdam, Elsevier, 2003, pp 127–140.
37 Cohen-Kettenis PT, Gooren LJ: Transsexualism: a review of etiology, diagnosis and treatment. J Psychosom Res 1999;46:315–333.
38 Zhou JN, Hofman MA, Gooren LJ, Swaab DF: A sex difference in the human brain and its relation to transsexuality. Nature 1995;378:68–70.
39 Kruijver FP, Zhou JN, Pool CW, Hofman MA, Gooren LJ, Swaab DF: Male-to-female transsexuals have female neuron numbers in a limbic nucleus. J Clin Endocrinol Metab 2000;85:2034–2041.
40 Chung WC, De Vries GJ, Swaab DF: Sexual differentiation of the bed nucleus of the stria terminalis in humans may extend into adulthood. J Neurosci 2002;22:1027–1033.
41 Cohen-Kettenis PT, van Goozen SH, Doorn CD, Gooren LJ: Cognitive ability and cerebral lateralisation in transsexuals. Psychoneuroendocrinology 1998;23:631–641.
42 Berglund H, Lindström P, Dhejne-Helmy C, Savic I: Male-to-female transsexuals show sex-atypical hypothalamus activation when smelling odorous steroids. Cereb Cortex 2008;18:1900–1908.
43 LeVay S: Queer Science. The Use and Abuse of Research into Homosexuality. MIT Press, Cambridge, 1996.
44 Kaiser S, Sachser N: Effects of prenatal social stress on offspring development. Curr Direction Psychol Sci 2009;18:118–121.
45 Green R: Sexual identity of 37 children raised by homosexual or transsexual parents. Am J Psychiatry 1978;135:692–697.
46 Swaab DF, Hofman MA: An enlarged suprachiasmatic nucleus in homosexual men. Brain Res 1990; 537:141–148.
47 Swaab DF: Sexual orientation and its basis in brain structure and function. Proc Natl Acad Sci USA 2008;105:10273–10274.
48 Savic I, Lindström P: PET and MRI show differences in cerebral asymmetry and functional connectivity between homo- and heterosexual subjects. Proc Natl Acad Sci USA 2008;105:9403–9408.
49 Kinnunen LH, Moltz H, Metz J, Cooper M: Differential brain activation in exclusively homosexual and heterosexual men produced by the selective serotonin reuptake inhibitor, fluoxetine. Brain Res 2004;1024:251–254.
50 Rahman Q, Cockburn A, Govier E: A comparative analysis of functional cerebral asymmetry in lesbian women, heterosexual women, and heterosexual men. Arch Sex Behav 2008;37:566–571.

Dick F. Swaab
Netherlands Institute for Neuroscience
Meibergdreef 47
NL–1105 BA Amsterdam ZO (The Netherlands)
Tel. +31 20 5665500, Fax +31 20 6966121, E-Mail d.f.swaab@nin.knaw.nl

Loche S, Cappa M, Ghizzoni L, Maghnie M, Savage MO (eds): Pediatric Neuroendocrinology.
Endocr Dev. Basel, Karger, 2010, vol 17, pp 36–43

Corticotropin-Releasing Hormone Receptor Antagonists: An Update

E. Zoumakis · G.P. Chrousos

Choremeion Research Laboratory, First Department of Pediatrics, Athens University Medical School, Aghia Sophia Children's Hospital, Athens, Greece

Abstract

The corticotropin-releasing hormone (CRH) family, CRH, CRH-related peptides and their receptors (R) play major roles in coordinating the behavioral, endocrine, autonomic, and immune responses to stress. The wide influence of the CRH system on physiologic processes in both brain and periphery implicates the respective peptides in the pathophysiology of numerous disorders characterized by dysregulated stress responses. CRH peptides and their receptors are being explored as therapeutic targets for intervention in stress-related disorders. Selective antagonists have been used experimentally to elucidate the role of CRH-related peptides in disease processes, such as anxiety and depression, sleep disorders, addictive disorders, inflammatory disorders, acute and chronic neurodegeneration and preterm labor. The development of effective antagonists with no significant side effects remains a challenge.

The 'CRH Family'

Corticotropin-releasing hormone (CRH) is a 41-amino acid neuropeptide secreted by the paraventricular nucleus of the hypothalamus [1]. CRH and its receptors are also found in many extrahypothalamic sites of the central nervous system (CNS). In the CNS, CRH plays a major coordinative role for the stress response, including activation of the arousal and sympathetic systems, central suppression of the immune system and elicitation of stress-related behaviors (fig. 1) [2]. CRH is the main member of a family of neuropeptides that includes the human urocortins (Ucn1, Ucn2 or stresscopin-related peptide, and Ucn3 or stresscopin), as well as fish urotensin I and frog sauvagine (table 1) [3].

CRH and CRH-related peptides actions are transduced across cell membranes via activation of two types of G-coupled CRH receptors, CRHR1 and CRHR2, encoded by different genes. Several splice variants of the mRNA CRHR1 have been identified, which encode different isoforms, termed R1β, R1c, R1d, R1e,

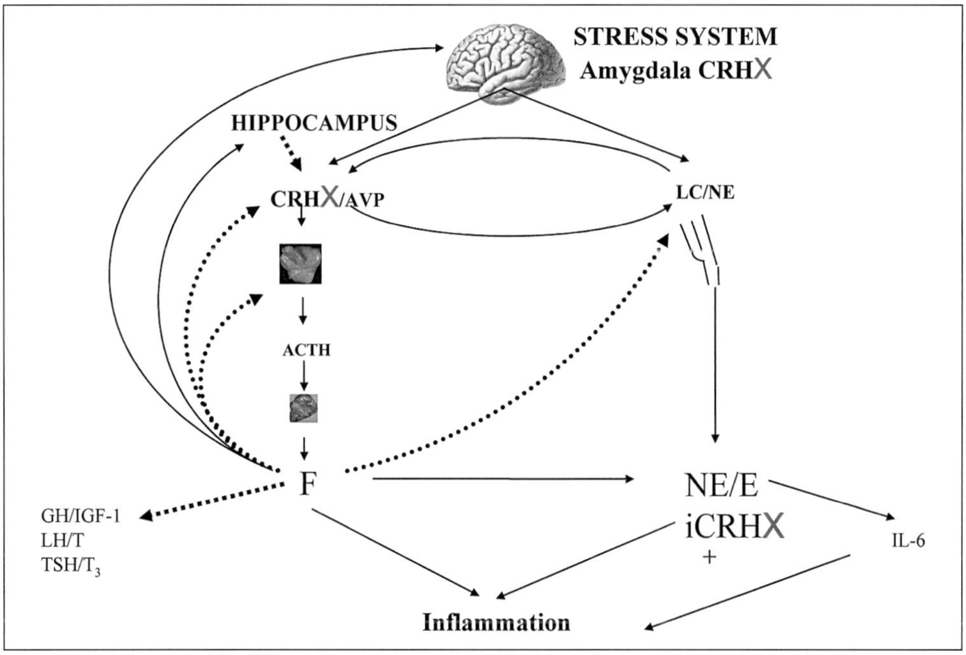

Fig. 1. Central and peripheral components of the stress system, their functional interrelations and their relations to other central systems involved in the stress response. X are the loci at which CRH antagonists block endogenous CRH actions. The CRH/AVP neurons and central catecholaminergic neurons of the LC/NE system reciprocally innervate and activate each other. The HPA axis is controlled by several feedback loops that tend to normalize the time-integrated secretion of cortisol, yet glucocorticoids stimulate the fear/anger centers in the amygdala. Activation of the HPA axis leads to suppression of the GH/IGF-1, LH/testosterone/E_2 and TSH/T_3 axes; activation of the sympathetic system increases IL-6 secretion. CRH = Corticotropin-releasing hormone; LC/NE sympathetic system = locus ceruleus/norepinephrine-sympathetic system; F = cortisol; AVP = arginine vasopressin; ACTH = adrenocorticotropic hormone; IL-6 = interleukin-6; solid lines = activation; dashed lines = inhibition.

Table 1. Sequence and homology of the CRH-peptide family

Peptide	Amino acid sequence	Length	Identity, %
Human CRH	SEEPPISLDLTFHLLREVLEMARAEQLAQQAHSNRKLMEII	41	100
Human Ucn1	DNPSLSIDLTFHLLRTLLELARTQSQRERAEQNRIIFDSV	40	43
Human Ucn2 (SRP)	IVLSLDVPIGLLQILLEQARARAAREQATTNARILARV	38	34
Human Ucn3 (SCP)	FTLSLDVPTNIMNLLFNIAKAKNLRAQAAANAHLMAQI	38	32
Frog sauvagine	ZGPPISIDLSLELLRKMIEIEKQEKEKQQAANNRLLLDTI	40	48
Fish urotensin I	NDDPPISIDLTFHLLRNMIEMARIENEREQAGLNRKYLDEV	41	54

R1f, R1g and R1h, whereas CRHR2 has three mRNA splice variants, encoding R2α, R2β and R2γ. Receptor subtypes have unique tissue distributions [4, 5]. Recently, a possible third CRH receptor (CRHR3) was identified in catfish brain and pituitary [6].

The CRH receptors exhibit unique pharmacological characteristics. CRHR1 binds CRH, Ucn, urotensin I and sauvagine, with approximately equal high affinity but does not recognize Ucn2 or Ucn3. On the other hand, CRHR2 binds Ucn1, Ucn2, Ucn3, sauvagine and urotensin I with significantly higher binding affinity than it does CRH, suggesting that these peptides might be its natural ligands. Finally, CRHR3 binds CRH with higher affinity than it does the other CRH-like peptides.

CRH and its receptors have been identified, not only throughout the CNS, but also in various organ systems, such as the immune and the female and male reproductive systems [7]. CRH-like immunoreactivity has been described in peripheral inflammatory sites [8] and in a number of reproductive organs. Thus, 'immune' and 'reproductive' CRH are forms of 'tissue' CRH, i.e. CRH found in peripheral tissues. 'Immune' CRH is secreted at inflammatory sites and possesses potent proinflammatory properties influencing innate and acquired immune processes. 'Reproductive' CRH is regulating reproductive functions with an inflammatory component. In addition, urocortins are widely distributed in immune and reproductive systems, suggesting important physiological roles in these tissues.

The recent development of a small molecule CRHR1 antagonist has provided important information on the contribution of this receptor to the development of stress-related diseases. Despite the high homology to the CRHR1 and the generation of peptide-based research tools, the physiological role of the CRHR2 is still unclear. This is due to different receptor expression patterns in rodents and primates and the lack of brain-penetrant CRHR2-selective antagonists.

CRH Receptor Antagonists

The first synthetic ligands for CRH receptors were peptide based. They do not penetrate the blood-brain barrier and no clinical applications have been pursued yet [9]. CRHR1 selective antagonists are small nonpeptide molecules, while nonselective and CRHR2 antagonists are peptides.

Patent claims have been made for nonpeptidic, selective CRHR1 antagonists with possible clinical potential [10]. Orally available nonpeptidic small molecules that are able to cross the blood-brain barrier have been discovered. Some of these have entered clinical development. Interest has been particularly focused on the following compounds: CP-154,526 and its methyl analog antalarmin, R-121919, R-278995, DMP-696 and DMP-904, SSR-125543A, NBI-35 965, NBI-30775/R121919 and NBI-34041.

Clinical Implications of CRHR Antagonists

Major depression and anxiety, conditions that are related to HPA hyperactivity are good targets for nonpeptidic CRH antagonists [11–13]. NBI-30775/R121919 was found to have a clinical profile comparable to that of paroxetine. Administration of NBI-34041 to healthy controls reduced the stress-elicited secretion of stress hormones. Neither compound impaired the CRH-induced ACTH and cortisol release. From these studies the authors conclude that both antagonists have psychotropic effects unrelated to their neuroendocrine action, in line with behavioral data obtained from transgenic mice with CRH gene deletions. In an open-label clinical trial, R121919 reduced measures of anxiety and depression in patients with major depression, which then relapsed when drug administration was discontinued. Based on these reports, NBI-34041 and other CRHR1 antagonists could be used to prevent development of stress-related disorders such as depression, anxiety, and posttraumatic stress disorder.

The promising completion of the first open-label clinical trial with the CRHR1 antagonist R121919 in severely depressed patients, along with the improvement of colonic motility and visceral perception by peripheral injection of the CRH antagonist α-helical CRH in irritable bowel syndrome (IBS) diarrhea-predominant patients, provides a strong basis for therapeutic use of CRHR1 antagonists to treat IBS, particularly given the high frequency of comorbid psychiatric disorders in IBS [14].

A possible therapeutic potential exists for conditions related to neurodegeneration, such as stroke or infantile seizures. The sites of degeneration have elevated levels of CRH expression [15]. CRHR1 antagonists exert anti-ischemic effects in rat models of permanent focal cerebral ischemia and reverse limbic seizures in neonatal rats [16]. Stress is associated with the activation of intracranial mast cells through the sequential action of CRH and sensory neuropeptides, suggesting implications in the treatment of neuroinflammatory disorders, such as migraines and cyclic vomiting syndrome.

The behavioral and physiological manifestations of drug withdrawal and the relapse to drug-taking behavior induced by environmental stressors, seems to be strongly related to the activity of extrahypothalamic brain CRH systems. CP-154,526 attenuates stress-induced relapse to drug seeking in rats induced by footshock [17]. These results extend previous reports on the role of CRH in reinstatement of drug seeking induced by stressors. Antalarmin reversed the place aversion produced by precipitated opiate withdrawal similar to buprenorphine [18], suggesting a therapeutic potential in opiate dependence.

During alcohol dependence, dysregulation of the CRH system may contribute to the basis of continued alcohol-seeking behavior [19], suggesting a possible effectiveness of CRHR1 antagonists. Increased CRH activity is a possible mechanism underlying the state of anxiety that develops in alcoholics and leads to mood disturbances and negative affect observed weeks after withdrawal. HPA axis activation is involved in all aspects of cocaine self-administration. CRH may be involved in the incentive motivation for the drug and in cue-induced reinstatement of extinguished cocaine-seeking behavior [20]. These preclinical data provide evidence for a CRH-based strategy for the treatment of compulsive drug use. CRHR1 were shown to control the expression of cocaine hyperactivation and sensitization as well as the cocaine-induced relapse behavior, whereas they did not seem to play any role in cocaine discrimination and self-administration. CRHR1 antagonists should be considered as possible medications in the treatment of cocaine addiction in humans.

The role of the CRH family of neuropeptides in inflammation, as well as experimental data supporting potential therapeutic applications of CRH compounds in various immune-related disorders have recently been reviewed [21]. CRH secretion in the hypothalamus is regulated by the cytokine IL-1β [22]. In parallel with the indirect influences of the CRH system on immune function through neuroendocrine activation of the HPA axis, a direct pathway exists through immune tissue-derived local inflammatory actions. Application of specific CRH antibodies or CRH antagonists attenuates the inflammatory reaction in in vivo models [23]. CRH endogenous neuropeptides are expressed in different immune cells, including macrophages, lymphocytes, and mast cells in proximity to their receptors and act as autocrine/paracrine modulators of inflammatory activity along with cytokines and other mechanisms.

In the mouse spleen, CRH appears to be necessary for the development of local inflammation induced by carrageenin or turpentine, for basal and inflammation-induced IL-6 expression and normal leukocyte function in vitro [24, 25]. Synthetic CRH R1 antagonists attenuate inflammation, indicating a CRH R1-mediated proinflammatory action. Chronic blockade of CRH R1 using antalarmin, significantly ameliorated adjuvant-induced arthritis in Lewis (LEW/N) rats, reducing the severity of inflammation in peripheral joints. Antalarmin prolonged survival of LPS-induced endotoxin shock and suppressed LPS-induced elevation of the macrophage-derived cytokines tumor necrosis factor (TNF), IL-1β, and IL-6, whereas it inhibited stress-induced gastric ulcerogenesis in rats.

Increased levels of CRH-related neuropeptides have been observed in several conditions associated with chronic inflammation, such as rheumatoid arthritis, ulcerative colitis, *Helicobacter pylori*-related gastritis, endometriosis and Hashimoto's thyroiditis [26–28].

Recently, CRH-deficient mice were shown to be resistant to experimental autoimmune encephalomyelitis (EAE) in a Th1-specific manner, whereas wild-type EAE mice treated with CRH antagonists showed a decrease in IFN-production by primed T cells in vitro, independent of corticosterone production. These suggest a proinflammatory role of peripheral CRH in EAE and might help in the treatment of Th1-mediated diseases such as multiple sclerosis [29].

CRH induced mast cell degranulation and vascular permeability in the skin, while antalarmin inhibited CRH-induced degranulation of mast cells and the secretion of vascular endothelial growth factor (VEGF), which is elevated in psoriasis [30]. CRH receptor antagonists have been suggested as adjunct agents to retinol and flavonoids for the inhibition of mast cell activation in chronic cutaneous inflammatory skin diseases exacerbated by stress, such as psoriasis and atopic dermatitis [31].

Hypothalamic CRH has a direct inhibitory effect on the female reproductive axis by suppression of gonadotropin-releasing hormone secretion [32]. Glucocorticoids inhibit gonadal axis function at the hypothalamic, pituitary, and uterine levels. CRH and its receptors have been identified in most female reproductive tissues, including the ovary, uterus, and placenta [33]. Endometrial implantation sites of the early pregnant rat uterus contain high concentrations of CRH [34]. CRH has been identified in human stromal endometrial cells exhibiting a decidual reaction, and has been shown to potentiate the decidualizing effect of progesterone on endometrial stromal cells in vitro [35]. Invasive trophoblasts induce apoptosis of activated Fas-expressing human T lymphocytes, an effect that can be inhibited by antalarmin. Subcutaneous administration of antalarmin in female rats in the first 6 days of gestation led to a dose-dependent decrease of endometrial implantation sites and live embryos, and markedly diminished endometrial FasL expression [36]. It is suggested that CRH participates in the process of both implantation and early pregnancy tolerance in a paradoxic combination of pro-inflammatory and antirejection activities. Therefore, antalarmin or its analogs might represent a novel class of nonsteroidal inhibitors of pregnancy at its very early stages. Furthermore, CRH was shown to inhibit interstitial trophoblast invasion in vitro, by decreasing the expression of CEACAM1 on extravillous trophoblasts. This effect was mediated by CRH-R1, suggesting that a defective CRH/CRHR1 system might be involved in the pathophysiology of clinical conditions characterized by impaired trophoblast invasion, such as preeclampsia and placenta accreta [37]. Given the promising future of CRH antagonists in the therapy of depression and anxiety disorders, their effects on reproductive physiology should be thoroughly examined.

In humans, placental CRH is secreted mostly during the latter half of pregnancy and is responsible for the physiologic hypercortisolism observed during this period. Placental CRH expression increases during the last week of pregnancy and drives the pituitary-adrenal axis to produce increased amounts of cortisol during the latter half of pregnancy. CRH may be the placental clock determining the onset of parturition [38]. Maternal CRH levels are significantly elevated in the plasma of women with preterm labor. This is further supported by findings showing that CRH infused into preterm fetal sheep precipitated early parturition. CRH-R1 antagonism in the late gestation of fetal sheep, using antalarmin, delays the onset of parturition. Finally, in rats, administration of antalarmin after the fifth day of gestation and until the end of pregnancy has no abortifacient or fetotoxic effect, suggesting that CRH antagonists could be used to protect the fetus from maternal stress and/or to prevent premature labor and delivery [36].

CRHR2 seems to be the major receptor type mediating stress and CRH-related gastric motor alterations, however, antalarmin can inhibit stress-induced gastric ulcerogenesis in rats, possibly by blockade of brain CRHR1 and vagal pathways. A prophylactic potential of CRHR1 antagonists against ulcer is anticipated.

Conditions such as chronic stress-induced metabolic syndrome and congenital adrenal hyperplasia, associated with elevations of CRH secretion, might benefit from therapy with CRH antagonists. Also, pituitary ACTH-secreting adenomas that are dependent upon CRH stimulation might be controlled by CRH antagonists.

References

1 Vale W, Spiess J, Rivier C, Rivier J: Characterization of a 41-residue ovine hypothalamic peptide that stimulates secretion of corticotropin and beta-endorphin. Science 1981;213:1394–1397.

2 Charmandari E, Tsigos C, Chrousos G: Endocrinology of the stress response. Annu Rev Physiol 2005;67:259–284.

3 Dautzenberg FM, Hauger RL: The CRF peptide family and their receptors: yet more partners discovered. Trends Pharmacol Sci 2002;23:71–77.

4 Grammatopoulos DK, Chrousos GP: Functional characteristics of CRH receptors and potential clinical applications of CRH-receptor antagonists. Trends Endocrinol Metab 2002;13:436–444.

5 Hillhouse EW, Grammatopoulos DK: The molecular mechanisms underlying the regulation of the biological activity of corticotropin-releasing hormone receptors: implications for physiology and pathophysiology. Endocr Rev 2006;27:260–286.

6 Arai M, Assil IQ, Abou-Samra AB: Characterization of three corticotropin-releasing factor receptors in catfish: a novel third receptor is predominantly expressed in pituitary and urophysis. Endocrinology 2001;142:446–454.

7 Kalantaridou SN, Zoumakis E, Makrigiannakis A, Godoy H, Chrousos GP: The role of corticotropin-releasing hormone in blastocyst implantation and early fetal immunotolerance. Horm Metab Res 2007;39:474–477.

8 J Karalis K, Muglia LJ, Bae D, Hilderbrand H, Majzoub JA: CRH and the immune system. Neuroimmunology 1997;72:131–136.

9 Christos TE, Arvanitis A: Corticotrophin-releasing factor receptor antagonists. Expert Opin Ther Patents 1998;8:143–152.

10 Zorrilla EP, Koob GF: The therapeutic potential of CRF1 antagonists for anxiety. Expert Opin Investig Drugs 2004;13:799–828.

11 Chen C: Recent advances in small molecule antagonists of the corticotropin-releasing factor type-1 receptor-focus on pharmacology and pharmacokinetics. Curr Med Chem 2006;13:1261–1282.

12 Ising M, Holsboer F: CRH-sub-1 receptor antagonists for the treatment of depression and anxiety. Exp Clin Psychopharmacol 2007;15:519–528.

13 Holsboer F, Ising M: Central CRH system in depression and anxiety: evidence from clinical studies with CRH1 receptor antagonists. Eur J Pharmacol 2008; 583:350–357.

14 Tache Y, Bonaz B: Corticotropin-releasing factor receptors and stress-related alterations of gut motor function. J Clin Invest 2007;117:33–40.

15 Bao AM, Meynen G, Swaab DF: The stress system in depression and neurodegeneration: focus on the human hypothalamus. Brain Res Rev 2008;57:531–553.

16 Stevens SL, Shaw TE, Dykhuizen E, Lessov NS, Hill JK, Wurst W, Stenzel-Poore MP: Reduced cerebral injury in CRH-R1 deficient mice after focal ischemia: a potential link to microglia and atrocytes that express CRH-R1. J Cereb Blood Flow Metab 2003;23:1151–1159.

17 Shaham Y, Erb S, Leung S, Buczek Y, Stewart J: CP-154,526, a selective, nonpeptide antagonist of the corticotropin-releasing factor1 receptor attenuates stress-induced relapse to drug seeking in cocaine- and heroin-trained rats. Psychopharmacology (Berl) 1998;137:184–190.

18 Stinus L, Cador M, Zorrilla EP, Koob GF: Buprenorphine and a CRF1 antagonist block the acquisition of opiate withdrawal-induced conditioned place aversion in rats. Neuropsychopharmacology 2005;30:90–98.

19 Sommer WH, Saavedra JM: Targeting brain angiotensin and corticotrophin-releasing hormone systems interaction for the treatment of mood and alcohol use disorders. J Mol Med 2008;86:723–728.

20 Goeders NE: Stress and cocaine addiction. Pharmacol Exp Ther 2002;301:785–789.

21 Gravanis A, Margioris AN: The corticotropin-releasing factor (CRF) family of neuropeptides in inflammation: potential therapeutic applications. Curr Med Chem 2005;12:1503–1512.

22 Chesnokova V, Melmed S: Minireview: neuro-immuno-endocrine modulation of the hypothalamic-pituitary-adrenal (HPA) axis by gp130 signaling molecules. Endocrinology 2002;143:1571–1574.

23 Webster EL, Torpy DJ, Elenkov IJ, Chrousos GP: Corticotropin-releasing hormone and inflammation. Ann NY Acad Sci 1998;840:21–32.

24 Karalis K, Sano H, Redwine J, Listwak S, Wilder RL, Chrousos GP: Autocrine or paracrine inflammatory actions of corticotropin-releasing hormone in vivo. Science 1991;254:421–423.

25 Venihaki M, Dikkes P, Carrigan A, Karalis KP: Corticotropin-releasing hormone regulates IL-6 expression during inflammation. J Clin Invest 2001; 108:1159–1166.

26 Chikanza IC, Petrou P, Chrousos G: Perturbations of arginine vasopressin secretion during inflammatory stress: pathophysiologic implications. Ann NY Acad Sci 2000;917:825–834.

27 Webster EL, Torpy DJ, Elenkov IJ, Chrousos GP: Corticotropin-releasing hormone and inflammation. Ann NY Acad Sci 1998;840:21–32.

28 Kempuraj D, Papadopoulou N, Stanford EJ, Christodoulou S, Madhappan B, Sant GR, Solage K, Adams T, Theoharides TC: Increased numbers of activated mast cells in endometriosis lesions positive for corticotropin-releasing hormone and urocortin. Am J Reprod Immunol 2004;52:267–275.

29 Heesen C, Gold SM, Huitinga I, Reul JM: Stress and hypothalamic-pituitary-adrenal axis function in experimental autoimmune encephalomyelitis and multiple sclerosis. Psychoneuroendocrinology 2007; 32:604–618.

30 Theoharides TC, Singh LK, Boucher W, Pang X, Letourneau R, Webster E, Chrousos G: Corticotropin-releasing hormone induces skin mast cell degranulation and increased vascular permeability, a possible explanation for its proinflammatory effects. Endocrinology 1998;139:403–413.

31 Singh LK, Pang X, Alexacos N, Letourneau R, Theoharides TC: Acute immobilization stress triggers skin mast cell degranulation via corticotropin releasing hormone, neurotensin, and substance P: a link to neurogenic skin disorders. Brain Behav Immun 1999;13:225–239.

32 Chrousos GP, Torpy DJ, Gold PW: Interactions between the hypothalamic-pituitary-adrenal axis and the female reproductive system: clinical implications. Ann Intern Med 1998;129:229–240.

33 Vitoratos N, Papatheodorou DC, Kalantaridou SN, Mastorakos G: 'Reproductive' corticotropin-releasing hormone. Ann NY Acad Sci 2006;1092:310–318.

34 Makrigiannakis A, Margioris AN, Le Goascogne C, Zoumakis E, Nikas G, Stournaras C, Psychoyos A, Gravanis A: Corticotropin-releasing hormone (CRH) is expressed at the implantation sites of early pregnant rat uterus. Life Sci 1995;57:1869–1875.

35 Kalantaridou SN, Zoumakis E, Weil S, Lavasidis LG, Chrousos GP, Makrigiannakis A: Reproductive corticotropin releasing hormone, implantation, and fetal immunotolerance. Crit Rev Clin Lab Sci 2007; 44:461–481.

36 Makrigiannakis A, Zoumakis E, Kalantaridou S, Coutifaris C, Margioris AN, Coukos G, Rice KC, Gravanis A, Chrousos GP: Corticotropin-releasing hormone promotes blastocyst implantation and early maternal tolerance. Nat Immunol 2001;2:1018–1024.

37 Bamberger AM, Minas V, Kalantaridou SN, Radde J, Sadeghian H, Loning T, Charalampopoulos I, Brummer J, Wagener C, Bamberger CM, Schulte HM, Chrousos GP, Makrigiannakis A: Corticotropin-releasing hormone modulates human trophoblast invasion through carcinoembryonic antigen-related cell adhesion molecule-1 regulation. Am J Pathol 2006;168:141–150.

38 McLean M, Bisits A, Davies J, Woods R, Lowry P, Smith R: A placental clock controlling the length of human pregnancy. Nat Med 1995;1:460–463.

G.P. Chrousos
Choremeion Research Laboratory, First Department of Pediatrics
Athens University Medical School, Aghia Sophia Children's Hospital
Athens 11527 (Greece)
Tel. +30 210 7794023, Fax +30 210 7759167, E-Mail chrousge@med.uoa.gr

Loche S, Cappa M, Ghizzoni L, Maghnie M, Savage MO (eds): Pediatric Neuroendocrinology.
Endocr Dev. Basel, Karger, 2010, vol 17, pp 44–51

New Concepts on the Control of the Onset of Puberty

Sergio R. Ojeda · Alejandro Lomniczi · Ursula Sandau · Valerie Matagne

Division of Neuroscience, Oregon National Primate Research Center, Beaverton, Oreg., USA

Abstract

The initiation of mammalian puberty requires an increased pulsatile release of gonadotropin-releasing hormone (GnRH) from the hypothalamus. This increase is brought about by changes in transsynaptic and glial-neuronal communication. Coordination of these cellular interactions likely requires the participation of sets of genes hierarchically arranged within functionally connected networks. Using high throughput, genetic, molecular and bioinformatics strategies, in combination with a systems biology approach, three transcriptional regulators of the pubertal process have been identified, and the structure of at least one hypothalamic gene network has been proposed. A genomewide analysis of hypothalamic DNA methylation revealed profound changes in methylation patterns associated with the onset of female puberty. Pharmacological disruption of two epigenetic marks associated with gene silencing (DNA methylation and histone deacetylation) resulted in pubertal failure, instead of advancing the onset of puberty, suggesting that disruption of these two silencing mechanisms leads to activation of repressor genes whose expression would normally decrease at puberty. These observations suggest that the genetic underpinnings of puberty are polygenic rather than specified by a single gene, and that epigenetic mechanisms may provide coordination and transcriptional plasticity to this genetic network.

General Aspects

Much has been learned in recent years about the neuroendocrine mechanisms controlling both the initiation and maintenance of female reproductive cycles. Both events require changes in the release of gonadotropin-releasing hormone (GnRH) from neurosecretory neurons mostly located in the medial basal hypothalamus of primates, and the preoptic region of rodents [1, 2]. These changes are, in turn, determined by modifications in transsynaptic [3] and glial [3, 4] inputs to the GnRH neuronal network. Studies in monkeys and rodents have shown that while the transsynaptic changes involve an increase in excitatory inputs and a reduction in inhibitory influences [1, 3, 5], the glial component of the system is predominantly facilitatory, and exerted by growth factors that directly or indirectly stimulate GnRH secretion [2, 4].

The general composition of each of these regulatory systems is also known. Thus, the excitatory transsynaptic regulation of GnRH secretion is provided by neurons that use glutamate [1, 2, 6], kisspeptin [2, 7], and, very likely, neurokinin B [8], as excitatory neurotransmitters/neuromodulators. The inhibitory counterpart of this circuitry depends principally on GABAergic neurons, but also on opiatergic neurons that employ different peptides and a variety of different receptors for inhibitory neurotransmission [reviewed in 5]. Adding complexity to this regulatory system, GABA not only inhibits GnRH secretion by acting on neuronal subsets connected to the GnRH neuronal network [2, 5], but can also excite GnRH neurons directly [9, 10].

Can the initiation of puberty be attributed to the activation of a single gene? On the surface, the answer to this question may be affirmative if one considers that rare mutations, such as those affecting *GNRHR* [11], *GPR54* [12, 13], *KiSS1* [14], *TAC3* and *TACR3* [8], result in pubertal failure. However, none of these genes appear to be in a commanding position to synchronize neuronal and glial networks involved in the initiation of puberty. Illustrating the general validity of this concept is the emerging consensus that – contrary to earlier expectations – KiSS1 is not a gene that sets in motion the pubertal process. Instead, KiSS1 neurons seem to be activated in response to developmental changes in estradiol production [15]. These observations and the recent demonstration that common genetic variation in a set of genes thought to play an essential role in puberty does not affect the timing of this process in humans [16] have made clear that no isolated pathway or cellular subset is responsible for the neuroendocrine control of puberty [17–19]. Instead, this control is likely exerted by complex regulatory gene networks composed of multiple functional modules [17].

'Upstream' Genes and the Transcriptional Control of Puberty

Studies from our laboratory have identified and functionally characterized several individual components of this regulatory system, including novel molecules required for glutamate release [20, 21], homeostatic maintenance of GnRH neuron excitability [22], unidirectional glia-to-GnRH neuron signaling [23], and glia-GnRH neuron adhesive communication [24]. We also identified 'upstream' genes involved in the transcriptional regulation of the pubertal process, including the POU-domain gene *OCT2* [25], the homeodomain gene *TTF1/NKX2.1* [26], and a novel gene provisionally termed chromosome 14 open reading frame 4 (C14ORF4), which we have now termed *EAP1* (Enhanced At Puberty1) [27]. Noteworthy, both *TTF1* and *EAP1* map to regions of chromosome 14 (14q13 and 14q24.3, respectively) implicated by linkage analysis in the control of puberty [28–30]. Based on a variety of experimental approaches, including the use of antisense oligodeoxynucleotides [25], Cre-loxP-mediated, neuron-specific conditional gene deletion [26] and siRNA-mediated, region-specific knock-down of gene expression [27] we have proposed that *OCT2, TTF1* and *EAP1* are upper-echelon (upstream) genes controlling the expression of subordinate genes that, differentially expressed in neurons and glial cells, are necessary for the neuron-to neuron and glia-to neuron regulation of GnRH secretion at puberty.

While advancing our knowledge, these findings have also made apparent the need for a global approach that can place these diverse components within the framework of a regulatory network (or set of networks) controlling puberty [17]. Until now, studies addressing this issue have not been forthcoming, essentially due to the lack of appropriate technologies, and the relative paucity of genetic and biochemical details that can be assimilated into a testable biological model. The emergence of high-throughput approaches and computational methods to create, organize, display and analyze the plethora of results derived from such approaches is rapidly changing this landscape, and giving us for the first time the opportunity of identifying functional genetic modules involved in the hierarchical control of puberty. Using a combination of gene expression microarrays, proteomics, 'guilt by association' (GBA), and 'retrospective' approaches we have singled out from the female rat and monkey hypothalamus a group of genes that appear to be representative members of one of the genetic networks involved in the neuroendocrine control of female puberty [31]. Although these genes have diverse cellular functions, they share the common feature of having been earlier identified as involved in tumor suppression/tumor formation.

A more detailed examination of this set of genes employing systems biology tools allowed us to construct a draft architectural model of a network predicting the existence of both controlling and subordinate nodes [31]. While the model is obviously imperfect, an integrated use of computational biology along with experimental verification, make it amenable to further refinement and restructuring. The ability of computational approaches to accurately estimate the hierarchical position of particular genes within the network can be illustrated by two examples. One of them is the prediction that a peripheral node would be composed of *KiSS1* and the gene encoding the kisspeptin receptor GPR54. There is unquestionable evidence now that activation of this system plays a critical role for the initiation of puberty [2, 7]. However, it also appears clear that such activation is a downstream event dependent upon the occurrence of prior events [15].The other example is provided by a tumor suppressor gene encoding an adhesion molecule known as SynCAM1, a protein previously implicated in synaptic organization. Our results showed that hypothalamic SynCAM1 expression is reduced in a mouse model of delayed puberty, and that this reduction is readily apparent in hypothalamic astrocytes, an unsuspected site of SynCAM1 production [Sandau et al., in revision]. Our results also showed that SynCAM1 functions as an adhesive substrate for both astrocytes and GnRH neurons. Ligand-dependent activation of astroglial erbB4 receptors results in rapid association of erbB4 to SynCAM1 and an abrupt, but transient increase in SynCAM1-mediated adhesiveness, followed later by increased SynCAM1 expression. These results suggest that erbB4 receptors regulate astroglial plasticity by modulating SynCAM1 adhesiveness, and that

SynCAM1 is an adhesion molecule used by the neuroendocrine brain for reciprocal glia-GnRH neuron communication. In additional studies, we generated transgenic mice expressing a mutated form of SynCAM1 targeted to astrocytes. The mutated SynCAM1 lacks the intracellular domain, which was replaced with a sequence encoding an enhanced green fluorescent protein. Both in vitro and in vivo experiments determined that the mutated protein is correctly targeted to the astrocytic cell membrane where it functions in a dominant negative fashion. The animals carrying this transgene have delayed vaginal opening, delayed ovulation and a disrupted estrous cycle. These observations indicate that genes predicted to play a subordinate role within a genetic network contribute significantly to the execution of the developmental program underlying the onset of puberty.

Essential for the experimental analysis of any gene network is the ability to perturb specific components of the system and analyze, using high-throughput and targeted approaches, the global response to these perturbations. The results can then be compared with those predicted by the model for validation and iterative refinement. Until only recently, there was a paucity of specific and reliable methods to deliver siRNAs to the brain to effect long-term gene silencing. The main limitations were the poor capability of in vitro transfection protocols to incorporate siRNAs into cells in situ without causing cell damage, the inability of a single siRNA administration to produce long-term effects, and the inability of conventional virus-based system to transduce nondividing cells. These difficulties were circumvented by the use of lentivirus-based systems capable of delivering siRNAs to mammalian tissues in vivo [32]. Because lentiviruses can infect non-dividing cells (like neurons) and the viral genome is stably incorporated into the cell's genome, this approach can be used to target specific brain regions for a long-lasting decrease in gene expression.

We have now used a lentivirus-mediated delivery system to silence *in* vivo, via RNA interference, expression of the EAP1 gene in the hypothalamus of prepubertal female rats [27]. Using this system, we targeted the medial preoptic area of 26-day-old juvenile female rats, and found that inhibition of *Eap1* expression in neurons of this region resulted in delayed puberty, disrupted estrous cyclicity, and unexpectedly, led to development of ovarian follicular and luteal cysts [27]. In a very recent report [33], again using female rats as the animal model, we showed that the pubertal increase in hypothalamic *Eap1* expression occurs independent of ovarian steroids, thereby suggesting that *EAP1* is a component of the increase in 'central drive' thought to initiate puberty in both rodents and primates.

Though revealing – and extensively used by us and many researchers in the field – the above findings are based on a purely genetic approach. As such, they cannot explain how inherited, permanent changes in DNA sequence can regulate gene expression dynamically, while simultaneously imposing an encompassing level of coordination and transcriptional plasticity to genetic networks, such as those postulated to control female reproductive development. It appears intuitively obvious that alternative mechanisms of control must exist.

Epigenetics and Puberty

A powerful biological regulatory system that meets these requirements is epigenetics, i.e. those heritable changes in gene expression that occur without changing the primary nucleotide sequence of a gene [34, 35]. Epigenetic mechanisms can not only provide gene-specific gate keeper functions [36], but are also endowed with a previously unsuspected degree of plasticity able to transiently change gene expression within hours [37], and even minutes [38]. Even more remarkable, epigenetic regulation of certain genes, including the gene encoding ERα [38], is unexpectedly cyclic, exhibiting a periodicity that results in a rapid, tight and dynamic control of gene expression. It is now clear that epigenetic information is also essential for a variety of neural functions, including memory formation [37], recovery of learning and memory [39], dendritic development [40], estrogen-induced gene expression [41], glial-neuronal interactions [42], and circadian rhythms [43].

There are two basic mechanisms conveying epigenetic information: (a) DNA methylation, a covalent modification found in cytosine residues of the dinucleotide sequence CpG [44], and (b) chromatin modifications, consisting of posttranslational modifications that alter the N-terminus tails of the so-called core histones (H2A, H2B, H3, and H4) in nucleosomes [45]. While basal DNA methylation is maintained by DNA methyltransferase1 (DNMT1), de novo methylation is a function of DNMT3a and DNMT3b, which target unmethylated and hemimethylated substrates with similar efficiencies [44]. DNA methylation is an epigenetic mark of gene repression: hypermethylation results in gene repression; conversely, hypomethylated genes are transcriptionally active. In contrast to this relative simplicity, core histones are subjected to at least nine types of transcriptional modifications, including acetylation, methylation, phosphorylation, ubiquitination, and sumoylation [45, 46]. Among these, acetylation by acetyltransferases (HATs), deacetylation by histone deacetylases (HDACs), and methylation by methyltransferases (HMTs) are the histone modifications most intimately involved in gene regulation. In general, acetylation is consistently associated with activation of transcription, whereas deacetylation is a hallmark of gene silencing [45]. Notwithstanding the importance of histone acetylation for gene regulation, promoter activation appears to require the combinatorial participation of acetylation and methylation, because acetylated H3 (acH3) and H3 trimethylated on lysine 4 (H3K4me3) are invariably associated to active promoters across the genome [47, 48]. In addition to methylation of lysine 4, H3 methylated at lysine 36 and 79 is also seen in active genes [35, 45]. In contrast, H3 methylation of lysine 9, 27 and 40 is a feature of silenced genes. Adding complexity to this scenario, DNA methylation and histone deacetylation work synergistically to silence genes [49], with DNMTs not only methylating DNA, but also associating with HDACs to bring about gene silencing [50]. The dynamic and encompassing nature of these mechanisms make epigenetic information ideally suited to provide temporal and spatial cues, not furnished by DNA sequence, to complex biological processes. The neuroendocrine regulation of puberty is one such process.

Initial studies aimed at examining the role of epigenetics in the control of female puberty have yielded fascinating results. These studies included: (a) a genome-wide analysis assessing the methylation status of known promoters and CpG islands of the female rat hypothalamus at different pre- and peripubertal developmental stages, (b) a pharmacological assessment of the consequences that blocking DNA methylation or histone deacetylation and a combination of both treatments have on the onset of puberty, and (c) a high-throughput Illumina array-mediated evaluation of the effect that each of these treatment has on hypothalamic gene expression. The results of the genomewide analysis of methylation were not only fascinating, but also entirely unexpected, as they show entire regions of different chromosomes becoming either more or less methylated with the advent of puberty. More specifically, the methylation status of DNA regions surrounding the transcriptional start site of individual genes decreases as puberty approaches, and these puberty-related changes in methylation are also seen in CpG islands. Not surprisingly, the results also showed that expression of selected genes predicted to be upstream regulators of the pubertal process, as well as that of several downstream is also regulated by DNA methylation and histone acetylation. More excitingly, blockade of these two processes resulted in pubertal failure, suggesting that epigenetic mechanisms are intimately involved in controlling the initiation of puberty.

Concluding Remarks

In closing, it is important to recognize that the concepts discussed above are still in their infancy. Extensive experimental validation will be necessary to either establish their validity or formulate alternative hypothesis. However, it is our belief that regardless of the particular players involved, and the relative contributions they may have to the control of puberty, the overall notion that genetic networks and epigenetic mechanisms control pubertal development will withstand future experimental scrutiny.

References

1. Plant TM, Witchel SF: Puberty in nonhuman primates and humans; in Neill JD (ed): The Physiology of Reproduction, ed 3. San Diego, Academic Press/Elsevier, 2006, pp 2177–2230.
2. Ojeda SR, Skinner MK: Puberty in the rat; in Neill JD (ed): The Physiology of Reproduction, ed 3. San Diego, Academic Press/Elsevier, 2006, pp 2061–2126.
3. Ojeda SR, Terasawa E: Neuroendocrine regulation of puberty; in Pfaff D, Arnold A, Etgen A, Fahrbach S, Moss R, Rubin R (eds): Hormones, Brain and Behavior. New York, Elsevier, 2002, vol 4, pp 589–659.
4. Ojeda SR, Prevot V, Heger S, Lomniczi A, Dziedzic B, Mungenast A: Glia-to neuron signaling and the neuroendocrine control of female puberty. Ann Med 2003;35:244–255.
5. Terasawa E, Fernandez DL: Neurobiological mechanisms of the onset of puberty in primates. Endocr Rev 2001;22:111–151.
6. Brann DW: Glutamate: A major excitatory transmitter in neuroendocrine regulation. Neuroendocrinology 1995;61:213–225.
7. Dungan HM, Clifton DK, Steiner RA: Minireview: kisspeptin neurons as central processors in the regulation of gonadotropin-releasing hormone secretion. Endocrinology 2006;147:1154–1158.

8 Topaloglu AK, Reimann F, Guclu M, Yalin AS, Kotan LD, Porter KM, Serin A, Mungan NO, Cook JR, Ozbek MN, Imamoglu S, Akalin NS, Yuksel B, O'Rahilly S, Semple RK: TAC3 and TACR3 mutations in familial hypogonadotropic hypogonadism reveal a key role for neurokinin B in the central control of reproduction. Nat Genet 2008;12:11.
9 DeFazio RA, Heger S, Ojeda SR, Moenter SM: Activation of A-type γ-aminobutyric acid receptors excites gonadotropin-releasing hormone neurons. Mol Endocrinol 2002;16:2872–2891.
10 Moenter SM, DeFazio RA: Endogenous gamma-aminobutyric acid can excite gonadotropin-releasing hormone neurons. Endocrinology 2005;146: 5374–5379.
11 Bedecarrats GY, Kaiser UB: Mutations in the human gonadotropin-releasing hormone receptor: insights into receptor biology and function. Semin Reprod Med 2007;25:368–378.
12 Seminara SB, Messager S, Chatzidaki EE, Thresher RR, Acierno JS Jr, Shagoury JK, Bo-Abbas Y, Kuohung W, Schwinof KM, Hendrick AG, Zahn D, Dixon J, Kaiser UB, Slaugenhaupt SA, Gusella JF, O'Rahilly S, Carlton MB, Crowley WF Jr, Aparicio SA, Colledge WH: The GPR54 gene as a regulator of puberty. N Engl J Med 2003;349:1614–1627.
13 de Roux N, Genin E, Carel J-C, Matsuda F, Chaussain J-L, Milgrom E: Hypogonadotropic hypogonadism due to loss of function of the KiSS1-derived peptide receptor GPR54. Proc Natl Acad Sci USA 2003;100:10972–10976.
14 Lapatto R, Pallais JC, Zhang D, Chan YM, Mahan A, Cerrato F, Le WW, Hoffman GE, Seminara SB: Kiss1-/- mice exhibit more variable hypogonadism than Gpr54–/– mice. Endocrinology 2007;148:4927–4936.
15 Herbison AE, Clarkson J: Kisspeptin regulation of puberty onset in the mouse. 1st World Conference Kisspeptin Signaling in the Brain, 2008.
16 Gajdos ZK, Butler JL, Henderson KD, He C, Supelak PJ, Egyud M, Price A, Reich D, Clayton PE, Le ML, Hunter DJ, Henderson BE, Palmert MR, Hirschhorn JN: Association studies of common variants in 10 hypogonadotropic hypogonadism genes with age at menarche. J Clin Endocrinol Metab 2008;93:4290–4298.
17 Ojeda SR, Lomniczi A, Mastronardi C, Heger S, Roth C, Parent AS, Matagne V, Mungenast AE: Minireview: the neuroendocrine regulation of puberty: Is the time ripe for a systems biology approach? Endocrinology 2006;147:1166–1174.
18 Krewson TD, Supelak PJ, Hill AE, Singer JB, Lander ES, Nadeau JH, Palmert MR: Chromosomes 6 and 13 harbor genes that regulate pubertal timing in mouse chromosome substitution strains. Endocrinology 2004;145:4447–4451.
19 Seminara SB, Crowley WF Jr: Perspective: the importance of genetic defects in humans in elucidating the complexities of the hypothalamic-pituitary-gonadal axis. Endocrinology 2001;142:2173–2177.
20 Ha CM, Choi J, Choi EJ, Costa ME, Lee BJ, Ojeda SR: NELL2, a neuron-specific EGF-like protein, is selectively expressed in glutamatergic neurons and contributes to the glutamatergic control of GnRH neurons at puberty. Neuroendocrinology 2008;88:199–211.
21 Choi J, Ha CM, Choi EJ, Jeong CS, Park JW, Baik JH, Park JY, Costa ME, Ojeda SR, Lee BJ: Kinesin superfamily-associated protein 3 is preferentially expressed in glutamatergic neurons and contributes to the excitatory control of female puberty. Endocrinology 2008;149:6146–6156.
22 Garcia-Rudaz C, Deng V, Matagne V, Ronnekleiv O, Bosch M, Han V, Percy AK, Ojeda SR: FXYD1, a modulator of Na(+),K(+)-ATPase activity, facilitates female sexual development by maintaining GnRH neuronal excitability. J Neuroendocrinol 2008;21: 108–122.
23 Lomniczi A, Cornea A, Costa ME, Ojeda SR: Hypothalamic tumor necrosis factor-α converting enzyme (TACE) mediates excitatory amino acid-dependent neuron-to-glia signaling in the neuroendocrine brain. J Neurosci 2006;26:51–62.
24 Parent AS, Mungenast AE, Lomniczi A, Sandau US, Peles E, Bosch MA, Ronnekleiv OK, Ojeda SR: A contactin-receptor-like protein tyrosine phosphatase beta complex mediates adhesive communication between astroglial cells and gonadotrophin-releasing hormone neurones. J Neuroendocrinol 2007;19:847–859.
25 Ojeda SR, Hill J, Hill DF, Costa ME, Tapia V, Cornea A, Ma YJ: The Oct-2 POU-domain gene in the neuroendocrine brain: a transcriptional regulator of mammalian puberty. Endocrinology 1999;140:3774–3789.
26 Mastronardi C, Smiley GG, Raber J, Kusakabe T, Kawaguchi A, Matagne V, Dietzel A, Heger S, Mungenast AE, Cabrera R, Kimura S, Ojeda SR: Deletion of the *Ttf1* gene in differentiated neurons disrupts female reproduction without impairing basal ganglia function. J Neurosci 2006;26:13167–13179.
27 Heger S, Mastronardi C, Dissen GA, Lomniczi A, Cabrera R, Roth CL, Jung H, Galimi F, Sippell W, Ojeda SR: Enhanced at puberty 1 (EAP1) is a new transcriptional regulator of the female neuroendocrine reproductive axis. J Clin Invest 2007;117:2145–2154.
28 Sutton VR, Shaffer LG: Search for imprinted regions on chromosome 14: comparison of maternal and paternal UPD cases with cases of chromosome 14 deletion. Am J Med Genet 2000;93:381–387.

29 Martin RA, Sabol DW, Rogan PK: Maternal uniparental disomy of chromosome 14 confined to an interstitial segment (14q23–14q24.2). J Med Genet 1999;36:633–636.
30 Tomkins DJ, Roux AF, Waye J, Freeman VC, Cox DW, Whelan DT: Maternal uniparental isodisomy of human chromosome 14 associated with a paternal t(13q14q) and precocious puberty. Eur J Hum Genet 1996;4:153–159.
31 Roth CL, Mastronardi C, Lomniczi A, Wright H, Cabrera R, Mungenast AE, Heger S, Jung H, Dubay C, Ojeda SR: Expression of a tumor-related gene network increases in the mammalian hypothalamus at the time of female puberty. Endocrinology 2007;148:5147–5161.
32 Tiscornia G, Singer O, Ilawa M, Verma IM: A general method for gene knockdown in mice by using lentiviral vectors expressing small interfering RNA. Proc Natl Acad Sci USA 2003;100:1844–1848.
33 Matagne V, Mastronardi C, Shapiro RA, Dorsa DM, Ojeda SR: Hypothalamic expression of *Eap1* is not directly controlled by ovarian steroids. Endocrinology 2008;150:1870–1878.
34 Wolffe AP, Matzke MA: Epigenetics: regulation through repression. Science 1999;286:481–486.
35 Herman JG, Baylin SB: Gene silencing in cancer in association with promoter hypermethylation. N Engl J Med 2003;349:2042–2054.
36 Garcia-Bassets I, Kwon YS, Telese F, Prefontaine GG, Hutt KR, Cheng CS, Ju BG, Ohgi KA, Wang J, Escoubet-Lozach L, Rose DW, Glass CK, Fu XD, Rosenfeld MG: Histone methylation-dependent mechanisms impose ligand dependency for gene activation by nuclear receptors. Cell 2007;128:505–518.
37 Miller CA, Sweatt JD: Covalent modification of DNA regulates memory formation. Neuron 2007;53:857–869.
38 Kangaspeska S, Stride B, Metivier R, Polycarpou-Schwarz M, Ibberson D, Carmouche RP, Benes V, Gannon F, Reid G: Transient cyclical methylation of promoter DNA. Nature 2008;452:112–115.
39 Fischer A, Sananbenesi F, Wang X, Dobbin M, Tsai LH: Recovery of learning and memory is associated with chromatin remodelling. Nature 2007;447:178–182.
40 Wu JI, Lessard J, Olave IA, Qiu Z, Ghosh A, Graef IA, Crabtree GR: Regulation of dendritic development by neuron-specific chromatin remodeling complexes. Neuron 2007;56:94–108.
41 Perillo B, Ombra MN, Bertoni A, Cuozzo C, Sacchetti S, Sasso A, Chiariotti L, Malorni A, Abbondanza C, Avvedimento EV: DNA oxidation as triggered by H3K9me2 demethylation drives estrogen-induced gene expression. Science 2008;319:202–206.
42 Shen S, Sandoval J, Swiss VA, Li J, Dupree J, Franklin RJM, Casaccia-Bonnefil P: Age-dependent epigenetic control of differentiation inhibitors is critical for remyelination efficiency. Nat Neurosci 2008;11:1024–1034.
43 Nakahata Y, Kaluzova M, Grimaldi B, Sahar S, Hirayama J, Chen D, Guarente LP, Sassone-Corsi P: The NAD+-dependent deacetylase SIRT1 modulates CLOCK-mediated chromatin remodeling and circadian control. Cell 2008;134:329–340.
44 Jaenisch R, Bird A: Epigenetic regulation of gene expression: how the genome integrates intrinsic and environmental signals. Nat Genet 2003;33(suppl):245–254.
45 Kouzarides T: Chromatin modifications and their function. Cell 2007;128:693–705.
46 Jenuwein T, Allis CD: Translating the histone code. Science 2001;293:1074–1080.
47 Berger SL: The complex language of chromatin regulation during transcription. Nature 2007;447:407–412.
48 Guttman M, Amit I, Garber M, French C, Lin MF, Feldser D, Huarte M, Zuk O, Carey BW, Cassady JP, Cabili MN, Jaenisch R, Mikkelsen TS, Jacks T, Hacohen N, Bernstein BE, Kellis M, Regev A, Rinn JL, Lander ES: Chromatin signature reveals over a thousand highly conserved large non-coding RNAs in mammals. Nature 2009;458:223–227.
49 Cameron EE, Bachman KE, Myohanen S, Herman JG, Baylin SB: Synergy of demethylation and histone deacetylase inhibition in the re-expression of genes silenced in cancer. Nat Genet 1999;21:103–107.
50 Robertson KD, it-Si-Ali S, Yokochi T, Wade PA, Jones PL, Wolffe AP: DNMT1 forms a complex with Rb, E2F1 and HDAC1 and represses transcription from E2F-responsive promoters. Nat Genet 2000;25:338–342.

Sergio R. Ojeda
Division of Neuroscience
Oregon National Primate Research Center/Oregon Health and Science University
505 N.W. 185th Avenue, Beaverton, OR 97006 (USA)
Tel. +1 503 690 5303, Fax +1 503 690 5384, E-Mail ojedas@ohsu.edu

Loche S, Cappa M, Ghizzoni L, Maghnie M, Savage MO (eds): Pediatric Neuroendocrinology.
Endocr Dev. Basel, Karger, 2010, vol 17, pp 52–62

Roles of Kisspeptins in the Control of Hypothalamic-Gonadotropic Function: Focus on Sexual Differentiation and Puberty Onset

Manuel Tena-Sempere

Department of Cell Biology, Physiology and Immunology, University of Córdoba, CIBER Fisiopatología de la Obesidad y Nutrición, and Instituto Maimonides de Investigaciones Biomédicas de Córdoba (IMIBIC), Córdoba, Spain

Abstract

Kisspeptins, a family of peptides encoded by the *Kiss1* gene that act via the G protein-coupled receptor 54 (GPR54 or Kiss1R), were initially catalogued as metastasis suppressors, but have recently emerged as pivotal gatekeepers of puberty onset and reproductive function. Indeed, since the seminal observations (in late 2003) that inactivating mutations of GPR54 are coupled to absence of puberty and hypogonadotropic hypogonadism in human and mice, a large number of experimental studies, conducted in different species, including humans, have substantiated the roles of kisspeptins and GPR54 as essential elements in the physiologic regulation of key aspects of reproductive maturation and function. These appear to include, among others, the process of brain sexual differentiation during critical (early) periods of maturation and the timing of puberty onset. Recent exciting developments in these particular areas will be comprehensively reviewed herein. These functions, together with the proven roles of kisspeptins in the control of GnRH neurons and the transmission of the regulatory actions of key signals, such as sex steroids, metabolic hormones and environmental cues, point out that the Kiss1 system is an indispensable player of the reproductive brain, whose discovery is now considered as (one of) the most important findings in reproductive physiology in the last decades.

In 2001, the *KISS1* gene, originally catalogued as metastasis suppressor, was found to encode a number of structurally related peptides, globally termed kisspeptins, which conduct their biological actions via the G protein-coupled receptor, GPR54 [1–3]. At that time, most of the attention devoted to this system lied in the field of cancer biology; indeed, the major product of KISS1 was named metastin due to its ability to inhibit tumor spread in different types of cancers [1]. However, it was not until late 2003 when the reproductive 'dimension' of kisspeptins and their receptor, now renamed KISS1 receptor (KISS1R) was disclosed, by the seminal observations from de Roux et al. [4]

and Seminara et al. [5] showing that humans and mice with genetic inactivation of GPR54 suffer hypogonadotropic hypogonadism. Such a striking phenotype, together with the original findings that pituitary responsiveness to exogenous GnRH as well as migration of GnRH neurons during early stages of development were grossly preserved in the absence of GPR54 [5], boosted an extraordinary interest among reproductive physiologists and clinicians, as they suggested for the first time the potential involvement of the so-called Kiss1 system in the physiological control of reproductive maturation and/or function. Nowadays, this contention has been firmly substantiated in a variety of mammalian and nonmammalian species, by an evergrowing number of molecular, physiologic and pharmacological studies [6, 7]. Indeed, the rapid expansion of the area makes it impossible to comprehensively condensate the state-of-the-art in this particular field within the limits of this brief review. In stead, in the present work, we will concentrate on recent developments in two exciting, and rapidly evolving facets of kisspeptin physiology: (1) the potential role of the Kiss1 system in sexual differentiation of the reproductive brain, and (2) the mechanisms whereby Kisspeptin neurons seemingly participate in the onset of puberty and its control by metabolic cues. Of important note, much of the progress in these areas has come from studies in laboratory rodents, as summarized herein. For nomenclature, we will partially adopt the recent proposal by Gottsch et al. [8], where *KISS1* and *Kiss1* are used to name the human and non-human genes, respectively. However, to keep the homogeneity with previous and current literature, the kisspeptin receptor will be termed GPR54 (usage of Kiss1R is fully valid as well). Finally, the term Kiss1 will be used for global reference to the ligand-receptor system, when no given species is alluded to.

Brain Sexual Differentiation and Puberty Onset

Puberty onset, as the period of full awakening of the hypothalamic-pituitary-gonadal (HPG) axis, is the end-point of a complex series of maturation events that allows the attainment of reproductive capacity and the acquisition of adult male and female phenotypes [9, 10]. Activation of the gonadotropic system at puberty, and its proper function later in life, critically depend on the adequate functional organization of the hypothalamic gonadotropin-releasing hormone (GnRH) network at the early stages of development [11]. In addition, the tempo of puberty is dictated by the dynamic interplay between central excitatory and inhibitory signals that impinge onto the GnRH system, and whose relative balance ranges from predominant restrain at early (infantile) periods to net activation at pre-pubertal stages of maturation. The nature and sources of such central regulators of puberty has been the subject of active investigation during the last years; identification of glia-to-neuron communication and the roles of kisspeptins being two clear examples of recent, exciting developments in the field [7, 12]. Besides these central factors, peripheral hormones participate also in this timely phenomenon, with sex steroids and metabolic factors (e.g. leptin) being key players in this process.

In rodents, brain sex differentiation takes place during a critical developmental window from late embryonic to early postnatal age [11, 13]. This is a sexually dimorphic phenomenon, mainly driven by gonadal steroids, whereby key neuronal networks at the hypothalamus become functionally organized in a permanent manner. This allows the timely activation of the reproductive axis at puberty, and the manifestation of sexually differentiated behaviors and neuroendocrine secretory patterns later on life [11, 13]. One of the neurohormonal traits that clearly displays sexual dimorphism is the cyclic secretory activity of the GnRH/gonadotropin system, together with the ability of estrogens to evoke the pre-ovulatory surge of gonadotropins from puberty onwards, which are detected only in the female [11]. Accordingly, experimental manipulations that alter the normal process of brain sex differentiation at early stages of development are capable to disrupt positive feedback and pre-ovulatory surges at adulthood. In addition, recent experimental data strongly suggest that puberty itself may define a second critical window for neuroendocrine development, as changes in sex steroid input during this period may result in permanent functional alterations of different neurohormonal axes (e.g. the corticotropic/stress axis) later in life [14].

Sexual Differentiation of Kiss1 Neurons: Functional Implications

Recent neuroanatomical studies, conducted mostly in laboratory rodents, but also in sheep and primates, have allowed the identification of discernible populations of Kiss1 neurons (and some of their projections) at the hypothalamus [6, 7, 15]. In the rat and mouse, these neurons are mostly located at the arcuate nucleus (ARC) and the anteroventral periventricular nucleus (AVPV) [6], although recent studies suggest that kisspeptin neurons at the latter site appear more as a continuum along the rostral periventricular area of the third ventricle (RP3V) [15]. Detailed description of the differential regulation of Kiss1/kisspeptin expression by sex steroids at these nuclei exceeds the scope of this review, and can be found elsewhere [6, 7]. For the purpose of this work, it is sufficient to stress that, based on the physiological profile of kisspeptins as potent elicitors of GnRH/gonadotropin secretion and their opposite patterns of response to sex steroids, it has been proposed that Kiss1 neurons at the ARC are involved in mediating the tonic negative feedback actions of androgens and estrogens on the gonadotropic axis in both males and females [6], whereas kisspeptin neurons at the AVPV seemingly participate in relaying the positive feedback actions of estradiol, which is mandatory for the generation of the pre-ovulatory surge of gonadotropins in the female only [6, 15].

Given the above features, characterization of the process of sexual differentiation of the hypothalamic Kiss1 system has been undertaken in rodents. In keeping with their putative physiological roles, Kiss1 neuronal population at the AVPV in the rat appear to be sexually dimorphic (much greater number in females vs. males), and sensitive to the organizing effects of sex steroids during the neonatal period of sexual maturation of the brain [16]. Indeed, neonatal exposure to high doses of androgen in female rats resulted in the complete 'masculinization' of the pattern of Kiss1 mRNA expression at the AVPV in adulthood since, contrary to cyclic females, neonatally androgenized female rats displayed negligible Kiss1 expression at this nucleus [16]. Moreover, exposure to estradiol as adults failed to increase Kiss1 mRNA levels at the AVPV of neonatally androgenized females; a response that was clearly detected in cyclic females [16]. Considering that neonatal androgenization of the female rat had been previously known to prevent the positive feedback effects of estradiol in terms of luteinizing hormone (LH) surges, these data strongly suggest that the mechanisms whereby the functional patterns of the GnRH/gonadotropic axis become sexually differentiated involve, at least in rodents, plastic changes in the population of Kiss1 neurons at the AVPV, which appear to be driven by sex steroid inputs at critical developmental periods. Those observations stress the sensitivity of the hypothalamic Kiss1 system to the organizing actions of endogenous (and eventually exogenous) sex steroids [17]. In this sense, analyses in α-fetoprotein (AFP) knock-out mice, where the congenital lack of this scavenger protein of circulating estrogens results in excessive estrogenic input during early development, have demonstrated that sexual differentiation and function of Kiss1 system is severely disrupted in these mice [18]. Similarly, we have recently shown that neonatal exposures to synthetic estrogens, known to disturb proper activation and function of the gonadotropic axis [19], persistently suppressed the hypothalamic expression of *Kiss1* gene at the expected time of puberty and adulthood in the rat [20, 21].

Of note, some of the above characteristics of the hypothalamic Kiss1 system in rodents might not be shared by other mammalian species. For instance, in the sheep, Kiss1 neurons responsible for mediating the negative and positive feedback effects of sex steroids appear to reside within different subareas of the ARC [22], but not in the AVPV/RP3V, whereas in primates (including humans), distribution of kisspeptin neurons at the hypothalamus seems to be mostly confined to the ARC/infundibular region [23, 24], where expression of *KISS1* gene is under the inhibitory regulation of androgens and estrogens. On the other hand, classical studies suggested decades ago that the mechanisms of sexual differentiation of gonadotropin control might be partially different between rodents and primates, as LH surges could be induced in male monkeys (even not subjected to hormonal manipulation at early stages of development), if provided with an appropriate ovarian (estrogen) signal as adults [25]. In this context, the nature and physiological relevance of the process of sexual differentiation of the hypothalamic kisspeptin system in non-rodent mammalian species, including humans, merit specific investigation.

Kiss1 System and the Timing of Puberty: Mechanisms and Physiological Relevance

The initial observations that the lack of functional GPR54 in humans and mice leads to absence of puberty and sexual immaturity pointed out the important physiological role of kisspeptin in the control of mammalian puberty [4, 5]; a contention that has been recently reinforced by analogous observations in Kiss1 KO mice [26, 27]. However, the underlying mechanisms subserving this critical function were not apparent on the basis of those original findings, and have attracted quite some attention in recent years. In fact, these mechanisms have been partially disclosed by expression and functional analyses, conducted mostly in laboratory rodents, which have documented the complex (and sophisticated) pattern of developmental activation of Kiss1 neurons along pubertal maturation. Integration of the available experimental evidence allows proposing that the mechanism whereby the Kiss1 system participates in the control of puberty onset in mammals are likely to include, at least, four major components:

(1) An increase in the endogenous kisspeptin tone, which seems to be sufficient *per se* to drive the GnRH/gonadotropin axis to a state of full activation – major evidence coming from studies in rats and monkeys [21, 28–30].

(2) An elevation in the sensitivity to the stimulatory effects of kisspeptin in terms of GnRH/LH responses – major evidence coming from studies in rats and mice [31, 32].

(3) An enhancement of GPR54 signaling efficiency, which is apparently coupled to a state of resistance to desensitization to kisspeptin stimulation – major evidence coming from studies in rats and mice [31, 33].

(4) An increase in the number of kisspeptin neurons (i.e. at the ARC and AVPV) and their projections to GnRH neurons from specific hypothalamic areas (i.e. AVPV) – major evidence coming from studies in mice [34].

An integral model for such a complex pattern of maturation and functions of the kisspeptin system in the context of the regulation of puberty onset is proposed in figure 1. Of important note, this multi-faceted process of maturation seems relevant for the precise timing of puberty, as the GnRH/LH axis is fully responsive to kisspeptin activation at earlier stages of postnatal development (e.g. neonatal/infantile period) [32, 35], which may otherwise render the system prone to precocious activation, especially considering that robust gonadotropic responses can be obtained in infantile rodents following administration of even modest doses of kisspeptin [32].

Also importantly, the above evidence raises the question of which signals are responsible for the array of maturational changes summarized above. Recent experimental evidence in female mice strongly suggests that the increase in kisspeptin expression at the hypothalamus at the time of puberty requires some degree of estrogenic input (from the ovary) [36]. This model implies that some sort of positive feedback loop between the ovary and the hypothalamus involving the Kiss1 system may exist before puberty and that, rather than genuine triggers, kisspeptin neurons would operate as estrogen-dependent amplifiers of GnRH neuron activity in the prepubertal period [36]. It remains to be defined which level of estrogenic input is required for the pubertal activation of the Kiss1 system. Likewise, the mechanisms and hypothalamic sites whereby Kiss1 neurons are activated and participate in the timing of puberty onset in males remain to be defined.

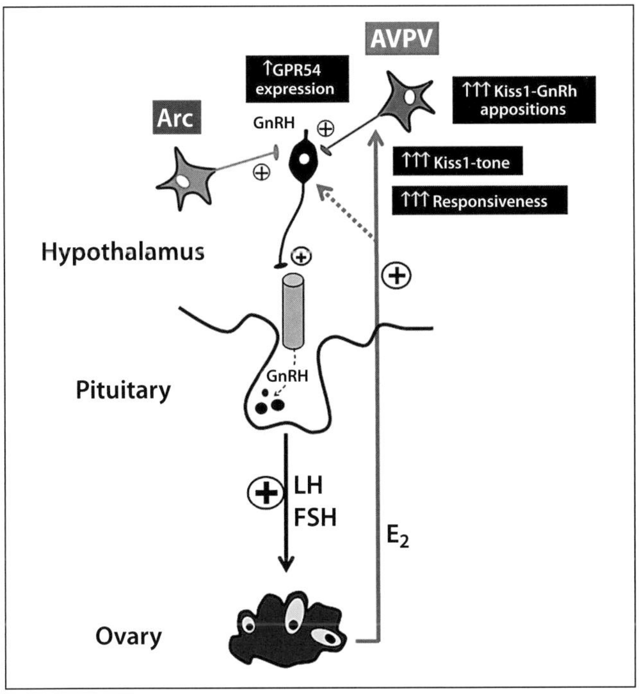

Fig. 1. Tentative model for the mechanisms involved in the predicted maturational and functional changes of kisspeptin/GPR54 system at the time of puberty in female rodents. These are likely to include: (1) the increase in endogenous kisspeptin tone at certain hypothalamic nuclei (mainly, at the AVPV); (2) the elevation of the expression of GPR54, which seems less consistent across the species than that of the ligand; (3) the rise in the sensitivity/responsiveness to the stimulatory effects of kisspeptin, together with enhanced efficiency of GPR54 coupling to its signaling systems, and (4) the increase in the number of projections/appositions between kisspeptin and GnRH neurons. Such a pubertal heightening of kisspeptin expression seems to require the permissive/driving effects of estrogens; Kiss1 neurons being estrogen-dependent amplifiers of GnRH neurosecretion at the time of puberty. Overall, the enhancement in the activity of Kiss1 system operates a major driving force for the full activation of the GnRH pulse generator (denoted by *arrows*), which in turn dictates gonadotropin secretion and gonadal function, at the time of puberty. The putative roles of Kiss1 neurons at the ARC in the timing/control of male and female puberty are less well characterized, and have not been schematized in the figure. Adapted from references [7, 36], with substantial modifications.

Kiss1 System as Transmitter for the Metabolic Regulation of Puberty and Fertility

Among different modulators, puberty onset is sensitive to the state of body fuel reserves; conditions of disturbed energy homeostasis being coupled to alterations in the timing of puberty and different degrees of subfertility later in life [37]. In recent years, compelling evidence, gathered in laboratory rodents, has strongly suggested that the hypothalamic Kiss1 system is under the regulation of metabolic cues; this being a tenable mechanism for the modulation of the timing of puberty by the energy status and nutritional factors. Indeed, conditions of negative energy balance induce variable degrees of inhibition of *Kiss1* mRNA expression in pubertal and adult rodents [38–42]. Moreover, the state of hypogonadotropism and lack of puberty induced by chronic subnutrition in female rats could be rescued (at least partially) solely by administration of exogenous kisspeptin [38]. Altogether, this experimental evidence supports the hypothesis that kisspeptin neurons at the hypothalamus operate as sensors and neuroendocrine conduit for conveying metabolic information onto reproductive centers (likely, GnRH neurons); a phenomenon which seems relevant for the tight relationship between body energy status and the onset of puberty [40, 43].

While the neuroendocrine mechanisms responsible for the metabolic regulation of Kiss1 neurons are yet to be fully characterized, compelling evidence has demonstrated that leptin, as adipose signal of energy abundance, plays a crucial role in this phenomenon. This has been exposed by studies in rodent models of rather 'extreme' metabolic alterations, such as the ob/ob mouse and the rat model of uncontrolled diabetes induced by streptozotocin administration [39, 42, 44]. In such conditions of severe hypogonadotropism and hypo-leptinemia, hypothalamic expression of Kiss1 mRNA was significantly suppressed; a condition that could be rescued by exogenous administration of leptin. In the same vein, leptin has been shown to significantly increase Kiss1 mRNA levels in the murine hypothalamic cell line, N6, which constitutively express the *Kiss1* gene [41]. Altogether, the above data document that leptin is a positive modulator of the kisspeptin system.

More relevant in terms of puberty control, preliminary studies from our group in pubertal female rats submitted to changes in perinatal food intake by means of manipulation of litter size further support a master role of leptin as modulator of hypothalamic Kiss1 system and puberty onset. In our experimental setting, female rats bred in small litters (SL: 4 pups/dam) show a persistent increase in body weight (BW) after weaning, with an earlier age of vaginal opening (standard index of puberty). In contrast, rats bred in large litters (LL: 20 pups/dam) display persistently lower body weights after weaning, with a modest delay in vaginal opening. In this model, there appears to exist a close correlation between body weight, age of vaginal opening and circulating leptin levels (SL>>LL). More interestingly, we have also observed a positive correlation between serum leptin concentrations and relative Kiss1 mRNA levels, as well as the number of kisspeptin-positive neurons, at the hypothalamus [Castellano and Tena-Sempere, in prep.]. These preliminary findings reinforce the contention that leptin is involved in the physiological control of hypothalamic Kiss1 neurons; thereby defining a discernible leptin-kisspeptin-GnRH pathway, with potential roles in the metabolic modulation of puberty onset. Importantly, the molecular mechanisms whereby leptin activates *Kiss1* gene expression have begun to be deciphered recently, as the Creb1 coactivator, Crtc1, has been pointed out as positive transcriptional regulator of *Kiss1* gene expression at discrete hypothalamic areas [45]. In the same line, we have recently obtained evidence that the sensor of the intracellular energy state, mammalian target of rapamycin (mTOR), is likely to play a crucial role in the central control of puberty onset, via modulation of *Kiss1* gene expression at the hypothalamus [Roa and Tena-Sempere, submitted]. Of note, both Crtc-1 and mTOR have been proposed as transducers of leptin effects in terms of energy homeostasis [45, 46]. In addition, they appear to serve an important, previously unnoticed function in the regulation of puberty onset and fertility, as crucial mediators of the effects of leptin on the expression of *Kiss1* gene.

Future Directions and Conclusions

Identification of the reproductive 'dimension' of the Kiss1/GPR54 system has revolutionized our understanding of the physiological mechanisms responsible for the control of key aspects of reproductive maturation and function. Among those facets, recent developments in the field have substantiated that, at least in rodents, Kiss1 neurons at the hypothalamus are the targets and important players of the process of brain sexual differentiation; proper functional organization of this neuronal population at early stages of development being mandatory for normal puberty onset and dynamic regulation of gonadotropin secretion (negative and positive feedbacks of sex steroids) later in life. Similarly, the hypothalamic Kiss1 system seems posed with a pivotal role in defining the timing of puberty onset, through a complex program of maturational changes, which might be driven, at least in the female mouse, by earlier changes in ovarian estrogen input and are influenced by the metabolic state of the organism, through a leptin-dependent mechanism. Altogether, these findings illustrate the physiological importance of kisspeptins, whose reproductive roles remained unnoticed for years, as one of the most fundamental players in the control of puberty and fertility.

However, despite the astonishing progress in the field, characterization of the physiological roles of kisspeptin is still at its infancy, and several key aspects of this system await further investigation. In this context, considerable excitement has been recently drawn by the identification of the reproductive consequences of inactivating mutations of TAC3 (encoding neurokin B; NKB) and TAC3R (encoding its putative receptor, NK3) genes [47]; patients which are an apparent phenocopy of GPR54 null humans. Intriguingly, in the sheep, kisspeptins and NKB are co-expressed in neurons at the ARC, which also express dynorphin [48]; NKB and dynorphin being previously recognized as putative modulators of the gonadotropic axis. Yet, the potential interplay of these three major regulators, its eventual co-expression in other mammalian species, and their roles, if any, in the modulation of sexual differentiation and puberty onset remain to be fully characterized. From a more general perspective, identification of the crucial functions of kisspeptin neurons in discrete hypothalamic areas has made it mandatory to re-assess the mechanisms of action, and potential interactions with kisspeptins, of many classical neurotransmitters and neuropeptides, already known to modulate GnRH function. Overall, it is anticipated that such research efforts will lead to a significant expansion of our current knowledge on the physiological roles of kisspeptin signaling in the brain, thereby allowing to better define how this novel ligand-receptor system participates in the dynamic regulation (and eventual alteration) of reproductive maturation and function along the life-span.

Acknowledgments

The author is indebted with the members of the research team at the Physiology Section of the University of Cordoba, who actively participated in the generation of experimental data discussed herein. The work from the author's laboratory reviewed in this article was supported by grants BFU 2005–07446 and BFU 2008–00984 (Ministerio de Ciencia e Innovación, Spain), funds from Instituto de Salud Carlos III (Red de Centros RCMN C03/08 and Project PI042082; Ministerio de Sanidad, Spain), Project P08-CVI-03788 (Junta de Andalucía, Spain), and EU research contracts EDEN QLK4-CT-2002–00603 and DEER FP7-ENV-2007–1. CIBER is an initiative of Instituto de Salud Carlos III (Ministerio de Sanidad, Spain).

References

1 Ohtaki T, Shintani Y, Honda S, Matsumoto H, Hori A, Kanehashi K, Terao Y, Kumano S, Takatsu Y, Masuda Y, Ishibashi Y, Watanabe T, Asada M, Yamada T, Suenaga M, Kitada C, Usuki S, Kurokawa T, Onda H, Nishimura O, Fujino M: Metastasis suppressor gene KiSS-1 encodes peptide ligand of a G-protein-coupled receptor. Nature 2001;411:613–617.

2 Muir AI, Chamberlain L, Elshourbagy NA, Michalovich D, Moore DJ, Calamari A, Szekeres PG, Sarau HM, Chambers JK, Murdock P, Steplewski K, Shabon U, Miller JE, Middleton SE, Darker JG, Larminie CG, Wilson S, Bergsma DJ, Emson P, Faull R, Philpott KL, Harrison DC: AXOR12, a novel human G protein-coupled receptor, activated by the peptide KiSS-1. J Biol Chem 2001;276:28969–28975.

3 Kotani M, Detheux M, Vandenbogaerde A, Communi D, Vanderwinden JM, Le Poul E, Brezillon S, Tyldesley R, Suarez-Huerta N, Vandeput F, Blanpain C, Schiffmann SN, Vassart G, Parmentier M: The metastasis suppressor gene KiSS-1 encodes kisspeptins, the natural ligands of the orphan G protein-coupled receptor GPR54. J Biol Chem 2001; 276:34631–34636.

4 de Roux N, Genin E, Carel JC, Matsuda F, Chaussain JL, Milgrom E: Hypogonadotropic hypogonadism due to loss of function of the KiSS1-derived peptide receptor GPR54. Proc Natl Acad Sci USA 2003;100: 10972–10976.

5 Seminara SB, Messager S, Chatzidaki EE, Thresher RR, Acierno JS Jr, Shagoury JK, Bo-Abbas Y, Kuohung W, Schwinof KM, Hendrick AG, Zahn D, Dixon J, Kaiser UB, Slaugenhaupt SA, Gusella JF, O'Rahilly S, Carlton MB, Crowley WF Jr, Aparicio SA, Colledge WH: The GPR54 gene as a regulator of puberty. N Engl J Med 2003;349:1614–1627.

6 Popa SM, Clifton DK, Steiner RA: The role of kisspeptins and GPR54 in the neuroendocrine regulation of reproduction. Annu Rev Physiol 2008;70: 213–238.

7 Roa J, Aguilar E, Dieguez C, Pinilla L, Tena-Sempere M: New frontiers in kisspeptin/GPR54 physiology as fundamental gatekeepers of reproductive function. Front Neuroendocrinol 2008;29:48–69.

8 Gottsch ML, Clifton DK, Steiner RA: From KISS1 to kisspeptins: an historical perspective and suggested nomenclature. Peptides 2009;30:4–9.

9 Ojeda SR, Skinner MK: Puberty in the rat; in Neill JD (ed): The Physiology of Reproduction. San Diego, Academic Press/Elsevier, 2006, pp 2061–2126.

10 Parent AS, Teilmann G, Juul A, Skakkebaek NE, Toppari J, Bourguignon JP: The timing of normal puberty and the age limits of sexual precocity: variations around the world, secular trends, and changes after migration. Endocr Rev 2003;24:668–693.

11 Gore AC: Developmental programming and endocrine disruptor effects on reproductive neuroendocrine systems. Front Neuroendocrinol 2008;29: 358–374.

12 Ojeda SR, Lomniczi A, Mastronardi C, Heger S, Roth C, Parent AS, Matagne V, Mungenast AE: Minireview: the neuroendocrine regulation of puberty: is the time ripe for a systems biology approach? Endocrinology 2006;147:1166–1174.
13 Morris JA, Jordan CL, Breedlove SM: Sexual differentiation of the vertebrate nervous system. Nat Neurosci 2004;7:1034–1039.
14 Evuarherhe O, Leggett JD, Waite EJ, Kershaw YM, Atkinson HC, Lightman SL: Organizational role for pubertal androgens on adult hypothalamic-pituitary-adrenal sensitivity to testosterone in the male Sprague Dawley rat. J Physiol 2009.
15 Herbison AE: Estrogen positive feedback to gonadotropin-releasing hormone (GnRH) neurons in the rodent: the case for the rostral periventricular area of the third ventricle (RP3V). Brain Res Rev 2008; 57:277–287.
16 Kauffman AS, Gottsch ML, Roa J, Byquist AC, Crown A, Clifton DK, Hoffman GE, Steiner RA, Tena-Sempere M: Sexual differentiation of Kiss1 gene expression in the brain of the rat. Endocrinology 2007;148:1774–1783.
17 Navarro VM, Tena-Sempere M: The KiSS-1/GPR54 system: putative target for endocrine disruption of reproduction at hypothalamic-pituitary unit? Int J Androl 2008;31:224–232.
18 Gonzalez-Martinez D, De Mees C, Douhard Q, Szpirer C, Bakker J: Absence of gonadotropin-releasing hormone 1 and Kiss1 activation in alpha-fetoprotein knockout mice: prenatal estrogens defeminize the potential to show preovulatory luteinizing hormone surges. Endocrinology 2008; 149:2333–2340.
19 Tena-Sempere M, Pinilla L, Gonzalez LC, Aguilar E: Reproductive disruption by exposure to exogenous estrogenic compounds during sex differentiation: lessons from the neonatally estrogenized male rat. Curr Top Steroid Res 2000;3:23–37.
20 Navarro VM, Sanchez-Garrido MA, Castellano JM, Roa J, Garcia-Galiano D, Pineda R, Aguilar E, Pinilla L, Tena-Sempere M: Persistent impairment of hypothalamic KiSS-1 system after exposures to estrogenic compounds at critical periods of brain sex differentiation. Endocrinology 2009;150:2359–2367.
21 Navarro VM, Castellano JM, Fernandez-Fernandez R, Barreiro ML, Roa J, Sanchez-Criado JE, Aguilar E, Dieguez C, Pinilla L, Tena-Sempere M: Developmental and hormonally regulated messenger ribonucleic acid expression of KiSS-1 and its putative receptor, GPR54, in rat hypothalamus and potent luteinizing hormone-releasing activity of KiSS-1 peptide. Endocrinology 2004;145:4565–4574.
22 Estrada KM, Clay CM, Pompolo S, Smith JT, Clarke IJ: Elevated KiSS-1 expression in the arcuate nucleus prior to the cyclic preovulatory gonadotrophin-releasing hormone/lutenising hormone surge in the ewe suggests a stimulatory role for kisspeptin in oestrogen-positive feedback. J Neuroendocrinol 2006;18:806–809.
23 Rometo AM, Krajewski SJ, Voytko ML, Rance NE: Hypertrophy and increased kisspeptin gene expression in the hypothalamic infundibular nucleus of postmenopausal women and ovariectomized monkeys. J Clin Endocrinol Metab 2007;92:2744–2750.
24 Shibata M, Friedman RL, Ramaswamy S, Plant TM: Evidence that down regulation of hypothalamic KiSS-1 expression is involved in the negative feedback action of testosterone to regulate luteinising hormone secretion in the adult male rhesus monkey (*Macaca mulatta*). J Neuroendocrinol 2007;19:432–438.
25 Norman RL, Spies HG: Cyclic ovarian function in a male macaque: additional evidence for a lack of sexual differentiation in the physiological mechanisms that regulate the cyclic release of gonadotropins in primates. Endocrinology 1986;118: 2608–2610.
26 d'Anglemont de Tassigny X, Fagg LA, Dixon JP, Day K, Leitch HG, Hendrick AG, Zahn D, Franceschini I, Caraty A, Carlton MB, Aparicio SA, Colledge WH: Hypogonadotropic hypogonadism in mice lacking a functional Kiss1 gene. Proc Natl Acad Sci USA 2007;104:10714–10719.
27 Lapatto R, Pallais JC, Zhang D, Chan YM, Mahan A, Cerrato F, Le WW, Hoffman GE, Seminara SB: Kiss1/ mice exhibit more variable hypogonadism than gpr54/mice. Endocrinology 2007;148:4927–4936.
28 Navarro VM, Fernandez-Fernandez R, Castellano JM, Roa J, Mayen A, Barreiro ML, Gaytan F, Aguilar E, Pinilla L, Dieguez C, Tena-Sempere M: Advanced vaginal opening and precocious activation of the reproductive axis by KiSS-1 peptide, the endogenous ligand of GPR54. J Physiol 2004;561:379–386.
29 Plant TM, Ramaswamy S, Dipietro MJ: Repetitive activation of hypothalamic G protein-coupled receptor 54 with intravenous pulses of kisspeptin in the juvenile monkey (*Macaca mulatta*) elicits a sustained train of gonadotropin-releasing hormone discharges. Endocrinology 2006;147:1007–1013.
30 Shahab M, Mastronardi C, Seminara SB, Crowley WF, Ojeda SR, Plant TM: Increased hypothalamic GPR54 signaling: a potential mechanism for initiation of puberty in primates. Proc Natl Acad Sci USA 2005;102:2129–2134.
31 Han SK, Gottsch ML, Lee KJ, Popa SM, Smith JT, Jakawich SK, Clifton DK, Steiner RA, Herbison AE: Activation of gonadotropin-releasing hormone neurons by kisspeptin as a neuroendocrine switch for the onset of puberty. J Neurosci 2005;25:11349–11356.

32 Castellano JM, Navarro VM, Fernandez-Fernandez R, Castano JP, Malagon MM, Aguilar E, Dieguez C, Magni P, Pinilla L, Tena-Sempere M: Ontogeny and mechanisms of action for the stimulatory effect of kisspeptin on gonadotropin-releasing hormone system of the rat. Mol Cell Endocrinol 2006;257–258:75–83.
33 Roa J, Vigo E, Garcia-Galiano D, Castellano JM, Navarro VM, Pineda R, Dieguez C, Aguilar E, Pinilla L, Tena-Sempere M: Desensitization of gonadotropin responses to kisspeptin in the female rat: analyses of LH and FSH secretion at different developmental and metabolic states. Am J Physiol Endocrinol Metab 2008;294:E1088–E1096.
34 Clarkson J, Herbison AE: Postnatal development of kisspeptin neurons in mouse hypothalamus; sexual dimorphism and projections to gonadotropin-releasing hormone neurons. Endocrinology 2006; 147:5817–5825.
35 Nazian SJ: Role of metastin in the release of gonadotropin-releasing hormone from the hypothalamus of the male rat. J Androl 2006;27:444–449.
36 Clarkson J, Boon WC, Simpson ER, Herbison AE: Postnatal development of an estradiol-kisspeptin positive feedback mechanism implicated in puberty onset. Endocrinology 2009;150:3214—3220.
37 Fernandez-Fernandez R, Martini AC, Navarro VM, Castellano JM, Dieguez C, Aguilar E, Pinilla L, Tena-Sempere M: Novel signals for the integration of energy balance and reproduction. Mol Cell Endocrinol 2006;254–255:127–132.
38 Castellano JM, Navarro VM, Fernandez-Fernandez R, Nogueiras R, Tovar S, Roa J, Vazquez MJ, Vigo E, Casanueva FF, Aguilar E, Pinilla L, Dieguez C, Tena-Sempere M: Changes in hypothalamic KiSS-1 system and restoration of pubertal activation of the reproductive axis by kisspeptin in undernutrition. Endocrinology 2005;146:3917–3925.
39 Castellano JM, Navarro VM, Fernandez-Fernandez R, Roa J, Vigo E, Pineda R, Dieguez C, Aguilar E, Pinilla L, Tena-Sempere M: Expression of hypothalamic KiSS-1 system and rescue of defective gonadotropic responses by kisspeptin in streptozotocin-induced diabetic male rats. Diabetes 2006;55:2602–2610.
40 Castellano JM, Roa J, Luque RM, Dieguez C, Aguilar E, Pinilla L, Tena-Sempere M: KiSS-1/kisspeptins and the metabolic control of reproduction: physiologic roles and putative physiopathological implications. Peptides 2009;30:139–145.
41 Luque RM, Kineman RD, Tena-Sempere M: Regulation of hypothalamic expression of KiSS-1 and GPR54 genes by metabolic factors: analyses using mouse models and a cell line. Endocrinology 2007;148:4601–4611.
42 Castellano JM, Navarro VM, Roa J, Pineda R, Sanchez-Garrido MA, Garcia-Galiano D, Vigo E, Dieguez C, Aguilar E, Pinilla L, Tena-Sempere M: Alterations in hypothalamic KiSS-1 system in experimental diabetes: early changes and functional consequences. Endocrinology 2009;150:784–794.
43 Tena-Sempere M: KiSS-1 and reproduction: focus on its role in the metabolic regulation of fertility. Neuroendocrinology 2006;83:275–281.
44 Smith JT, Acohido BV, Clifton DK, Steiner RA: KiSS-1 neurones are direct targets for leptin in the ob/ob mouse. J Neuroendocrinol 2006;18:298–303.
45 Altarejos JY, Goebel N, Conkright MD, Inoue H, Xie J, Arias CM, Sawchenko PE, Montminy M: The Creb1 coactivator Crtc1 is required for energy balance and fertility. Nat Med 2008;14:1112–1117.
46 Cota D, Proulx K, Smith KA, Kozma SC, Thomas G, Woods SC, Seeley RJ: Hypothalamic mTOR signaling regulates food intake. Science 2006;312:927–930.
47 Topaloglu AK, Reimann F, Guclu M, Yalin AS, Kotan LD, Porter KM, Serin A, Mungan NO, Cook JR, Ozbek MN, Imamoglu S, Akalin NS, Yuksel B, O'Rahilly S, Semple RK: TAC3 and TACR3 mutations in familial hypogonadotropic hypogonadism reveal a key role for neurokinin B in the central control of reproduction. Nat Genet 2009;41:354–358.
48 Goodman RL, Lehman MN, Smith JT, Coolen LM, de Oliveira CV, Jafarzadehshirazi MR, Pereira A, Iqbal J, Caraty A, Ciofi P, Clarke IJ: Kisspeptin neurons in the arcuate nucleus of the ewe express both dynorphin A and neurokinin B. Endocrinology 2007;148:5752–5760.

Manuel Tena-Sempere
Department of Cell Biology, Physiology and Immunology
Faculty of Medicine, University of Córdoba
Avda. Menéndez Pidal s/n, ES–14004 Córdoba (Spain)
Tel. +34 957 218280, Fax +34 957 218 288; E-Mail fi1tesem@uco.es

Loche S, Cappa M, Ghizzoni L, Maghnie M, Savage MO (eds): Pediatric Neuroendocrinology.
Endocr Dev. Basel, Karger, 2010, vol 17, pp 63–76

Role of the Growth Hormone/Insulin-Like Growth Factor 1 Axis in Neurogenesis

N. David Åberg

Center of Brain Research and Rehabilitation, Institute of Physiology and Neuroscience, and Laboratory of Experimental Endocrinology, Department of Internal Medicine, Institute of Medicine, Sahlgrenska University Hospital, University of Gothenburg, Gothenburg, Sweden

Abstract

The growth hormone/insulin-like growth factor 1 (GH/IGF-1) axis is not only involved in brain growth, development and myelination, but also in brain plasticity as indexed by neurogenesis. This may have links to various cognitive effects of GH and IGF-1. GH and IGF-1 affect the genesis of neurons, astrocytes, endothelial cells and oligodendrocytes. Specifically, IGF-1 increases progenitor cell proliferation and numbers of new neurons, oligodendrocytes, and blood vessels in the dentate gyrus of the hippocampus. In the adult cerebral cortex IGF-1 only affects oligodendrogenesis. Recently, GH therapy has also been shown to induce cell genesis in the adult brain. The profile of effects by GH therapy may be somewhat different than that of IGF-1. In addition, GH secretagogues (GHS) also have neuroprotective and cell regenerative effects per se in the brain. Finally, transgenic disruptions in GH signaling pathways affect neuron and astrocyte cell numbers during development and during adulthood. Altogether, data suggest that both exogenous and endogenous GH and/or IGF-1 may be used as agents to enhance cell genesis and neurogenesis in the adult brain. Theoretically these substances could be used to enhance recovery after brain injuries. However, further experiments with specific animal models for brain injuries are needed before clinical trials can be started.

The subject of growth hormone (GH) and insulin-like growth factor-1 (IGF-1) in neurogenesis requires the attention of two scientific fields to come together, i.e. neurobiology and endocrinology. For a number of years it has been known that GH has positive cognitive effects in adult patients with GH deficiency (GHD) [1, 2]. Also in children with GHD intellectual properties are decreased, and it appears that GH treatment improves cognitive function at least in girls with the Turner syndrome [3]. It was shown already forty years ago, that GH treatment in rats affected brain structure [4]. Later on it was shown that GH affected other biochemical parameters in the brain, for example neurotransmitter abundance [5]. Positive cognitive effects of GH treatment have been further characterized in both humans and animals. Specifically,

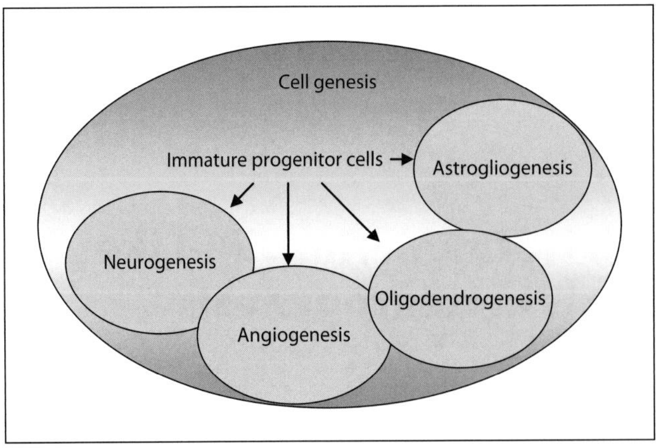

Fig. 1. The conceptual relations between neurogenesis and other de novo cell genesis in the brain. Sometimes neurogenesis is emphasized at the expense of other types of cell genesis in both the young and old brain. However, it appears that formation of new oligodendrocytes and new blood vessels (angiogenesis) and even new astrocytes contribute to the regeneration in the adult brain. GH and IGF-1 have been shown to enhance de novo genesis of all these four types of cell renewal in various brain regions in different animal models.

it appears that mental alertness and hippocampal-dependent memory functions are positively affected by GH [2].

Since it was rediscovered that neurogenesis actually occurred in the adult mammalian brain in the early 1980s [6, 7], the scientific field of cell genesis has received exponentially more interest. An important hallmark in the field was when Peter Eriksson discovered that neurogenesis occurs both in the adult human hippocampus [8] and subventricular zone and olfactory bulb [9]. As neurogenesis has gained increasing interest, other cell genesis has also come into focus (fig. 1). Especially, oligodendrogenesis is an important contributor to positive effects in the brain. During the last years, neurogenesis and cell genesis has become more integrated into a general view including many mechanisms of plasticity in the brain such as for example synapse density, neurophysiology, cell communication, and neuroendocrinology.

The role of GH and IGF-1 in neurogenesis includes some important issues that need to be highlighted, as GH and IGF-1 may have different effects under different conditions. Very important is the difference between systemic and local GH and IGF-1. Another important issue is whether experiments using transgenic constructs to alter GH-IGF-1 systemic and local expression differ to defined systemic treatments. In addition, it appears that there are quite profound differences between the effects of GH-IGF-1 in the development as compared to adult and old ages. Finally, there are also brain region-specific effects of GH and IGF-1, as well as specific effects of GH and IGF-1, respectively. The goal of this chapter is to bring some light to these issues.

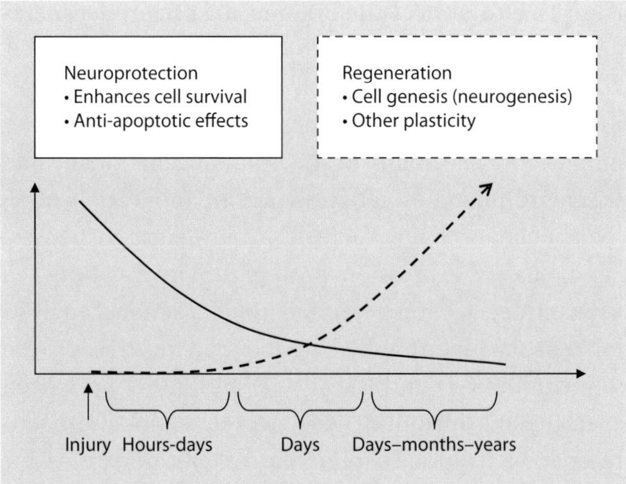

Fig. 2. Neuroprotection and regeneration. GH and IGF-1 was first studied in the brain with respect to protecting the brain against injury, mostly hypoxic-ischemic injuries. Later it has been observed that the time window for treating with GH and IGF-1 can be expanded for longer time periods (more than a week). The long-term beneficial effects of GH and IGF-1 treatment after an injury likely partly depends on the birth of new cells, including neurogenesis, that replaces damaged brain tissue. This process is part of the regenerative response. While the neuroprotective responses of GH and IGF-1 are comparatively well known in experimental animals, there is still a need of further studies to explore the exact nature and time windows of the long-term regenerative effects of GH and IGF-1 after an injury in the brain.

Neurogenesis, Neuroprotection and Plasticity

Neurogenesis has gained progressively increasing interest in terms of brain plasticity in the last 15–20 years [for reviews, see 6, 7]. The reason for this is to a large degree that neurogenesis is relatively easy to monitor with histological techniques [6]. Also, newborn cells are easy to track for long times of follow-up and newborn cells can also be easily analyzed for other markers of differentiation. Finally, neurogenesis appears to have direct significance for memory formation and brain function [10, 11]. The concept of neuroprotection has been partly changed by with the advent of studies focusing on neurogenesis. As the CNS was not capable of regenerating new neurons, studies were largely focusing on protecting or saving brain tissue from damage after an injury (neuroprotection; fig. 2). However, clinically it was evident that there was a functional healing of the CNS after various injuries, and when adult neurogenesis was rediscovered in the 1980s, the concept of regeneration came into focus in parallel with the concept of neuroprotection. Interestingly, during the last 10 years it has become clear that many of the substances that can 'protect' the CNS also are the same substances that actively 'regenerate' the brain. This certainly appears to be the case of both GH secretagogues (GHS, GH and IGF-1) [for reviews, see 12, 13]. Also, neuroprotection sometimes takes place to protect the brain against neurodegenerative diseases, acting by various plasticity mechanisms.

Although adult neurogenesis and genesis of other cell types such as astrocytes, oligodendrocytes and blood vessels in the brain contributes to brain plasticity, other types of changes are also very important. The ability of the brain to functionally and structurally adapt to a new task, environment, or consequences of an injury is often referred to as brain plasticity. This includes changes in mRNA, proteins, post-translational modifications, cellular and regional expression, protein activity function, cell physiology (e.g. ions and neurotransmitters, action potentials), and functional analysis of memory, behavior, and motor-sensory function. During the years this has proven to be true for many substances, including GH and IGF-1. GH and IGF-1 have been shown to affect a multitude of mechanisms, including neurogenesis, oligodendrogenesis, angiogenesis, glutamate receptor activation, cholinergic system, dopaminergic reward system, monoamine abundance, dendritic arborization, astrocyte communication via connexin 43, and opioid receptor abundance [for review, see 13]. Plasticity in the brain has even in humans been extended to include macrostructural changes in the brain. A well-known example is the study of London taxi drivers whose anterior and posterior hippocampal diameters were changed with more years in duty [14]. Within this concept of brain plasticity, a description of cellular mechanisms of action for GH and IGF-1 will be presented.

The Growth Hormone and Insulin-Like Growth Factor 1 System in the Brain

GH receptors (GH-R) and IGF-1 receptors are present in wide parts of the brain. GH receptor immunoreactivity is found in both neurons, astrocytes and oligodendrocytes [15] (for review, see table 1, Åberg et al. [13]). Abundant GH-R expression is found in the choroid plexus, hippocampus and the hypothalamus in both rodents [15] and humans [16]. IGF-1-R is expressed in neuronal stem cells [17], but is also present in neurons and glial cells throughout the brain [18, 19]. Like GH-R, the IGF-1-R is highly abundant in the choroid plexus as shown in both ligand-binding experiments [20] and from IGF-1 receptor mRNA studies [21].

Apart from GH and IGF-1 in the circulation there is also a local synthesis of both GH and IGF-1 in the brain outside the pituitary. Evidence of extrapituitary GH synthesis was demonstrated already around 1980 in hypophysectomized rats and primates [22, 23] and extrapituitary GH-like material was found long after hypophysectomy with levels about 10^6 less than in the anterior pituitary [22]. Also, GH mRNA has been reported in the caudate putamen, the striatum, the ventral thalamus, the formatio reticularis, the outer part of hippocampus and the basal cortex [24]. Although controversial for a number of years, additional data have added support for at least a low-level expression of extrapituitary GH [25, 26]. IGF-1 immunoreactivity is also widespread in all types of neurons in the brain [27]. IGF-1 expression in the CNS is particularly high during fetal development and peaks during the first 2 postnatal weeks, predominantly in neurons but also in glial progenitors [28–31]. Moreover, IGF-1 expression is partly transient corresponding to regions and periods of axon outgrowth, dendritic maturation and synaptogenesis [32].

Circulating IGF-1 is bound to different IGF binding proteins (IGFBPs), of which six (IGFBP1–6), have been characterized to date [for review of CNS function, see 13]. At the cell surface or in the extracellular cell matrix, IGFBPs can either inhibit or enhance the presentation of IGF-1 to its receptor. In addition, it appears that there are IGF-1 independent actions of the IGFBPs [for review, see 33]. Altogether, the exact roles of the different IGFBPs in the CNS [for reviews, see 34, 35] are largely unknown, especially in the context of brain injury and repair.

GH is taken up from the bloodstream into the brain parenchyma through different routes. First, GH-R is present in the choroid plexus and it has been suggested to play a role in the transport of GH across the blood-CSF barrier [16]. Moreover, when GH was administered peripherally to patients with GH deficiency, a tenfold increase in cerebrospinal fluid levels of GH was reported [36]. It appears that GH passes the capillary bed blood-brain barrier (BBB) into both the mouse and rat brain in vivo and experiments in endothelial cell cultures in vitro favors the idea of an influx of GH by simple diffusion, despite the absence of a specific transport system [37]. It is not clear whether there is another specific transport in the blood-CSF barrier than in the choroid plexus. In addition, the BBB (both blood-CSF barrier and capillary bed BBB) might be compromised in different pathological conditions such as after a hypoxic-ischemic event [38] or even by hypophysectomy itself [39]. Taken together, there is growing support of a passage of GH over the BBB, although the exact mechanisms and extent of passage remains to be further elucidated.

IGF-1 also reaches the brain via both the capillary bed BBB and via the blood-CSF barrier. It appears that IGF-1 uptake is mediated by a specific carrier both in the capillary bed BBB [40] and in the blood-CSF barrier [41, 42]. Moreover, IGF-1 transport across the BBB can be either increased, such as by exercise [43], or by injuries such as after hypoxic-ischemic injury [44]. Thus, although not fully characterized, there appear to be mechanisms for transport of both GH and IGF-1 across the BBB.

Age-Related Effects of Growth Hormone and Insulin-Like Growth Factor 1 on Neurogenesis

The GH-IGF-1 system clearly has some similar effects but there are also differences in significance for the brain in different parts of life. Early in embryonic life it is important to note that local brain GH appears to be earlier expressed than pituitary GH [for review see, 45]. Therefore, early in life, it is only local extrapituitary GH that affects the brain. The importance of embryonic local GH expression is best reflected by transgenic animals with GH signaling defects that are not primarily pituitary-dependent.

In results from two studies in mice with suppressor of cytokine signaling-2 (SOCS2) –/– which exhibit increased GH signaling and in mice with GH receptor (GHR) –/– which have reduced GH signaling [46, 47], it appears that during prenatal and postnatal development GH plays a role for a relative suppression in the formation on new neurons with a subsequent decrease in the neuron:glia index. In other words, local GH signaling appears to promote the proliferation and survival of astrocytes in brain development. Interestingly, a higher astrocyte number (i.e. a lower neuron:glia index) is thought to be associated with a higher cognitive function when comparing different species [48]. As a curiosity, areas 9 and 39 had more astrocytes in the brain of Albert Einstein, as compared to control brains [49]. In addition to local GH signaling, administration of systemic GH also appears to stimulate brain growth in early prenatal development [50].

Postnatal brain development days 6–27 is also favored by GH administration in rats, in that brain growth is enhanced [4]. During postnatal development, the importance of circulating pituitary GH increases, which affect brain size and myelination in the animal model with pituitary GH defects. In Little mice which are monodeficient in circulating GH and IGF-1 (due to GHRH-receptor mutation), brain weights were less than controls starting at postnatal day 20 [51]. Conversely, in Ames dwarf mice which are deficient in all anterior pituitary hormones [26], there is an actual increase in the number of neurons in the hippocampus. However, that is likely due to an upregulation of IGF-1 expression locally in the hippocampus [26], which underscores the importance of differences in therapeutic effects and transgenic manipulation of the GH-IGF-1 system. Although very intriguing the effects of GH or IGF-1 therapy on neurogenesis (and other cell genesis) in naïve young animals have not been studied so far. This is an area of research which is very important, as the plasticity of the CNS is believed to be larger in younger individuals. As circulating IGF-1 has been shown to mediate the effects of physical exercise in adults rodents in terms of cell genesis in the adult brain [52, 53], it would certainly be plausible with similar but more pronounced effects in young prepubertal individuals.

In adult animals, GH also has distinct effects in the brain. GH treatment increases cell proliferation in wide parts of the brain except the subventricular zone [54]. Also in the hippocampus the numbers of newborn neurons were increased [54]. The effect of circulating GH appears to be largely mediated by liver-derived circulating IGF-1 [13, 55, 56]. Interestingly, exercise is a factor known to enhance cell genesis in the brain, and it appears that IGF-1 is a key mediator of the effect of exercise in terms of cell genesis in the adult brain [52, 53]. In adult transgenic animals, local GH signaling appears to enhance cell survival in SOCS-2 transgenic animals (these animals exhibit enhanced GH signaling, see also above) in the granule cell layer of the hippocampus as compared to WT and GH-R–/– animals in both control housing and after voluntary running [57]. As opposed to these results, it appears that circulating GH and IGF-1 has both cell proliferative and cell-survival promoting effects in different conditions [13, 54–56]. While GH treatment has been only been studied to enhance adult neurogenesis [54], IGF-1 treatment enhances neurogenesis [52, 53, 55], oligodendrogenesis [56, 58] and angiogenesis [59]. However, it is plausible that GH has similar effects, and indeed GH treatment enhances CNPase abundance in the cerebral cortex of adult hypophysectomized rats [unpubl. obs., our laboratory].

Late in life GH secretion from the pituitary decreases, a condition named the somatopause. Naturally, this leads to the question whether substitution therapy may ameliorate age-related cognitive decline and age-related brain diseases. Therefore, in old animals, foremost the effect of GH therapy has been investigated leaving the effects of GH signaling uninvestigated. Interestingly, GH therapy attenuated the age-related loss of neurons that occurs in the rat hippocampus between 22 and 24 months of age [60]. The authors conclude that GH primarily had an effect on increased cell survival, but they did not investigate cell markers of either cell proliferation or cell-survival, and the effect could partly derive from stimulation of cell genesis. Interestingly, IGF-1 treatment has been shown to attenuate cell loss and cognitive function in mice with transgenic amyloid-beta (Abeta) precursor protein (APP) and presenilin (PS) 2 expression, a model for the Alzheimer disease [61].

Endogenous and Local Growth Hormone and Insulin-Like Growth Factor 1 versus Therapy

It appears that the effect of GH-IGF-1 is dependent on two major factors: the amount of GH-IGF-1 in the circulation and secondly the efficacy of local GH-IGF-1 transduction. This is likely the major reason for the discrepancy between animal models with GH-IGF-1 disruption (increasing gliogenesis comparatively more) as compared to treatments with GH (increasing mostly neurogenesis, see above for details). Another factor when considering the effects on GH treatment is whether there is a lack of circulating GH-IGF-1 which is supplemented. Clearly, GH treatment likely has a much more robust effect if it used to supplement a deficiency. Still, it appears that GH therapy, even in normal young rats may augment cell proliferation in the hippocampus [unpubl. obs., our laboratory]. Also, in a physiological setting with normal GH and IGF-1 levels, such as after physical exercise, circulating IGF-1 appears to be necessary to enhance neurogenesis in the hippocampus [52, 53].

In long-term settings, especially in animal models with life-long disruptions of the GH-IGF-1 signaling (both transgenic animals and mutated animal models), there may often arise difficulties in interpretation of the effects of GH and IGF-1 due to local compensatory mechanisms. For example, Ames dwarf mice deficient in all anterior pituitary [26], there is an actual paradoxical increase in the number of neurons in the hippocampus which is likely due to an upregulation of IGF-1 expression locally [26]. However, it appears that local expression of IGF-1 in the cerebral cortex is not affected by treatment with IGF-1 in a more medium-term setting (= 3 weeks [56]). Perhaps at least 1 or 2 months of long-term disruption may be needed to change local expression of the GH and IGF-1 system, as indicated by the increase in local GH-like material found in rats after about 24–48 days post-hypophysectomy [22]. Clearly, exogenous gene therapy affecting long-term GH-IGF-1 signaling should be used with caution, as many of these long-term secondary effects may be difficult to foresee.

Brain Region-Specific Effects

While some effects of GH appears to be global in the brain, other effects are more brain region specific and cell type specific. With respect to cell genesis in the adult brain, it appears that GH primarily increases cell proliferation in one of the two neurogenic brain regions, i.e. the hippocampus, whereas the subventricular zone (SVZ) is unaffected [54]. Although the proliferative rate is not affected in the SVZ by GH treatment, it appears that the long-term pool of surviving proliferating cells may still be increased by GH [54]. This phenomenon was not observed for the hippocampus. A clear effect of IGF-1 treatment on cell survival has been observed in the cerebral cortex [56] as opposed to the hippocampus [55], further indicating brain-region specific effects of the GH-IGF-1 system. In addition, IGF-1 has been shown to enhance angiogenesis or blood vessel density in the hippocampus and cerebellum [59], while the cerebral cortex parenchyma was not shown to be affected in these parameters by IGF-1 treatment [56, 59]. However, GH treatment has been found to increase cerebrocortical surface capillary density in aged rodents [62]. This may be of importance if GH/IGF-1 is used for treating focal brain diseases. GH-IGF-1 could perhaps be used to induce neurogenesis in hippocampal lesions but not in cerebrocortical, while cerebrocortical lesions could perhaps be ameliorated by de novo genesis of oligodendrocytes and angiogenesis.

Treatment of Disease and Neurogenesis

In the treatment of clinical diseases GH has been used mainly for the treatment of GHD, whereas in experimental animal models both GH and IGF-1 have been used to treat a wider range of diseases. Below there is a short summary of conditions that may have a relation to neurogenesis whereas treatments of GHD will be only briefly mentioned.

For quite some years GHS, GH and IGF-1 have been used to protect against experimental hypoxic-ischemic events. IGF-1 has been most extensively studied in terms of protecting against hypoxic-ischemic damage [for reviews, see 63, 64]. Both the brains of perinatal [65], young [66] and adult animals [67] are protected, and IGF-1 may be administered peripherally [68] or centrally [67]. In addition, GH treatment during the early phase of ischemia appears to protect nervous tissue from damage in both neonatal and perinatal [69], young [70] while adult and old animals have not been studied in these aspects. Lately, there is also a report of neuroprotection against ischemia using ICV administration of the GH secretagogue hexarelin [71]. With the advent of adult persistence of neurogenesis as part of CNS regeneration [7], additional studies have shown functional and histological regeneration using long-term treatment of IGF-1 after hypoxic-ischemic events [68, 72]. However, the effects of GH therapy have not been investigated using long-term treatments after such injuries.

Traumatic brain injury (TBI) is characterized by mental fatigue, decreased quality of life, depressive symptoms [73] and problems with cognitive concentration. In about 12% of the patients, a GHD syndrome develops [74], and in recent years GH therapy has been used to supplement the patients that can be diagnosed with a severe GHD [75]. It is tempting to speculate that several mechanisms of brain plasticity occur simultaneously, of which neurogenesis may also be active. To my knowledge there are no experimental studies that have evaluated GH therapy on neurogenesis after severe TBI.

In the old population various neurodegenerative diseases become progressively more frequent, sometimes complicated by being a mixture between post-stroke-related dementia and the Alzheimer disease. However, there is also a more typical Alzheimer dementia that is clearly separated from the stroke-related injuries. Both GH [76] and IGF-1 [42] treatment has proven to protect the experimental animals against progression in Alzheimer disease models. Also, IGF-1 delivery to experimental animals with the Parkinson disease has been proven to be successful [77]. GH therapy to patients with multiple systemic atrophy (MSA) has also shown tendencies of beneficial cognitive effects [78]. The effects of GH and IGF-1 in these studies are probably a mixture between protective and regenerative effects.

Finally, the positive cognitive effects of long-term GH- and lately IGF-1 treatment of GHD in both young [79] and adult [2, 80] and elderly [81] patients may also be at least partly associated with neurogenesis. This is supported by the observation that GHD caused by hypophysectomy in rats exhibit reduced cell genesis in the hippocampus, a condition that was reversed by IGF-1 treatment [55].

Experimental Validity for Human Clinical Use

The use of laboratory animals is obvious for exploring the effects of the GH-IGF-1 system on neurogenesis and general neurobiology. However, there are now three major lines of evidence that support the notion of similar effects by GH-IGF-1 on the human brain. First, the presence of the GH and IGF-1 system in the human brain has a similar appearance as compared to rodents [for review, see Åberg et al., 13]. Second, accumulating studies show positive beneficial cognitive effects of GH substitution in GH-deficient patients [for review, see 2]. Third, with respect to neurogenesis, this exciting phenomenon has been shown to be present in the adult human hippocampus [8] as well as in the subventricular zone [9], even in 68-year-old humans. Also, there is support that neurogenesis may be activated after CNS injury in humans, as a post-mortem study has observed increased neurogenesis after ischemic stroke [82]. Interestingly, it appears that MR spectroscopy may semi-quantitatively identify the pool and size of neural progenitor cells in living humans [83]. This may be a tool to study longitudinal effects of various treatments and conditions in humans.

As GH therapy appears to be safe and nontoxic in the treatment of GH deficiency, it will be exciting in the next years whether it can be used in other human diseases, such as preventing Alzheimer disease progression, neuroprotective agents in acute stroke both in infants and in adults, and in long-term rehabilitation after stroke and other injuries of the brain.

Conclusion

GH and IGF-1 and possibly GHS treatment have effects on brain cell genesis. There are differences between the effects of endogenous GH-IGF-1 local signal transduction and effects caused by changes in circulating GH-IGF-1. Also, it appears that GH and IGF-1 have partly different effects in the growing CNS where GH promotes genesis of astrocytes relatively more than neurogenesis as opposed to the adult CNS, where GH and IGF-1 therapy primarily promotes neurogenesis. While GH (and IGF-1) has been clinically used mostly for patients with GHD, experimentally it appears that both hormones have profound effects in both protecting the CNS from damage, as well as in regenerating damaged brain tissue. As physical exercise has positive effects in many diseases as well as in normal health, it is of interest that circulating IGF-1 as been shown to be one of the mediators of enhanced neurogenesis in the hippocampus. Altogether, it appears that there is a future potential for using both of these hormones for additional indications in clinical medicine.

References

1 Burman P, Deijen JB: Quality of life and cognitive function in patients with pituitary insufficiency. Psychother Psychosom 1998;67:154–167.

2 Falleti MG, Maruff P, Burman P, Harris A: The effects of growth hormone (GH) deficiency and GH replacement on cognitive performance in adults: A meta-analysis of the current literature. Psychoneuroendocrinology 2006;31:681–691.

3 Ross JL: Effects of growth hormone on cognitive function. Horm Res 2005;64(suppl 3):89–94.

4 Diamond MC: The effects of early hypophysectomy and hormone therapy on brain development. Brain Res 1968;7:407–418.

5 Stern WC, Miller M, Jalowiec JE, Forbes WB, Morgane PJ: Effects of growth hormone on brain biogenic amine levels. Pharmacol Biochem Behav 1975;3:1115–1118.

6 Gage FH: Mammalian neural stem cells. Science 2000;287:1433–1438.

7 Gross CG: Neurogenesis in the adult brain: death of a dogma. Nat Rev Neurosci 2000;1:67–73.

8 Eriksson PS, Perfilieva E, Björk-Eriksson T, Alborn A-M, Nordborg C, Peterson DA, Gage FH: Neurogenesis in the adult human hippocampus. Nat Med 1998;4:1313–1317.

9 Curtis MA, Kam M, Nannmark U, Anderson MF, Axell MZ, Wikkelso C, Holtås S, van Roon-Mom WM, Björk-Eriksson T, Nordborg C, Frisen JF, Dragunow M, Faull RL, Eriksson PS: Human Neuroblasts Migrate to the Olfactory Bulb via a Lateral Ventricular Extension. Science 2007;315: 1243–1249.

10 Saxe MD, Battaglia F, Wang JW, Malleret G, David DJ, Monckton JE, Garcia AD, Sofroniew MV, Kandel ER, Santarelli L, Hen R, Drew MR: Ablation of hippocampal neurogenesis impairs contextual fear conditioning and synaptic plasticity in the dentate gyrus. Proc Natl Acad Sci USA 2006;103:17501–17506.

11 Shors TJ, Miesegaes G, Beylin A, Zhao M, Rydel T, Gould E: Neurogenesis in the adult is involved in the formation of trace memories. Nature 2001;410: 372–376.

12 Isgaard J, Åberg D, Nilsson M: Protective and regenerative effects of the GH/IGF-1 axis on the brain. Minerva Endocrinol 2007;32:103–113.

13 Åberg ND, Brywe KG, Isgaard J: Aspects of growth hormone and insulin-like growth factor-I related to neuroprotection, regeneration, and functional plasticity in the adult brain. Scientific World J 2006;6:53–80.

14 Maguire EA, Gadian DG, Johnsrude IS, Good CD, Ashburner J, Frackowiak RS, Frith CD: Navigation-related structural change in the hippocampi of taxi drivers. Proc Natl Acad Sci USA 2000;97:4398–4403.

15 Lobie PE, Garcia Aragon J, Lincoln DT, Barnard R, Wilcox JN, Waters MJ: Localization and ontogeny of growth hormone receptor gene expression in the central nervous system. Brain Res Dev Brain Res 1993;74:225–233.

16 Lai ZN, Emtner M, Roos P, Nyberg F: Characterization of putative growth hormone receptors in human choroid plexus. Brain Res 1991;546:222–226.

17 Åberg MAI, Åberg ND, Palmer TD, Alborn AM, Carlsson-Skwirut C, Bang P, Rosengren LE, Olsson T, Gage FH, Eriksson PS: IGF-1 has a direct proliferative effect in adult hippocampal progenitor cells. Mol Cell Neurosci 2003;24:23–40.

18 Chung YH, Shin CM, Joo KM, Kim MJ, Cha CI: Region-specific alterations in insulin-like growth factor receptor type I in the cerebral cortex and hippocampus of aged rats. Brain Res 2002;946:307–313.

19 Werther GA, Abate M, Hogg A, Cheesman H, Oldfield B, Hards D, Hudson P, Power B, Freed K, Herington AC: Localization of insulin-like growth factor-I mRNA in rat brain by in situ hybridization–relationship to IGF-1 receptors. Mol Endocrinol 1990;4:773–778.

20 Araujo DM, Lapchak PA, Collier B, Chabot JG, Quirion R: Insulin-like growth factor-1 (somatomedin-C) receptors in the rat brain: distribution and interaction with the hippocampal cholinergic system. Brain Res 1989;484:130–138.

21 Aguado F, Rodrigo J, Cacicedo L, Mellström B: Distribution of insulin-like growth factor-I receptor mRNA in rat brain. Regulation in the hypothalamo-neurohypophysial system. J Mol Endocrinol 1993; 11:231–239.

22 Hojvat S, Baker G, Kirsteins L, Lawrence AM: Growth hormone (GH) immunoreactivity in the rodent and primate CNS: distribution, characterization and presence posthypophysectomy. Brain Res 1982;239:543–557.

23 Pacold ST, Kirsteins L, Hojvat S, Lawrence AM: Biologically active pituitary hormones in the rat brain amygdaloid nucleus. Science 1978;199:804–806.

24 Gossard F, Dihl F, Pelletier G, Dubois PM, Morel G: In situ hybridization to rat brain and pituitary gland of growth hormone cDNA. Neurosci Lett 1987; 79:251–256.

25 Flavell DM, Wells T, Wells SE, Carmignac DF, Thomas GB, Robinson IC: Dominant dwarfism in transgenic rats by targeting human growth hormone (GH) expression to hypothalamic GH-releasing factor neurons. EMBO J 1996;15:3871–3879.

26 Sun LY, Evans MS, Hsieh J, Panici J, Bartke A: Increased neurogenesis in dentate gyrus of long-lived Ames dwarf mice. Endocrinology 2005;146: 1138–1144.

27 D'Ercole AJ, Ye P, Calikoglu AS, Gutierrez Ospina G: The role of the insulin-like growth factors in the central nervous system. Mol Neurobiol 1996;13:227–255.

28 Bach MA, Shen Orr Z, Lowe WL Jr, Roberts CT Jr, LeRoith D: Insulin-like growth factor I mRNA levels are developmentally regulated in specific regions of the rat brain. Brain Res Mol Brain Res 1991;10:43–48.

29 Bartlett WP, Li XS, Williams M: Expression of IGF-1 mRNA in the murine subventricular zone during postnatal development. Brain Res Mol Brain Res 1992;12:285–291.

30 Daughaday WH, Rotwein P: Insulin-like growth factors I and II. Peptide, messenger ribonucleic acid and gene structures, serum, and tissue concentrations. Endocr Rev 1989;10:68–91.

31 Sara VR, Hall K: Insulin-like growth factors and their binding proteins. Physiol Rev 1990;70:591–614.

32 Bondy C, Werner H, Roberts CT Jr, LeRoith D: Cellular pattern of type-I insulin-like growth factor receptor gene expression during maturation of the rat brain: comparison with insulin-like growth factors I and II. Neuroscience 1992;46:909–923.

33 Monzavi R, Cohen P: IGFs and IGFBPs: role in health and disease. Best Pract Res Clin Endocrinol Metab 2002;16:433–447.

34 Werther GA, Russo V, Baker N, Butler G: The role of the insulin-like growth factor system in the developing brain. Horm Res 1998;49(suppl 1):37–40.

35 Zumkeller W: IGFs and IGF-binding proteins as diagnostic markers and biological modulators in brain tumors. Expert Rev Mol Diagn 2002;2:473–477.

36 Johansson J-O, Larson G, Andersson M, Elmgren A, Hynsjö L, Lindahl A, Lundberg P-A, Isaksson OGP, Lindstedt S, Bengtsson B-Å: Treatment of growth hormone-deficient adults with recombinant human growth hormone increases the concentration of growth hormone in the cerebrospinal fluid and affects neurotransmitters. Neuroendocrinology 1995;61:57–66.

37 Pan W, Yu Y, Cain CM, Nyberg F, Couraud PO, Kastin AJ: Permeation of growth hormone across the blood-brain barrier. Endocrinology 2005;46: 4898–4904.

38 Lin CY, Chang C, Cheung WM, Lin MH, Chen JJ, Hsu CY, Chen JH, Lin TN: Dynamic changes in vascular permeability, cerebral blood volume, vascular density, and size after transient focal cerebral ischemia in rats: evaluation with contrast-enhanced magnetic resonance imaging. J Cereb Blood Flow Metab 2008;28:1491–1501.

39 Scheepens A, Sirimanne E, Beilharz E, Breier BH, Waters MJ, Gluckman PD, Williams CE: Alterations in the neural growth hormone axis following hypoxic-ischemic brain injury. Brain Res Mol Brain Res 1999;68:88–100.

40 Duffy KR, Pardridge WM, Rosenfeld RG: Human blood-brain barrier insulin-like growth factor receptor. Metabolism 1988;37:136–140.

41 Armstrong CS, Wuarin L, Ishii DN: Uptake of circulating insulin-like growth factor-I into the cerebrospinal fluid of normal and diabetic rats and normalization of IGF-1I mRNA content in diabetic rat brain. J Neurosci Res 2000;59:649–660.

42 Carro E, Spuch C, Trejo JL, Antequera D, Torres-Aleman I: Choroid plexus megalin is involved in neuroprotection by serum insulin-like growth factor I. J Neurosci 2005;25:10884–10893.

43 Carro E, Nunez A, Busiguina S, Torres-Aleman I: Circulating insulin-like growth factor I mediates effects of exercise on the brain. J Neurosci 2000; 20:2926–2933.

44 Guan J, Skinner SJ, Beilharz EJ, Hua KM, Hodgkinson S, Gluckman PD, Williams CE: The movement of IGF-1 into the brain parenchyma after hypoxic-ischaemic injury. Neuroreport 1996;7:632–636.

45 Harvey S, Hull K: Neural growth hormone: an update. J Mol Neurosci 2003;20:1–14.

46 Ransome MI, Goldshmit Y, Bartlett PF, Waters MJ, Turnley AM: Comparative analysis of CNS populations in knockout mice with altered growth hormone responsiveness. Eur J Neurosci 2004;19: 2069–2079.

47 Turnley AM, Faux CH, Rietze RL, Coonan JR, Bartlett PF: Suppressor of cytokine signaling 2 regulates neuronal differentiation by inhibiting growth hormone signaling. Nat Neurosci 2002;5:1155–1162.

48 Reichenbach A: Glia:neuron index: review and hypothesis to account for different values in various mammals. Glia 1989;2:71–77.

49 Diamond MC, Scheibel AB, Murphy GM Jr, Harvey T: On the brain of a scientist: Albert einstein. Exp Neurol 1985;88:198–204.

50 Zamenhof S, Mosley J, Schuller E: Stimulation of the proliferation of cortical neurons by prenatal treatment with growth hormone. Science 1966; 152:1396–1397.

51 Morisawa K, Sugisaki T, Kanamatsu T, Aoki T, Noguchi T: Factors contributing to cerebral hypomyelination in the growth hormone-deficient little mouse. Neurochem Res 1989;14:173–177.

52 Carro E, Trejo JL, Busiguina S, Torres-Aleman I: Circulating insulin-like growth factor I mediates the protective effects of physical exercise against brain insults of different etiology and anatomy. J Neurosci 2001;21:5678–5684.

53 Trejo JL, Carro E, Torres-Aleman I: Circulating insulin-like growth factor I mediates exercise-induced increases in the number of new neurons in the adult hippocampus. J Neurosci 2001;21:1628–1634.

54 Åberg ND, Johansson I, Åberg M, Lind J, Johansson U, Cooper-Kuhn C, Kuhn HG, Isgaard J: Peripheral administration of GH induces cell proliferation in the brain of adult hypophysectomized rats. J Endocrinol 2009;201:141–150.

55 Åberg MAI, Åberg ND, Hedbäcker H, Oscarsson J, Eriksson PS: Peripheral infusion of IGF-1 selectively induces neurogenesis in the adult rat hippocampus. J Neurosci 2000;20:2896–2903.

56 Åberg ND, Johansson UE, Åberg MAI, Hellström NAK, Lind J, Bull C, Isgaard J, Anderson M, Oskarsson J, Eriksson PS: Peripheral infusion of insulin-like growth factor-I increases the number of newborn oligodendrocytes in the cerebral cortex of adult hypophysectomized rats. Endocrinology 2007; 148:3765–3772.

57 Ransome MI, Turnley AM: Growth hormone signaling and hippocampal neurogenesis: Insights from genetic models. Hippocampus 2008;18:1034–1050.

58 Hsieh J, Aimone JB, Kaspar BK, Kuwabara T, Nakashima K, Gage FH: IGF-1 instructs multipotent adult neural progenitor cells to become oligodendrocytes. J Cell Biol 2004;164:111–122.

59 Lopez-Lopez C, LeRoith D, Torres-Aleman I: Insulin-like growth factor I is required for vessel remodeling in the adult brain. Proc Natl Acad Sci USA 2004;101:9833–9838.

60 Azcoitia I, Perez-Martin M, Salazar V, Castillo C, Ariznavarreta C, Garcia-Segura LM, Tresguerres JA: Growth hormone prevents neuronal loss in the aged rat hippocampus. Neurobiol Aging 2005;26: 697–703.

61 Carro E, Trejo JL, Gerber A, Loetscher H, Torrado J, Metzger F, Torres-Aleman I: Therapeutic actions of insulin-like growth factor I on APP/PS2 mice with severe brain amyloidosis. Neurobiol Aging 2005; 27:1250–1257.

62 Sonntag WE, Lynch C, Thornton P, Khan A, Bennett S, Ingram R: The effects of growth hormone and IGF-1 deficiency on cerebrovascular and brain ageing. J Anat 2000;197(Pt 4):575–585.

63 Gluckman PD, Guan J, Williams C, Scheepens A, Zhang R, Bennet L, Gunn A: Asphyxial brain injury–the role of the IGF system. Mol Cell Endocrinol 1998;140:95–99.

64 Guan J, Bennet L, Gluckman PD, Gunn AJ: Insulin-like growth factor-1 and post-ischemic brain injury. Prog Neurobiol 2003;70:443–462.

65 Brywe KG, Mallard C, Gustavsson M, Hedtjärn M, Leverin A-L, Wang X, Blomgren K, Isgaard J, Hagberg H: IGF-1 neuroprotection in the immature brain after hypoxia-ischemia, involvement of Akt and GSK3b. Eur J Neurosci 2005;21:1489–1502.

66 Sizonenko SV, Sirimanne ES, Williams CE, Gluckman PD: Neuroprotective effects of the N-terminal tripeptide of IGF-1, glycine-proline-glutamate, in the immature rat brain after hypoxic-ischemic injury. Brain Res 2001;922:42–50.

67 Guan J, Williams C, Gunning M, Mallard C, Gluckman P: The effects of IGF-1 treatment after hypoxic-ischemic brain injury in adult rats. J Cereb Blood Flow Metab 1993;13:609–616.

68 Schäbitz WR, Hoffmann TT, Heiland S, Kollmar R, Bardutzky J, Sommer C, Schwab S: Delayed neuroprotective effect of insulin-like growth factor-I after experimental transient focal cerebral ischemia monitored with MRI. Stroke 2001;32:1226–1233.

69 Gustafson K, Hagberg H, Bengtsson B-Å, Brantsing C, Isgaard J: Possible protective role of growth hormone in hypoxia-ischemia in neonatal rats. Pediatr Res 1999;45:318–323.

70 Scheepens A, Sirimanne ES, Breier BH, Clark RG, Gluckman PD, Williams CE: Growth hormone as a neuronal rescue factor during recovery from CNS injury. Neuroscience 2001;104:677–687.

71 Brywe KG, Leverin AL, Gustavsson M, Mallard C, Granata R, Destefanis S, Volante M, Hagberg H, Ghigo E, Isgaard J: Growth hormone-releasing peptide hexarelin reduces neonatal brain injury and alters Akt/glycogen synthase kinase-3beta phosphorylation. Endocrinology 2005;146:4665–4672.

72 Dempsey RJ, Sailor KA, Bowen KK, Tureyen K, Vemuganti R: Stroke-induced progenitor cell proliferation in adult spontaneously hypertensive rat brain: effect of exogenous IGF-1 and GDNF. J Neurochem 2003;87:586–597.

73 Kelly DF, McArthur DL, Levin H, Swimmer S, Dusick JR, Cohan P, Wang C, Swerdloff R: Neurobehavioral and quality of life changes associated with growth hormone insufficiency after complicated mild, moderate, or severe traumatic brain injury. J Neurotrauma 2006;23:928–942.

74 Schneider HJ, Kreitschmann-Andermahr I, Ghigo E, Stalla GK, Agha A: Hypothalamopituitary dysfunction following traumatic brain injury and aneurysmal subarachnoid hemorrhage: a systematic review. JAMA 2007;298:1429–1438.

75 Kreitschmann-Andermahr I, Poll EM, Reineke A, Gilsbach JM, Brabant G, Buchfelder M, Fassbender W, Faust M, Kann PH, Wallaschofski H: Growth hormone deficient patients after traumatic brain injury–baseline characteristics and benefits after growth hormone replacement–an analysis of the German KIMS database. Growth Horm IGF Res 2008;18:472–478.

76 Ling FA, Hui DZ, Ji SM: Protective effect of recombinant human somatotropin on amyloid beta-peptide induced learning and memory deficits in mice. Growth Horm IGF Res 2007;17:336–341.

77 Ebert AD, Beres AJ, Barber AE, Svendsen CN: Human neural progenitor cells over-expressing IGF-1 protect dopamine neurons and restore function in a rat model of Parkinson's disease. Exp Neurol 2007;209:213–223.

78 Holmberg B, Johansson JO, Poewe W, Wenning G, Quinn NP, Mathias C, Tolosa E, Cardozo A, Dizdar N, Rascol O, Slaoui T: Safety and tolerability of growth hormone therapy in multiple system atrophy: a double-blind, placebo-controlled study. Mov Disord 2007;22:1138–1144.

79 Creyghton WM, van Dam PS, Koppeschaar HP: The role of the somatotropic system in cognition and other cerebral functions. Semin Vasc Med 2004;4:167–172.

80 McGauley GA: Quality of life assessment before and after growth hormone treatment in adults with growth hormone deficiency. Acta Paediatr Scand Suppl 1989;356:70–72.
81 Feldt-Rasmussen U, Wilton P, Jonsson P: Aspects of growth hormone deficiency and replacement in elderly hypopituitary adults. Growth Horm IGF Res 2004;14(suppl A):S51–S58.
82 Jin K, Wang X, Xie L, Mao XO, Zhu W, Wang Y, Shen J, Mao Y, Banwait S, Greenberg DA: Evidence for stroke-induced neurogenesis in the human brain. Proc Natl Acad Sci USA 2006;103:13198–13202.
83 Manganas LN, Zhang X, Li Y, Hazel RD, Smith SD, Wagshul ME, Henn F, Benveniste H, Djuric PM, Enikolopov G, Maletic-Savatic M: Magnetic resonance spectroscopy identifies neural progenitor cells in the live human brain. Science 2007;318:980–985.

Dr. N. David Åberg
Laboratory of Experimental Endocrinology, Department of Internal Medicine
Sahlgrenska University Hospital, Göteborg University
Gröna Stråket 16, SE–413 45 Göteborg (Sweden)
Tel. +46 31 3428422, Fax +46 31 82 53 30, E-Mail david.aberg@medic.gu.se

Loche S, Cappa M, Ghizzoni L, Maghnie M, Savage MO (eds): Pediatric Neuroendocrinology.
Endocr Dev. Basel, Karger, 2010, vol 17, pp 77–85

Sex Steroids, Growth Hormone, Leptin and the Pubertal Growth Spurt

Alan D. Rogol

Riley Hospital for Children, Indianapolis, Ind., and University of Virginia, Charlottesville, Va., USA

Abstract

A normal rate for the linear growth of a child or adolescent is a strong statement for the good general health of that child. Normal growth during childhood is primarily dependent on adequate nutrition, an adequate psychosocial environment, the absence of disease and adequate amounts thyroid hormone and growth hormone (and its downstream product, IGF-1). At adolescence there is the reawakening of the hypothalamic-pituitary-gonadal axis and its interaction with the GH/IGF-1 axis to subserve the pubertal growth spurt. The fat tissue-derived hormone, leptin and its receptor are likely involved in at least two aspects of pubertal development – sexual development itself and the alterations in body composition including the regional distribution of fat and bone mineralization. During the prepubertal years the male female differences in body composition are quite modest, but change remarkably during pubertal development with boys showing a relative decrement in fat percentage and girls a marked increase in concert with rising levels of circulating leptin. The boys show a much greater increase in lean body tissue and the relative proportions of water, muscle and bone. These may be observed as the differential growth of the shoulders and hips. The net effect of these pubertal changes is that the young adult woman has ~25% body fat in the 'gynoid' distribution while the male has much more muscle, especially in the shoulders and upper body but only ~13% body fat.

A normal rate for the linear growth of a child is a strong statement for the good general health of that child. On a population basis just knowing the mid-arm circumference of a large cohort of children denotes similar information concerning the nutritional status of the children (and the gross national product of the nation). Growth during childhood is characterized by a relatively constant rate averaging 5–6 cm/year and 2.5 kg/year for both boys and girls after the fourth year of life [1]. Normal growth during childhood is primarily dependent on adequate nutrition, an adequate psychosocial environment, and absence of disease. From the hormonal point of view one must have adequate levels of thyroid hormone and sufficient levels of insulin-like growth factor 1 (IGF-1) as the stable pharmacodynamic marker of growth hormone

(GH) function. The hypothalamic-pituitary-gonadal (HPG) axis operates at a very low activity until late childhood [2] when early (re)activation occurs well before the outward signs of pubertal development – testicular enlargement in boys and glandular breast tissue in girls.

Linear growth progresses at a virtually constant rate until very late childhood when there may be a slight decrease before the inflection to an increase ('take off'), when height velocity accelerates [3]. Some, but certainly not all, children show a minor growth spurt (Mid-growth spurt) in stature and weight during late childhood. Adrenal androgens (adrenarche) may be responsible for this 'mini'-spurt which may be missed if very infrequent measurements are obtained.

Most healthy children are measured approximately yearly at this age and the usual growth chart represent 'smoothed' growth data. Linear growth is actually a saltatory (episodic with stepwise jumps) at least as noted by daily measurements over time in both newborns and adolescents [4–6].

The Hypothalamic-Pituitary-Gonadal Axis

Pulsatile gonadotropin-releasing hormone (GnRH) secretion (as detected by pulsatile LH release) is present at all ages, but particularly prominent just after birth (mini-puberty) and during adolescent development [2, 7]. The relatively robust secretion of LH and gonadal steroid hormones in the first few months of life is damped, likely by an alteration in the hypothalamic feedback system for gonadal steroids on GnRH secretion. During the vast majority of the rest of childhood the small, but now measurable concentrations of sex steroids (by modern chromatography/mass spectrometry methods) are able to restrain the GnRH neurons from making very much peptide product. Very likely the first alteration is a change in feedback sensitivity so that these same levels of gonadal steroids are no longer capable of inhibiting GnRH secretion. Thus, GnRH is secreted in greater amounts at first only at night, likely coincident with the first episode of deep sleep. Since the gonadotropes are capable of responding to GnRH, LH is secreted and coaxes the testis or ovary to produce testosterone or estradiol. The increase in the concentrations of the gonadal steroids is once again able to inhibit GnRH secretion for the rest of the night and during the entire day. This process continues with decreasing levels of sensitivity at the hypothalamus and then more LH secretion during the night and finally during the day [7]. The system comes into a steady state with secretion of both LH (and FSH) and gonadal steroid hormones during the night and day with an imbalance favoring the nighttime until at least late mid-puberty. Gonadal steroid hormone levels promote the development and growth of the secondary sexual characteristics and the changes in body composition (see below) characteristic of pubertal development.

GH/IGF-1 Axis

During childhood GH secretion patterns are very much alike for boys and girls with a marked night/day rhythm favoring early nighttime (after the first episode of deep sleep). GH secretion is thus maximal during the early hours of sleep. Additional bursts of GH release occur throughout the rest of the night/day, but with smaller amplitude. There is virtually no GH circulating between secretory episodes, although levels can be measured using very sensitive immunoassays. However, the effector for many, but not all, of GH actions is circulating IGF-1 produced under the direction of this pattern of GH secretion. Exercise, food intake, and emotional factors can modify the pattern of GH release. After an individual peak one has an absolute and then a relative refractory period before the next burst of GH secretion.

Puberty is heralded by a dramatic activation of the GH/IGF-1 axis. The rise in mean 24-hour GH levels results from an increase in the amplitude of the secretory burst and in the mass of the GH release per burst rather than in the number of secretory events [8]. The differential increase between boys and girls during pubertal development follows the pattern of change in height velocity noting that that is biologically anchored rather than being related to one's chronological age. Girls show a significant increase in GH secretory dynamics (GH and IGF-1 levels) beginning at Tanner breast stage 2, with the highest circulating levels at Tanner breast stage 3/4. In boys the increases of GH and IGF-1 concentrations occur later during pubertal development, peaking at Tanner genital stage 4. After full sexual development (but before the adult body composition is attained) the levels of GH and IGF-1 fall to those of the young adult.

Leptin and Central Peptide Hormones

The fat-derived hormone, leptin, and its receptor are likely involved in at least two aspects of pubertal development – sexual development itself and the alterations in body composition including bone. Normosmic idiopathic hypogonadotropic hypogonadism is clearly linked to defects in the leptin (LEP) or the leptin receptor (LEPR) genes [9, 10]. The linkage of the leptin signaling system to normal pubertal development has yet to be proven. It is possible that common variants in LEP or LEPR may contribute to the variation of pubertal development (timing and/or tempo) within the normal population of adolescents [11].

The onset of puberty is almost certainly polygenic. At least one major upstream regulator of GnRH release is the kisspeptin/GPR54 system [12]. Kisspeptin from some arcuate and periventricular (hypothalamic) nuclei interacts with its cognate receptor, GPR54 on the cell membranes of GnRH neurons. In some mammals kisspeptin levels increase during pubertal development. In the prepubertal macacque repetitive administration of an intravenous infusion of kisspeptin-10 (2 μg in 1 ml as a pulse of 1 min duration once every hour for 48 h) was able to induce GnRH release as measured by circulating levels of LH. This was consistent with advancing the start of puberty. This response was abrogated by concomitant treatment with a GnRH antagonist. These findings are consistent with the concept that in primates the transition from the juvenile (prepubertal) period (attenuated GnRH release) to the pubertal state is controlled by a process that includes KISS-1 gene product activating the GPR54 on hypothalamic GnRH neurons [13].

In the human the activity of the kisspeptin/GPR54 system is likely activated during puberty, since inactivating mutations of either the ligand or the receptor are associated with delayed pubertal development [12] and activating mutations with central precocious puberty [14]. Although upstream regulators of the kisspeptin/GPR54 system have yet to be convincingly demonstrated, recently IGF-1 has been proposed as a positive regulator of KISS-I gene expression in the anteroventral periventricular (AVPV) nucleus of the prepubertal female rat. This was true whether the IGF-1 was delivered into the third ventricle or systemically through the jugular vein. The specificity of the effect was clarified when it was noted that the IGF-1 receptor antagonist, JB-1 blocked the IGF-1-induced increase in KISS-1 gene expression [15]. It is clear from these animal studies that the kisspeptin/GP54R system is necessary for pubertal development (tonic GnRH release); however, it may very well be that other aspects of HPG axis physiology, such as positive feedback of estradiol on the hypothalamus and pituitary to release the surge of LH, are not [16].

Leptin/LEPR may be one of the conduits linking pubertal development with central energy regulation (homeostasis). The center for this integration is likely the arcuate nucleus (infundibular in the human) for it integrates neural, metabolic and humoral signals from all parts of the body. It is likely that the 'sum' of these inputs is a signal to control appetite as well as energy stores [17, 18]. The central melanocortin system, as defined by MC3R and MC4R on distinct subsets of neurons within the arcuate nucleus, is the primary sensor for the whole body energy homeostasis. The orexigenic peptides neural peptide Y (NPY) and agouti-related protein (AgRP) are secreted from cells within the arcuate nucleus. The latter (AgRP) is a potent MC3R and MC4R antagonist. Since the proopiomelanocortin (POMC) neurons acting on MC3R and MC4R decrease food intake, the NPY and AgRP neurons act as part of the orexigenic pathway by silencing the POMC system (fig. 1).

Taken together the reciprocal activity of the two potent systems, NPY and AgRP (orexigenic) and POMC (anorexic) can control energy homeostasis at puberty (and other stages of development) to sense whether pubertal development should advance, as well as to fine tune alterations in body composition and likely the regional distribution of body fat. In the excess energy state POMC neurons are activated and release melanocortins that activate MCR4, suppressing food intake and perhaps increasing energy expenditure. Concurrently, activity within the AgRP/NPY system is suppressed. That has the effect of removing inhibitory activity of α-MSH on MC4R. The opposite occurs during times of energy deficit – the activity

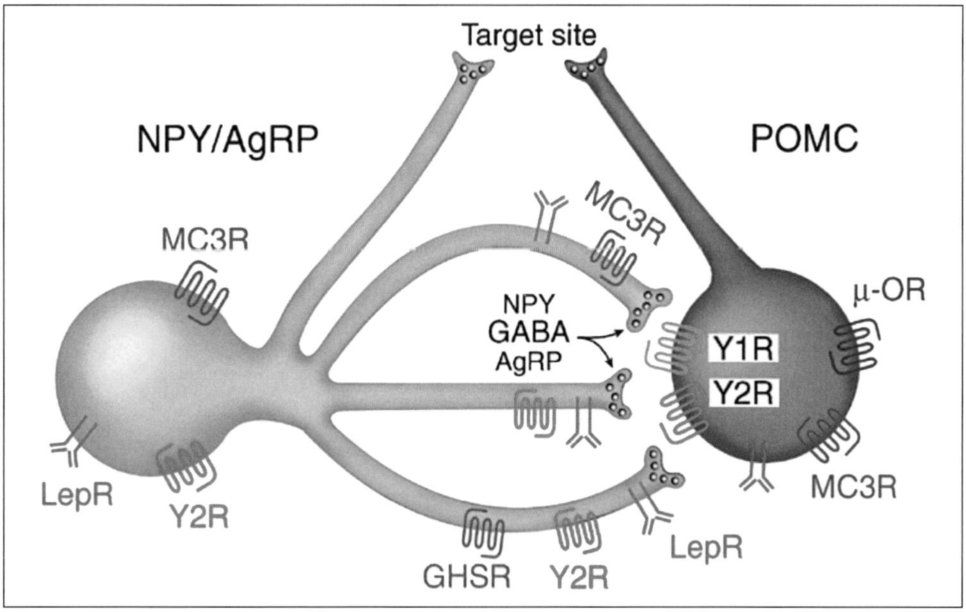

Fig. 1. Schematic of the melanocortin system within the arcuate nucleus of the hypothalamus. NPY/AgRP and POMC neurons within the arcuate nucleus form a coordinately regulated network because of dense NPY/AgRP fibers projecting to POMC cell bodies. Some receptors for the large numbers of hormones and neuropeptides known to regulate the network are indicated. LepR, leptin receptor, μ-OR, μ opioid receptor, Y2R, type 2 NPY receptor. In most cases, whether the receptors are presynaptic or postsynaptic is not known. From Cone [17], with permission.

of the anorexigenic POMC neurons is decreased and the activity of the orexigenic NPY/AgRP system is increased. The 'goal' is to bring the organism back to energy homeostasis. The previously noted LEP and LEPR system is intimately involved with receptors on NPY/AgRP neurons that have the reciprocal relationship with POMC neurons (fig. 1).

We [19] and others [20] have observed a very close relationship between subcutaneous fat and serum LEP levels with those with higher degrees of fatness (and LEP levels) perhaps entering puberty earlier [21], at least in girls. Bandini et al. [22] took this concept one step further using as a biological anchor the age at menarche and noting the body compositional and hormonal relationships over time both before and after menarche. At menarche the girls averaged 24.6% body fat (bioelectrical impedance, not a criterion method). Leptin levels rose from 8.4 ng/ml at menarche to approximately 12 ng/ml after menarche as the percent body fat increased to approximately 27. One cannot determine causation from these data; however, the change in leptin concentration closely paralleled the change in percent body fat. Thus, there are associated changes in both adolescent development, the hormones of the hypothalamic-pituitary-gonadal and GH/IGF-1 axes and the central neuroendocrine

Table 1. Parameters of the adolescent growth spurt in Swiss and British children

	Girls		Boys	
	mean	range	mean	range
Age at takeoff, years				
Swiss	9.6	6.6–12.9	11.0	7.8–13.5
British	9.0	7.7–10.0	10.7	8.6–12.4
Age at PHV, years				
Swiss	12.2	9.3–15.0	13.9	12.0–15.8
British	11.9	10.3–13.2	14.2	11.9–16.2
PHV				
Swiss	7.1	5.0–10.1	9.0	6.7–12.4
British	7.5	601–9.3	8.2	5.6–10.0

Note: Swiss data are adapted from Largo et al. [28] for 110 girls and 112 boys; British data are adapted from Preece and Baines [29] for 23 girls and 35 boys.

regulation of energy homeostasis through the reciprocal activation of the NPY/AgRP and POMC neuronal systems. There are many too many unknowns to identify the primary driver for the onset and progression of pubertal development. Suffice it to say that there are extensive connections among the regulators of central energy homeostasis, including the control of appetite and body composition as well as the timing and tempo of pubertal development. These are the familiar HPG and GH/IGF-1 axes.

Linear Growth and Adolescent Development

Although virtually all growth curves for adolescents have the same appearance, variation in the timing and tempo of pubertal development may be detected from several parameters that provide useful information about the adolescent growth spurt and provide an indicator of sexual maturation [3]. The two primary parameters are takeoff, or initiation of the spurt (often after a slight deceleration or 'dip' in height velocity) and peak height velocity. The age, size and rate of growth at takeoff and peak height velocity can be derived from the growth curves, either graphically or mathematically by curve fitting. The age at peak height velocity is an indicator of somatic maturity, specifically related to the timing of pubertal development. The peak height velocity (cm/year) itself provides an estimate of the tempo. Estimates of these parameters of the adolescent growth spurt for mainly European are shown in table 1. Since these are for individuals and not populations of adolescents, the range is quite broad, for these normal populations. Similarly broad ranges apply to the development of the secondary sexual characteristics.

Body Composition and Adolescent Development

Body composition may be described with a series of methods from two, three and four compartment models to molecular and anatomic ones [23]. All are approximations that indirectly estimate body composition, some with very large sets of assumptions. The major issue at puberty is the changing state of hydration of the fat-free mass, the largest source of metabolically active tissue. Methods that use a fixed value (rather than an experimentally determined one) may lead to significant systematic errors in that determination, and thus in the appropriate basal energy expenditure as part of the calculation of energy homeostasis.

During the prepubertal years the male-female differences in body composition are quite modest. Children of both genders have relative decreases in body fat between 1 and 6 years of age. Girls then begin to increase in fatness again whereas the boys primarily gain lean body mass as they gain weight [24]. There are marked differences in the regional distribution of fat mass emerge at puberty with boys losing relative fat mass in comparison with the marked gain in lean body mass. For girls the gain in lean body mass is more modest than that of fat mass with a predominance on the trunk compared to peripheral sites [24]. In girls there are epidemiological data to indicate that BMI *z*-score at 36 months, the rate of change of BMI between 36 months and grade 1 in school (~age 6 years) are associated with earlier pubertal development [25]. From a population perspective the data suggest that the increasing rate of obesity may result in an earlier average age on onset of pubertal development. It should be noted that often those girls who begin pubertal development at an earlier age have a slower *tempo* of sexual development and do not have menarche much earlier than those girls starting with breast development at an average age [26].

The marked changes in body composition [27], including alterations in the relative proportions of water, muscle, fat and bone are characteristic of pubertal maturation and the result of not only the hypothalamic-pituitary-gonadal axis (male-female differences), but also the GH/IGF-1 and hypothalamic-pituitary-adrenal axes and the relevant upstream (hypothalamic) hormones [27]. The end points are the increases in lean body, fat, and bone mineralization attained within the third decade (attainment of the adult body composition several years after reaching adult height). Differential growth of the shoulders and hips and differences in lean tissue accrual highlight the sexually dimorphic alterations in body composition during pubertal development. The net effect of all of these factors is that the young adult female has ~25% body fate and the male ~13%.

References

1 Rallison ML: Growth Disorders in Infants, Children and Adolescents, New York, Wiley, 1986.

2 Mitamura, R, Yano K, Suzuki N, Ito Y, Makita Y, Okuno A: Diurnal rhythms of luteinizing hormone, follicle-stimulating hormone, testosterone and estradiol secretion before the onset of female puberty in short children. J Clin Endocrinol Metab 2000;85: 1074–1080.

3 Malina RM, Bouchard C, Bar-Or O: Growth, Maturation, and Physical Activity, ed 2. Champaign, Human Kinetics Press, 2004, pp 277–305.

4 Lampl M, Veldhuis J, Johnson ML: Saltation and stasis: a model of human growth. Science 1992;258: 801–803.

5 Lampl M: Evidence of salutatory growth in infancy. Am J Hum Biol 1993;5:641–52.

6 Lampl M, Johnson ML: A case study in daily growth during adolescence: a single spurt or changes in the dynamics of salutatory growth? Ann Hum Biol 1997;20:595–603.

7 Apter D, Butzow, T, Laughlin G, Yen S: Gonadotropin-releasing hormone pulse generator activity during pubertal transition in girls: pulsatile and diurnal patterns of circulating gonadotropins. J Clin Endocrinol Metab 1993;76:940–949.

8 Clark PA, Rogol AD: Growth hormone and sex steroid interactions at puberty. Endocrinol Metab Clin N Am 1996;3:665–681.

9 Farooqi IS, Jebb SA, Langmark G, Lawrence E, Cheetham CH, Prentice AM, Hughes IA, McCamish MA, O'Rahilly S: Effects of recombinant leptin therapy in a child with congenital leptin deficiency. N Engl J Med 1999;341:879–884.

10 Farooqi IS, Wangensteen T, Collins S, Kimber W, Matarese G, Keogh JM, Lank E, Bottomley B, Lopes-Fernandez J, Ferraz-Amaro I, Dattani MT, Ercan O, Myhre AG, Retterstol L, Stanhope R, Edge JA, McKenzie S, Lessan N, Ghosdi M, De Rosa V, Perna F, Fontana S, Barroso I, Undlein DE, O'Rahilly S: Clinical and molecular genetic spectrum of congenital deficiency of the leptin receptor. N Engl J Med 2007;356:237–247.

11 Kaminski BA, Palmert MR: Genetic control of pubertal timing. Curr Opin Pediatr 2008;20:458–464.

12 Seminara SB, Messager S, Chatzidake EE, Thresher RR, Acierno JS, Shagoury JK, Bo-Abbas Y, Kuohung W, Schwinor KM, Hendrick AG, Zahn D, Dixon J, Kaiser UB, Slaugenhaupt SA, Gusella JF, O'Rahilly S, Carlton MBL, Crowley WF Jr, Aparicio SAJR, Colledge WH: The GPR54 gene as a regulator of puberty. N Engl J Med 2003;349:1614–1627.

13 Plant TM, Ramaswamy S, Pietro MJ: Repetitive activation of hypothalamic G protein-coupled receptor 54 with intravenous pulses of kisspeptin in the juvenile monkey (*Macaca mulatta*) elicits a sustained train of gonadotropins-releasing hormone discharges. Endocrinology 2006;147:1007–1013.

14 Teles MG, Bianco SD, Brito VN, Trarbach EB, Kuohung Wm Xu S, Seminara SB, Mendonca BB, Kaiser UB, Latronica AC: A GPR54-activating mutation in a patient with central precocious puberty. N Engl J Med 2008;358:709–715.

15 Hiney JK, Srivastava VK, Pine MD, Dees WL: Insulin-like growth factor-1 activates KISS-1 gene expression in the brain of the prepubertal female rat. Endocrinology 2009;150:376–384.

16 Dungan HM, Gottsch ML Zeng H, Gragerov A, Bergmann JE, Vassilatis DK, Clifton DK, Steiner RA: The role of kisspeptin-GPR54 signaling in the tonic regulation and surge release of gonadotropin-releasing hormone/luteinizing hormone. J Neurosci 2007;27:12088–12095.

17 Cone RD: Anatomy and regulation of the central melanocortin system. Nature Neurosci 2005;8:571–578.

18 Coll AP, Farooqi IS, Challis BG, Yeo GS, O'Rahilly S: Proopiomelanocortin and energy balance: Insights from human and murine genetics. J Clin Endocrinol Metab 2004;89:2557–2562.

19 Roemmich JN, Clark PA, Berr SS, Mai V, Mantzoros CS, Flier JS, Weltman A, Rogol AD: Gender differences in leptin levels during puberty are related to subcutaneous fat distribution and sex steroids. Am J Physiol 1998;275:35:E543–E551.

20 Ahmed ML, Ong KKL, Morrell DJ, Cox L, Drayer N, Perry L, Preece MA, Dunger DB: Longitudinal study of leptin concentrations during puberty: sex differences and relationship to changes in body composition. J Clin Endocrinol Metab 1999;84:899–905.

21 Matkovic V, Ilich JZ, Skugor M, Badenhop NE, Goel P, Clairmont A, Klisovich D, Nahhas RW, Landoll JD: Leptin is inversely related to age at menarche in human females. J Clin Endocrinol Metab 1997;82: 3239–3245.

22 Bandini LG, Must A, Naumova EN, Anderson S, Caprio S, Spadano-Gasbarro JI, Dietz WH: Change in leptin, body composition and other hormones around menarche: a visual representation. Acta Paediatr 2008;97:1454–1459.

23 Roemmich JN, Clarke PA, Weltman A, Rogol AD: Alterations in growth and body composition during puberty. I. Comparing multicompartment body composition models. J Appl Physiol 1997;83:927–935.

24 Wells JCK: Sexual dimorphism of body composition. Best Pract Res Clin Endocrinol Metab 2007; 21:415–430.
25 Lee JM, Appugliese D, Kaciroti N, Corwyn RF, Bradley RH: Weight status in young girls and the onset of puberty. Pediatrics 2007;119:e624–e630.
26 Rosenfield RL, Lipton RB, Drum ML: Thelarche, pubarche, and menarche attainment in children with normal and elevated body mass index. Pediatrics 2009;123:84–88.
27 Veldhuis JD, Roemmich JN, Richmond EJ, Rogol AD, Lovejoy JC, Scheffield-Moore M, Mauras N, Bowers CY: Endocrine control of body composition in infants, children and puberty. Endocr Rev 2005; 26:114–146.
28 Largo RH, Gasser T, Prader A, Stuetzie W, Huber PJ: Analysis of the adolescent growth spurt using smoothing spine functions. Ann Hum Biol 1978;5: 421–434.
29 Preece MA, Baines MJ: A new family of mathematical models describing the human growth curve. Ann Hum Biol 1978;5:1–24.

Dr. Alan D. Rogol, MD, PhD
Department of Pediatrics, University of Virginia
685 Explorers Road
Charlottesville, 2291–8441 VA (USA)
Tel. +1 804 971 6687, Fax +1 804 971 1147, E-Mail adrogol@comcast.net., arogol@cstone.net

Loche S, Cappa M, Ghizzoni L, Maghnie M, Savage MO (eds): Pediatric Neuroendocrinology.
Endocr Dev. Basel, Karger, 2010, vol 17, pp 86–95

Endocrine and Metabolic Actions of Ghrelin

Valentina Gasco · Guglielmo Beccuti · Filippa Marotta · Andrea Benso · Riccarda Granata · Fabio Broglio · Ezio Ghigo

Division of Endocrinology, Diabetology and Metabolism, University of Turin, Turin, Italy

Abstract

The acylated form of ghrelin (GRLN) has been discovered as the natural ligand of the GH secretagogue (GHS) receptor-1a (GHS-R1a). This peptide, whose acylation is performed by a specific octanoyl-transferase, is predominantly produced by the stomach, although expressed by many other endocrine and nonendocrine, peripheral and central tissues. Also GHS-R1a shows wide distribution, being distributed in several central and peripheral tissues. GRLN displays strong GH-releasing activity but its action is not specific for GH exhibiting other neuroendocrine activities such as stimulation of PRL and ACTH and inhibition of LH. GRLN is now mostly recognized as a potent orexigenic factor stimulating food intake and modulating energy expenditure. At the peripheral level, GRLN modulates gastrointestinal motility and secretion and also exerts cardiovascular actions. Mostly, at the peripheral level, GRLN exerts probably its major physiological action regulating glucose and lipid metabolism. In fact, GRLN in its acylated form has a diabetogenic action while in its non-acylated form it has a favorable influence on glucose, lipid metabolism and insulin sensitivity as well as the inhibition of lipolysis. GRLN receptors have been well demonstrated either in the endocrine pancreas or the adipose tissue; at these levels there are receptors that bind GRLN independently of its acylation (therefore a non-GHS-R1a, still undefined receptor). In all, the products of the GRLN gene, i.e. acylated and nonacylated GRLN, as well as obestatin, play a major role in regulating peripheral metabolism and it is not by chance that their secretion is mostly under metabolic regulation.

The acylated form of ghrelin (GRLN) has been discovered as the natural ligand of the GH secretagogue (GHS) receptor-1a (GHS-R1a) [1–4]. This peptide, whose acylation is performed by a specific octanoyl-transferase (GOAT) [5], is predominantly produced by the stomach, although expressed by many other endocrine and nonendocrine, peripheral and central tissues [2].

Also, GHS-R1a shows a widespread distribution, being concentrated in the hypothalamus-pituitary area but also distributed in several central and peripheral tissues [6, 7].

The widespread distribution of either GRLN or GHS-R1a predicts a wide spectrum of biological actions instead that have a specificity for GH.

Indeed, GRLN displays strong GH-releasing activity but also exhibits other neuroendocrine activities [3, 4]. GRLN is now mostly recognized as potent orexigenic factor stimulating appetite and food intake while modulating energy expenditure [8–11]; however, at the CNS level, it also influences sleep and behavior [3, 4]. At the peripheral level, as a gastroenteropancreatic hormone, GRLN modulates gastrointestinal motility and secretion [3, 4] but also exerts significant cardiovascular actions [3, 4]. Most of all, at the peripheral level, GRLN contributes to the regulation of glucose and lipid metabolism [3, 4, 12]. In this context it has now been clearly demonstrated that GRLN in its acylated form (AG) has a diabetogenic action [13, 14] while in its nonacylated form (UAG) it has a favorable influence on glucose and lipid metabolism including improvement of insulin synthesis, secretion and sensitivity as well as inhibition of lipolysis [12, 15, 16]. The presence in either the endocrine pancreas or the adipose tissue of both GHS-R1a and GRLN receptors binding GRLN independently of its acylation (thus, non-GHS-R1a) [4] represents the rational basis for understanding GRLN as a hormone with the major role of regulating peripheral metabolism.

The aim of this paper is to provide a brief review of GRLN, focusing on its neuroendocrine and peripheral metabolic actions.

Neuroendocrine Actions

GH-Releasing Activity

GRLN as well as synthetic GHSs possess strong and dose-related GH-releasing effects [1, 3, 17, 18]. Natural and synthetic GHSs stimulate GH release from somatotrope cells in vitro, probably depolarizing the somatotrope membrane and by increasing the amount of GH secreted per cell [1, 19]. GRLN and GHRH have a synergistic effect indicating that they act, at least partially, via different mechanisms [17, 20]. Nevertheless, GHSs need GHRH activity to fully elicit their GH-releasing effect and probably act by triggering GHRH-secreting neurones, being strongly inhibited by a GHRH antagonist as well as by hypothalamus-pituitary disconnection [21, 22]. GRLN probably also acts as a functional somatostatin antagonist at both the pituitary and the hypothalamic level [22]. In humans, the GH response to GRLN is partially refractory to exogenous somatostatin or cortistatin [23, 24]. The GH response to GRLN and GHSs is also partially refractory to other factors known to affect somatotrope secretion, such as glucose, lipids, arginine, cholinergic agonists and antagonists, IGF-I and GH itself [3, 25, 26]. The somatotrope response to GRLN and GHSs administration is independent of gender while it undergoes marked age-related variations increasing at puberty, persisting similary in adulthood and decreasing with aging [3, 18]; variations in estrogenic levels, GHRH hypoactivity, somatostatinergic hyperactivity and a reduced expression of the hypothalamic GHS-R1a in the aged human brain would explain these age-related changes and theoretically play a role in the age-related decrease of GH secretion [3, 18].

It now seems clear that GRLN does not play a major role in the physiological control of GH secretion; in fact, mice KO for GRLN or GHS-R1a are not dwarf [27]. Likely, GRLN has some role in the physiological control of GH pulsatility being able to amplify pulse amplitude, as indicated by studies using GRLN antagonists [28].

GRLN would, however, play some role in the GH response to energy restriction; in fact, the GH hyper- and hyposecretion that connote anorexia and obesity, respectively, could reflect GRLN hyper- and hyposecretion [29–31]. Interestingly, the GH response to GRLN is reduced not only in obesity but, at variance with that to GHRH, also in anorexia nervosa [32, 33]; thus, chronic hyperghrelinemia could induce some desensitization to exogenous GRLN actions in anorexia nervosa.

AG as well as synthetic GHSs could have diagnostic implications based on the strong and reproducible GH-releasing effects. Particularly when combined with GHRH, GRLN and GHSs could be used as potent and reliable provocative test to evaluate the capacity of the pituitary to release GH for the diagnosis of GHD [3, 4].

The potential therapeutic perspectives for GRLN and synthetic GHSs (replacement of rhGH for treatment of GHD or as anabolic intervention in aging and cachexia) have never been demonstrated [4, 8].

PRL- and ACTH-Releasing Activity

GRLN modulates also lactotrope and corticotrope secretion in humans as well as in animals [3, 4]. The stimulatory effect of GRLN and GHSs on PRL secretion in humans is slight, independent of both gender and age and probably involving both direct action on somatomammotrope cells and indirect hypothalamic actions [17, 18]. The magnitude of the PRL-releasing action of GRLN in humans is far lower than that of dopaminergic antagonists and TRH but similar to that of arginine [3, 4].

The acute stimulatory effect of GRLN and GHSs on the activity of the hypothalamic-pituitary-adrenal (HPA) axis in humans is similar to that after naloxone, AVP and even corticotropin-releasing hormone (CRH) [3, 4]. The ACTH-releasing activity of GHSs depends totally on CNS-mediated mechanisms and probably involves CRH, AVP, neuropeptide Y (NPY) and gamma-aminobutyric acid (GABA) neurones [3, 4].

The GHSs-induced ACTH release is independent of gender but shows peculiar age-related variations, increasing at puberty, then showing a reduction in adulthood and, again, a trend toward an increase in aging [18, 34].

The ACTH response to GHSs is generally sensitive to the negative cortisol feedback mechanism [3]. However, the stimulatory effect of GRLN and GHSs on corticotrope secretion is surprisingly enhanced and higher than that of hCRH in patients with pituitary ACTH-dependent Cushing's disease, probably reflecting an action on neoplastic ACTH-secreting cells where both GRLN and GHS-R are expressed [35].

Influence on Gonadotrope Secretion

Several in vitro and in vivo animal studies suggest that the GRLN system negatively influences the gonadal axis [36–39]. In animals intracerebroventricular injection of GRLN has been reported to be able to decrease the frequency of pulsatile LH secretion leading to a decrease in LH concentration [36, 37]. Also in humans, it has been reported that a prolonged infusion of AG inhibited LH mean concentration and pulsatility but not FSH secretion in healthy young males [40]. These findings probably reflect a modulation of the activity of the GnRH pulse generator and indicate that GRLN also plays a role in the central control of gonadotrope function [36]. In contrast with in vitro data showing that GRLN reduces the LH response to GnRH in rodents [39], in humans the LH response to this neurohormone is not modified by the exposure to AG; these findings are therefore against the hypothesis that GRLN plays any direct inhibitory role on pituitary gonadotropic cells. As AG inhibits the gonadotropin response to naloxone in humans, this clearly points toward a CNS-mediated inhibitory action on the human gonadal axis [40]. GRLN could, however, also play a role in the control of the gonadal axis at the peripheral level [4].

Ghrelin, Appetite and Energy Expenditure

GRLN is now mostly recognized as major orexigenic factor [8–11]. In fact, GRLN stimulates appetite through both central orexigenic and anorexigenic pathways, by acting mainly on the hypothalamic arcuate nucleus (ARC). The ARC contains two neuronal population: the neurons expressing neuropeptide Y (NPY) and agouti-related protein (AgRP), which have orexigenic action, and the neurons expressing pro-opiomelanocortin (POMC, the precursor to α-melanocyte-stimulating hormone – αMSH) and cocaine- and amphetamine-regulated transcript (CART), which have anorexigenic action [8]. GRLN stimulates NPY and AgRP neurons expressing GHS-R1a and its orexigenic action functionally depend on the presence of NPY and AgRP. In fact, GRLN-induced feeding is abolished in both NPY-null and AgRP-null mice or when endogenous NPY and AgRP are inhibited by anti-NPY and anti-AgRP antibodies [9].

Also, GRLN inhibits POMC neurons and the release of anorexigenic αMSH; the hypothalamic melanocortin tone is reduced also through the GRLN induced increase of AgRP that is an antagonist of hypothalamic melanocortin receptors [8]. Vagal, dopaminergic and cannabinoid pathways are also involved in GRLN-induced food intake [8, 10]. More recently, it has been demonstrated that the orexigenic action of GRLN is mediated by the uncoupling protein 2 (UCP2); this is needed to modulate on NPY/AgRP neurons and is driven by a hypothalamic fatty acid oxidation pathway involving AMPK, carnitine palmitoyltransferase 1 and free radicals [41]. In fact, the orexigenic action of GRLN involves specific inhibition of fatty acid biosynthesis induced by AMPK resulting in decreased hypothalamic levels of malonyl-CoA and CPT1 activity [42].

GRLN and its receptors are expressed mostly within the ARC nucleus but also in other CNS areas [4, 8]; this distribution allows to one understand why GRLN is involved in the control of synaptic plasticity, spatial learning and memory, sleep [4, 8].

The orexigenic action of GRLN has been demonstrated also in humans [43] and this evidence further prompted the enormous interest about this hormone. However, KO animal models demonstrated that GRLN and GHS-R1a KO mice are not anorectic dwarf [27]. Moreover, there is a negative relationship between multiple measures of adiposity in humans and circulating GRLN levels that are generally reduced in obese patients [10]. Also, increased signaling through GHS-R1a has not been shown to be the cause for most form of human obesity [10].

It remains that some authors demonstrated that the GRLN-null mice have a phenotype similar to that of wild type mice, but, when fed with high-fat diet, eat less food, store less of their consumed calories, preferentially use fat as an energy substrate, and accumulate less body weight and adiposity than control mice [10, 44]. Moreover, young mice are protected from the rapid weight gain induced by early exposure to a high-fat diet, in association to a decreased adiposity, increased energy expenditure and locomotor activity [10, 44]. These data suggest that endogenous GRLN has an important role in the metabolic adaptation to nutrient availability and absence of GRLN protects against early-onset obesity [45]. In this context, it is of major importance to notice that GRLN / GHS-R1a double KO mice exhibit decreased body weight, increased energy expenditure and increased motor activity on a standard diet without exposure to a high caloric environment [46].

Thus, it is clear that GRLN has an important role in the energy homeostasis and in long-term body weight regulation. This obviously predicts an impact of GRLN on peripheral metabolism. It has to be emphasized, however, that the ablation of GRLN was found able to improve the diabetic but not obese phenotype of ob/ob mice [47]. This evidence pointed toward direct, peripheral metabolic actions of GRLN. In agreement with this hypothesis there were old observations indicating that synthetic GHSs and GRLN would play a diabetogenic action: (a) synthetic GHSs stimulate the HPA axis and are diabetogenic in the Zucker diabetic fatty rat [48]; (b) prolonged daily oral administration of a GHS (MK-677) in healthy elderly subjects produces significant increase in fasting glucose and worsened insulin sensitivity [49]; (c) GRLN counteracts the inhibitory effect of insulin on gluconeogenesis from hepatoma cells [14]; (d) GRLN inhibits insulin secretion stimulated by glucose, arginine and carbachol from the perifused rat pancreas [50]. As discussed in the following paragraph, it is now clear that the direct, peripheral metabolic action of GRLN on glucose metabolism is likely to be its most important role.

Peripheral Metabolic Actions of Ghrelin

Glucose Metabolism and Insulin Secretion

The rational basis for an involvement of GRLN in the glucose metabolism is the existence of a new islet GRLN-producing ε-cell population in the endocrine pancreas where GHS-R1a and also specific binding sites that recognize GRLN independently of its acylation have been demonstrated [51, 52]. Interestingly, the pancreas has been shown as the most important GRLN source during fetal life [53]. Thus, that GRLN would play, at least, a paracrine/autocrine action within the endocrine pancreas is well based.

Noteworthy, the ablation of GRLN gene is associated to clear-cut improvement of glucose metabolism reflecting clear improvement in glucose sensitivity [47]. This evidence clearly indicates that the GRLN gene 'negatively' affects glucose metabolism. However, it is now clear that it must be distinguished between AG and UAG.

AG has been shown to regulate glucose homeostasis by modulating sensitivity of glucose-sensing neurons in the brain [54], insulin secretion and hepatic glucose production [12]. In humans, AG plays a negative role in glucose metabolism, inducing hyperglycemia and reducing insulin secretion [13]. Moreover, AG has been shown to induce lipolysis and insulin resistance independently of GH and cortisol [55]. In rodents AG, but not UAG, elevates blood glucose levels, through GHS-R1a-mediated signaling [56].

However, transgenic overexpressing UAG, under the control of the rat insulin II promoter in pancreatic islets, showed reduced glucose-stimulated insulin secretion, reduced blood glucose levels and increased insulin sensitivity, suggesting a role for UAG in glucose homeostasis [57]. UAG also prevents AG-induced increase of serum insulin and plasma glucose levels and co-administration of AG and UAG improves insulin sensitivity [15]. In hepatocytes, AG stimulates, whereas UAG inhibits glucose production and counteracts AG stimulatory effect [12]. In human hepatoma cells, AG exerts either insulin-like action or anti-insulin action through suppression of Akt activity and upregulation of gluconeogenesis [14]. Depending on the different experimental conditions, AG and UAG have been shown to both inhibit [13, 50, 56, 58] and stimulate [52, 59, 60] insulin secretion in humans and animals.

The localization of GRLN within the endocrine pancreas [53, 60] suggested its role also in the regulation of β-cell fate and function. Interestingly, either AG or UAG have been shown able to prevent diabetes in streptozotocin-treated rats, by increasing β-cell mass and insulin secretion [16]. In agreement with these findings, AG and even more UAG have been shown to promote proliferation and inhibit apoptosis of β-cells and human pancreatic islets through cAMP/PKA-, ERK1/2- and PI3K/Akt-mediated mechanisms. Both peptides were found to even stimulate glucose-induced insulin secretion in β-cells and human islets. As UAG is not bound by the GHS-R1a, this evidence implies the existence of a new GRLN receptor subtype that is still waiting to be discovered [52].

Conclusions

The story of GRLN was born with synthetic GHSs in late 1970s; the first dream was that synthetic GHSs would replace rhGH for treatment of GH deficiency. Evidence indicating that GRLN is a major orexigenic factor suggested the following dream, i.e. that GRLN antagonists and agonists would have therapeutic implications for treatment of obesity and cachexia, respectively. Although it is widely accepted that GRLN display a wide spectrum of biological actions (central and peripheral, endocrine and nonendocrine actions), the most recent findings in this field of research indicate that the most important physiological role for GRLN is likely to be represented by the regulation of glucose and lipid metabolism. Whether GRLN analogues would have therapeutic perspectives for treatment of diabetes and metabolic syndrome is likely the new dream related to this gastroenteropancreatic hormone.

References

1 Kojima M, Hosoda H, Date Y, Nakazato M, Matsuo H, Kangawa K: Ghrelin is a growth-hormone-releasing acylated peptide from stomach. Nature 1999; 402:656–660.
2 Kojima M, Hosoda H, Matsuo H, Kangawa K: Ghrelin: discovery of the natural endogenous ligand for the growth hormone secretagogue receptor. Trends Endocrinol Metab 2001;12:118–122.
3 Van der Lely AF, Tschop M, Heiman ML, Ghigo E: Biological, physiological, pathophysiological, and pharmacological aspects of ghrelin. Endocr Rev 2004;25:866–866.
4 Ghigo E, Broglio F, Arvat E, Maccario M, Papotti M, Muccioli G: Ghrelin: more than a natural gh secretagogue and/or an orexigenic factor. Clin Endocrinol 2005;62:1–17.
5 Gutierrez JA, Solenberg PJ, Perkins DR, Willency JA, Knierman MD, Jin Z, Witcher DR, Luo S, Onyia JE, Hale JE: Ghrelin octanoylation mediated by an orphan lipid transferase. Proc Natl Acad Sci USA 2008;105:6320–6325.
6 Papotti M, Ghe C, Cassoni P, Catapano F, Deghenghi R, Ghigo E, Muccioli G: Growth hormone secretagogue binding sites in peripheral human tissues. J Clin Endocrinol Metab 2000;85:3803–3807.
7 Gnanapavan S, Kola B, Bustin SA, Morris DG, McGee P, Fairclough P, Bhattacharya S, Carpenter R, Grossman AB, Korbonits M: The tissue distribution of the mRNA of ghrelin and subtypes of its receptor, GHS-R, in humans. J Clin Endocrinol Metab 2002;87:2988.
8 Wiedmer P, Nogueiras R, Broglio F, D'Alessio D, Tschop MH: Ghrelin, obesity and diabetes. Nat Clin Pract Endocrinol Metab 2007;3:705–712.
9 De Vriese C, Delporte C: Influence of ghrelin on food intake and energy homeostasis. Curr Opin Clin Nutr Metab Care 2007;10:615–619.
10 Nogueiras R, Tschop MH, Zigman JM: Central nervous system regulation of energy metabolism: ghrelin versus leptin. Ann NY Acad Sci 2008;1126; 14–19.
11 Cummings DE: Ghrelin and the short- and long-term regulation of appetite and body weight. Physiol Behav 2006;89:71–84.
12 Gauna C, Delhanty PJ, Hofland LJ, Janssen JA, Broglio F, Ross RJ, Ghigo E, van der Lely AJ: Ghrelin stimulates, whereas des-octanoyl ghrelin inhibits, glucose output by primary hepatocytes. J Clin Endocrinol Metab 2005;90:1055–1060.
13 Broglio F, Arvat E, Benso A, Gottero C, Muccioli G, Papotti M, van der Lely AJ, Deghenghi R, Ghigo E: Ghrelin, a natural GH secretagogue produced by the stomach, induces hyperglycemia and reduces insulin secretion in humans. J Clin Endocrinol Metab 2001;86:5083–5086.
14 Murata M, Okimura Y, Iida K, Matsumoto M, Sowa H, Kaji H, Kojima M, Kangawa K, Chihara K: Ghrelin modulates the downstream molecules of insulin signaling in hepatoma cells. J Biol Chem 2002;277:5667–5674.
15 Gauna C, Meyler FM, Janssen JA, Delhanty PJ, Abribat T, van Koetsveld P, Hofland LJ, Broglio F, Ghigo E, van der Lely AJ: Administration of acylated ghrelin reduces insulin sensitivity, whereas the combination of acylated plus unacylated ghrelin strongly improves insulin sensitivity. J Clin Endocrinol Metab 2004;89:5035–5042.

16 Irako T, Akamizu T, Hosoda H, Iwakura H, Ariyasu H, Tojo K, Tajima N, Kangawa K: Ghrelin prevents development of diabetes at adult age in streptozotocin-treated newborn rats. Diabetologia 2006;49: 1264–1273.
17 Arvat E, Maccario M, Di Vito L, Broglio F, Benso A, Gottero C, Papotti M, Muccioli G, Dieguez C, Casanueva FF, Deghenghi R, Camanni F, Ghigo E: Endocrine activities of ghrelin, a natural growth hormone secretagogue (GHS), in humans: comparison and interactions with hexarelin, a nonnatural peptidyl GHS, and GH-releasing hormone. J Clin Endocrinol Metab 2001;86:1169–1174.
18 Broglio F, Benso A, Castiglioni C, Gottero C, Prodam F, Destefanis S, Gauna C, van der Lely AJ, Deghenghi R, Bo M, Arvat E, Ghigo E: The endocrine response to ghrelin as a function of gender in humans in young and elderly subjects. J Clin Endocrinol Metab 2003;88:1537–1542.
19 Goth MI, Lyons CE, Canny BJ, Thorner MO: Pituitary adenylate cyclase activating polypeptide, growth-hormone (GH)-releasing peptide and GH-releasing hormone stimulate GH release through distinct pituitary receptors. Endocrinology 1992;130:939–944.
20 Hataya Y, Akamizu T, Takaya K, Kanamoto N, Ariyasu H, Saijo M, Moriyama K, Shimatsu A, Kojima M, Kangawa K, Nakao K: A low dose of ghrelin stimulates growth hormone (GH) release synergistically with GH-releasing hormone in humans. J Clin Endocrinol Metab 2001;86:4552.
21 Popovic V, Miljic D, Micic D, Damjanovic S, Arvat E, Ghigo E, Dieguez C, Casanueva FF: Ghrelin main action on the regulation of growth hormone release is exerted at hypothalamic level. J Clin Endocrinol Metab 2003;88:3450–3453.
22 Tannenbaum GS, Epelbaum J, Bowers CY: Interrelationship between the novel peptide ghrelin and somatostatin/growth hormone-releasing hormone in regulation of pulsatile growth hormone secretion. Endocrinology 2003;144:967–974.
23 Broglio F, Arvat E, Benso A, Gottero C, Prodam F, Grottoli S, Papotti M, Muccioli G, van der Lely AJ, Deghenghi R, Ghigo E: Endocrine activities of cortistatin-14 and its interaction with GHRH and ghrelin in humans. J Clin Endocrinol Metab 2002;87: 3783–3790.
24 Di Vito L, Broglio F, Benso A, Gottero C, Prodam F, Papotti M, Muccioli G, Dieguez C, Casanueva FF, Deghenghi R, Ghigo E, Arvat E: The GH-releasing effect of ghrelin, a natural GH secretagogue, is only blunted by the infusion of exogenous somatostatin in humans. Clin Endocrinol 2002;56:643–648.
25 Broglio F, Benso A, Gottero C, Prodam F, Grottoli S, Tassone F, Maccario M, Casanueva FF, Dieguez C, Deghenghi R, Ghigo E, Arvat E: Effects of glucose, free fatty acids or arginine load on the GH-releasing activity of ghrelin in humans. Clin Endocrinol 2002; 57:265–271.
26 Broglio F, Gottero C, Benso A, Prodam F, Casanueva FF, Dieguez C, van der Lely AJ, Deghenghi R, Arvat E, Ghigo E: Acetylcholine does not play a major role in mediating the endocrine responses to ghrelin, a natural ligand of the GH secretagogue receptor, in humans. Clin Endocrinol 2003;58:92–98.
27 Sun Y, Wang P, Zheng H, Smith RG: Ghrelin stimulation of growth hormone release and appetite is mediated through the growth hormone secretagogue receptor. Proc Natl Acad Sci USA 2004;101: 4679–4684.
28 Zizzari P, Halem H, Taylor J, Dong JZ, Datta R, Culler MD, Epelbaum J, Bluet-Pajot MT: Endogenous ghrelin regulates episodic growth hormone (GH) secretion by amplifying GH pulse amplitude: evidence from antagonism of the GH secretagogue-R1a receptor. Endocrinology 2005;146:3836–3842.
29 Ariyasu H, Takaya K, Tagami T, Ogawa Y, Hosoda K, Akamizu T, Suda M, Koh T, Natsui K, Toyooka S, Shirakami G, Usui T, Shimatsu A, Doi K, Hosoda H, Kojima M, Kangawa K, Nakao K: Stomach is a major source of circulating ghrelin, and feeding state determines plasma ghrelin-like immunoreactivity levels in humans. J Clin Endocrinol Metab 2001;86:4753–4758.
30 Tschop M, Weyer C, Tataranni PA, Devanarayan V, Ravussin E, Heiman ML: Circulating ghrelin levels are decreased in human obesity. Diabetes 2001;50: 707–709.
31 Shiiya T, Nakazato M, Mizuta M, Date Y, Mondal MS, Tanaka M, Nozoe S, Hosoda H, Kangawa K, Matsukura S: Plasma ghrelin levels in lean and obese humans and the effect of glucose on ghrelin secretion. J Clin Endocrinol Metab 2002;87:240–244.
32 Tassone F, Broglio F, Destefanis S, Rovere S, Benso A, Gottero C, Prodam F, Rossetto R, Gauna C, van der Lely AJ, Ghigo E, Maccario M: Neuroendocrine and metabolic effects of acute ghrelin administration in human obesity. J Clin Endocrinol Metab 2003;88:5478–5483.
33 Broglio F, Gianotti L, Destefanis S, Fassino S, Abbate Daga G, Mondelli V, Lanfranco F, Gottero C, Gauna C, Hofland L, Van der Lely AJ, Ghigo E: The endocrine response to acute ghrelin administration is blunted in patients with anorexia nervosa, a ghrelin hypersecretory state. Clin Endocrinol (Oxf) 2004; 60:592–599.

34 Arvat E, Ramunni J, Bellone J, Di Vito L, Baffoni C, Broglio F, Deghenghi R, Bartolotta E, Ghigo E: The GH, prolactin, ACTH and cortisol responses to hexarelin, a synthetic hexapeptide, undergo different age-related variations. Eur J Endocrinol 1997; 137:635–642.
35 Leal-Cerro A, Torres E, Soto A, Dios E, Deghenghi R, Arvat E, Ghigo E, Dieguez C, Casanueva FF: Ghrelin is no longer able to stimulate growth hormone secretion in patients with Cushing's syndrome but instead induces exaggerated corticotropin and cortisol responses. Neuroendocrinology 2002;76: 390–396.
36 Furuta M, Funabashi T, Kimura F: Intracerebroventricular administration of ghrelin rapidly suppresses pulsatile luteinizing hormone secretion in ovariectomized rats. Biochem Biophys Res Commun 2001;288:780–785.
37 Fernandez-Fernandez R, Tena-Sempere M, Aguilar E, Pinilla L: Ghrelin effects on gonadotropin secretion in male and female rats. Neurosci Lett 2004; 362:103–107.
38 Vulliemoz NR, Xiao E, Xia-Zhang L, Germond M, Rivier J, Ferin M: Decrease in luteinizing hormone pulse frequency during a five-hour peripheral ghrelin infusion in the ovariectomized rhesus monkey. J Clin Endocrinol Metab 2004;89:5718–5723.
39 Fernandez-Fernandez R, Tena-Sempere M, Navarro VM, Barreiro ML, Castellano JM, Aguilar E, Pinilla L: Effects of ghrelin upon gonadotropin-releasing hormone and gonadotropin secretion in adult female rats: in vivo and in vitro studies. Neuroendocrinology 2005;82:245–255.
40 Lanfranco F, Bonelli L, Baldi M, Me E, Broglio F, Ghigo E: Acylated ghrelin inhibits spontaneous luteinizing hormone pulsatility and responsiveness to naloxone but not that to gonadotropin-releasing hormone in young men: evidence for a central inhibitory action of ghrelin on the gonadal axis. J Clin Endocrinol Metab 2008;93:3633–3639.
41 Andrews ZB, Liu ZW, Walllingford N, Erion DM, Borok E, Friedman JM, Tschop MH, Shanabrough M, Cline G, Shulman GI, Coppola A, Gao XB, Horvath TL, Diano S: UCP2 mediates ghrelin's action on NPY/AgRP neurons by lowering free radicals. Nature 2008; 454; 846–851.
42 Lopez M, Lage R, Saha AK, Perez-Tilve D, Vazquez MJ, Varela L, Sangiao-Alvarellos S, Tovar S, Raghay K, Rodriguez-Cuenca S, Deoliveira RM, Castaneda T, Datta R, Dong JZ, Culler M, Sleeman MW, Alvarez CV, Gallego R, Lelliott CJ, Carling D, Tschop MH, Dieguez C, Vidal-Puig A: Hypothalamic fatty acid metabolism mediates the orexigenic action of ghrelin. Cell Metab 2008;7:389–399.
43 Wren AM, Seal LJ, Cohen MA, Brynes AE, Frost GS, Murphy KG, Dhillo WS, Ghatei MA, Bloom SR: Ghrelin enhances appetite and increases food intake in humans. J Clin Endocrinol Metab 2001;86:5992.
44 Dimaraki EV, Jaffe CA: Role of endogenous ghrelin in growth hormone secretion, appetite regulation and metabolism. Rev Endocr Metab Disord 2006;7: 237–249.
45 Ukkola O: Ghrelin and metabolic disorders. Curr Protein Pept Sci 2009;10; 2–7.
46 Pfluger PT, Kirchner H, Gunnel S, Schrott B, Perez-Tilve D, Fu S, Benoit SC, Horvath T, Joost HG, Wortley KE, Sleeman MW, Tschop MH: Simultaneous deletion of ghrelin and its receptor increases motor activity and energy expenditure. Am J Physiol Gastrointest Liver Physiol 2008;294:G610–G618.
47 Sun Y, Asnicar M, Saha PK, Chan L, Smith RG: Ablation of ghrelin improves the diabetic but not obese phenotype of ob/ob mice. Cell Metab 2006; 3:379–386.
48 Clark RG, Thomas GB, Mortensen DL, Won WB, Ma YH, Tomlinson EE, Fairhall KM, Robinson IC: Growth hormone secretagogues stimulate the hypothalamic-pituitary-adrenal axis and are diabetogenic in the Zucker diabetic fatty rat. Endocrinology 1997;138:4316–4323.
49 Chapman IM, Bach MA, vanCauter E, Farmer M, Krupa D, Taylor AM, Schilling LM, Cole KY, Skiles EH, Pezzoli SS, Hartman ML, Veldhuis JD, Gormley GJ, Thorner MO: Stimulation of the growth hormone (GH)-insulin-like growth factor I axis by daily oral administration of a GH secretogogue (MK-677) in healthy elderly subjects. J Clin Endocrinol Metab 1996;81:4249–4257.
50 Egido EM, Rodriguez-Gallardo J, Silvestre RA, Marco J: Inhibitory effect of ghrelin on insulin and pancreatic somatostatin secretion. Eur J Endocrinol 2002;146:241–244.
51 Prado CL, Pugh-Bernard AE, Elghazi L, Sosa-Pineda B, Sussel L: Ghrelin cells replace insulin-producing beta cells in two mouse models of pancreas development. Proc Natl Acad Sci USA 2004;101:2924–2929.
52 Granata R, Settanni F, Biancone L, Trovato L, Nano R, Bertuzzi F, Destefanis S, Annunziata M, Martinetti M, Catapano F, Ghe C, Isgaard J, Papotti M, Ghigo E, Muccioli G: Acylated and unacylated ghrelin promote proliferation and inhibit apoptosis of pancreatic beta-cells and human islets: involvement of 3′,5′-cyclic adenosine monophosphate/protein kinase A, extracellular signal-regulated kinase 1/2, and phosphatidyl inositol 3-kinase/Akt signaling. Endocrinology 2007;148:512–529.
53 Wierup N, Svensson H, Mulder H, Sundler F: The ghrelin cell: a novel developmentally regulated islet cell in the human pancreas. Regul Pept 2002;107:63–69.

54 Wang WG, Chen X, Jiang H, Jiang ZY: Effects of ghrelin on glucose-sensing and gastric distension sensitive neurons in rat dorsal vagal complex. Regul Pept 2008;146:169–175.
55 Vestergaard ET, Gormsen LC, Jessen N, Lund S, Hansen TK, Moller N, Jorgensen JO: Ghrelin infusion in humans induces acute insulin resistance and lipolysis independent of growth hormone signaling. Diabetes 2008;57:3205–3210.
56 Dezaki K, Hosoda H, Kakei M, Hashiguchi S, Watanabe M, Kangawa K, Yada T: Endogenous ghrelin in pancreatic islets restricts insulin release by attenuating Ca^{2+} signaling in beta-cells: implication in the glycemic control in rodents. Diabetes 2004;53: 3142–3151.
57 Iwakura H, Hosoda K, Son C, Fujikura J, Tomita T, Noguchi M, Ariyasu H, Takaya K, Masuzaki H, Ogawa Y, Hayashi T, Inoue G, Akamizu T, Hosoda H, Kojima M, Itoh H, Toyokuni S, Kangawa K, Nakao K: Analysis of rat insulin II promoter-ghrelin transgenic mice and rat glucagon promoter-ghrelin transgenic mice. J Biol Chem 2005;280:15247–15256.
58 Broglio F, Gottero C, Benso A, Prodam F, Destefanis S, Gauna C, Maccario M, Deghenghi R, van der Lely AJ, Ghigo E: Effects of ghrelin on the insulin and glycemic responses to glucose, arginine, or free fatty acids load in humans. J Clin Endocrinol Metab 2003;88:4268–4272.
59 Date Y, Nakazato M, Hashiguchi S, Dezaki K, Mondal MS, Hosoda H, Kojima M, Kangawa K, Arima T, Matsuo H, Yada T, Matsukura S: Ghrelin is present in pancreatic alpha-cells of humans and rats and stimulates insulin secretion. Diabetes 2002;51: 124–129.
60 Lee HM, Wang G, Englander EW, Kojima M, Greeley GH Jr: Ghrelin, a new gastrointestinal endocrine peptide that stimulates insulin secretion: enteric distribution, ontogeny, influence of endocrine, and dietary manipulations. Endocrinology 2002;143:185–190.

Ezio Ghigo, MD
Division of Endocrinology, Diabetology and Metabolism
Department of Internal Medicine, University of Turin
Corso Dogliotti 14, IT–10126 Torino (Italy)
Tel. +39 011 6334317, Fax +39 011 6647421, E-Mail ezio.ghigo@unito.it

Loche S, Cappa M, Ghizzoni L, Maghnie M, Savage MO (eds): Pediatric Neuroendocrinology.
Endocr Dev. Basel, Karger, 2010, vol 17, pp 96–107

Pitfalls in the Diagnosis of Central Adrenal Insufficiency in Children

Rasa Kazlauskaite[a] · Mohamad Maghnie[b]

[a]Department of Preventive Medicine, Rush University Medical Center, Chicago, Ill., USA; [b]IRCCS Giannina Gaslini Clinica Pediatrica Università di Genova, Genova, Italy

Abstract

The diagnosis of central adrenal insufficiency relies heavily on laboratory testing of cortisol levels in the systemic circulation. The lack of cortisol assay standardization challenges the reliability of dynamic tests of the hypothalamic-pituitary adrenal axis. Although the insulin-induced hypoglycemia or metyrapone tests remain the accepted standards for evaluating central adrenal insufficiency in children their associated risks and inconvenience make them unattractive for routine use. Corticotropin testing is an effective first step to evaluate for chronic central adrenal insufficiency for children older than 2 years who are ambulatory, have normal sleep-wake cycle and normal serum protein levels. The low-dose (1 μg) corticotropin test may be superior to standard-dose (250 mcg) for patients with suspected hypothalamic-pituitary disease.

Chronic central adrenal insufficiency (CAI) is characterized by the impaired synthesis and release of adrenocorticotropic hormone (ACTH) from the pituitary gland, impaired release or effect of corticotropin-releasing factor (CRH) from the hypothalamus, due to disease or injury to the hypothalamus-pituitary area or from prolonged exogenous glucocorticoid administration that exceeds physiological doses. The consequence of ACTH or CRH deficiency is reduced synthesis and release of cortisol. One of the cardinal differences distinguishing CAI from primary adrenal insufficiency is that CAI does not significantly affect the mineralocorticoid axis, as mineralocorticoids are primarily regulated by the renin-angiotensin system, and only partially by ACTH.

The reference tests for establishing the integrity of the hypothalamic-pituitary-adrenal (HPA) axis require assessing the response to either a strong stimulus (e.g. insulin-induced hypoglycemia) or an interruption of the negative feedback from cortisol (overnight metyrapone test). However, these reference tests have major drawbacks. The insulin tolerance test is contraindicated in children with a history of seizures and requires continuous physician supervision to monitor for serious adrenergic or neurological symptoms [1]. The overnight metyrapone test carries a risk of adrenal crisis, and errors can occur from other drugs affecting metyrapone clearance [2]. Thus, there is a great clinical demand for alternative tests that are quicker, cheaper, and safer.

The rationale for using the corticotropin stimulation test is the assumption that in chronic endogenous corticotropin deficiency, acute responsiveness of the adrenal zona fasciculata is diminished and fails to mount an adequate cortisol response [3]. We examined the published literature for evidence on two tests – using either a standard (250 μg) or low-dose (1 μg) corticotropin analog – and summarized the results in a quantitative meta-analysis [4] in the 'gold-standard' diagnosis of central adrenal insufficiency, defined by results of the insulin tolerance test or overnight metyrapone test. In this paper, we examine the results for studies evaluating pediatric patients.

Methods

Data Collection

We searched the PubMed (www.PubMed.gov) database from 1966 to 2006 for articles with the key words 'adrenal insufficiency' and 'diagnosis' and limited the search to human studies published in English. We selected studies with at least 10 subjects with suspected CAI and required that the disease be verified with either the insulin tolerance test or the metyrapone test. We then contacted the principal investigator of each relevant study to request their patient-level data on the following variables: results of the integrated HPA axis reference test, baseline cortisol value, and cortisol values after the standard-dose and low-dose corticotropin tests.

To be eligible for inclusion, subjects had to be suspected of CAI from disease or injury to the pituitary or hypothalamus or from prolonged exogenous glucocorticoid administration in supraphysiological doses. Patients had to be affected by hypothalamic-pituitary disease for at least 4 weeks in order to exclude acute hypothalamic or pituitary disorders. A normal sleep-wake cycle was required (or assumed, if no information) as cortisol secretion has a diurnal cycle. We did not include data from studies performed in the critical care setting.

In actual clinical practice, testing is performed when there is some suspicion for CAI. We therefore investigated the performance of the tests in at-risk patients in order to avoid the problem of spectrum bias [5], which occurs when tests are evaluated among patients who are different from the ones who will be tested in practice. Thus, we excluded those studies that included control subjects who were described as normal healthy children ('healthy volunteers' in whom there was no suspicion of pituitary disease based on signs, symptoms, or imaging).

The main reason for HPA axis testing was growth hormone deficiency or multiple pituitary hormone deficiencies, although some children were investigated after the treatment of brain tumors, leukemia, and other central nervous system malignancies [6].

Reference Tests

The diagnosis of CAI was based on an abnormal response to one of the two reference standards for evaluating the integrity of the HPA axis: insulin tolerance test or overnight metyrapone test. We relied on individual study investigators to correctly dichotomize the reference test results into CAI present or absent.

For the overnight metyrapone test in children, a single oral dose of metyrapone was administered at 24.00 h [6] or at 23.00 h [7]. Metyrapone was given orally in a dose of 1 g/m^2 for children weighing 30 kg or less, 2–3 g/m^2 for 30–60 kg, and 3 g/m^2 for those weighing above 60 kg [6], which approximates doses of 30–40 mg/kg used in another study [7]. Blood glucose was monitored hourly during the night and serum cortisol and 11-deoxycortisol were measured on the following morning at 08:00 h. Response to metyrapone was defined as low if serum 11-deoxycortisol was ≤7 μg/dl (200 nmol/l) with serum cortisol ≤5 μg/dl (140 nmol/l).

For the insulin tolerance test [8], 0.1 U/kg of human regular insulin was injected and serum cortisol and glucose were measured at baseline and at 30, 60, 90 and 120 min after insulin administration. The test was positive if the cortisol was <20 μg/dl (550 nmol/l) when the glucose was below 40 mg/dl (2.2 nmol/l) with glucopenic symptoms.

Cortisol Assay

Cortisol assays are not standardized and vary across hospitals and studies [9–11]. The cortisol assay methods used in various studies included commercially available radioimmunoassays or immunometric methods.

Standard-Dose Corticotropin Stimulation Test

One of the two available synthetic corticotropin analogs – cosyntropin (Cortrosyn, Amphastar Pharmaceuticals, Inc.) or tetracosactrin (Synacthen, Novartis Pharma, Switzerland) – was administered intravenously at a dose of 250 μg, and serum cortisol levels were obtained at baseline and at least once after injection (most commonly at 30 or 60 min).

A standard-dose corticotropin stimulation test involves a dose of 250 μg (0.25 mg) of either cosyntropin or tetracosactrin, which are equivalent to 25 USP units of corticotropin. For brevity, we use the term 'corticotropin' for both analogs, while acknowledging that Synacthen and Cortrosyn are synthetic corticotropin analogs, different from the native ACTH molecule.

Low-Dose Corticotropin Stimulation Test

The low-dose test was performed in the morning with patients fasting. One of the two synthetic corticotropin analogs (cosyntropin or tetracosactrin) was administered intravenously after being prepared using the method of Dickstein et al. [12]. The dose for children varies by study. Maghnie et al. [8] used a 1-μg dose, Gonc et al. [7] used 0.5 μg/m^2, and Rose et al. [6] used 1 μg/m^2 body surface area. Serum cortisol was measured at baseline and at 30 min postinjection, except for the study by Rose et al. [6], where it was measured at 20 min.

Basal Cortisol

All studies measured serum cortisol between 08.00 h and 10.00 h after an overnight fast (basal cortisol).

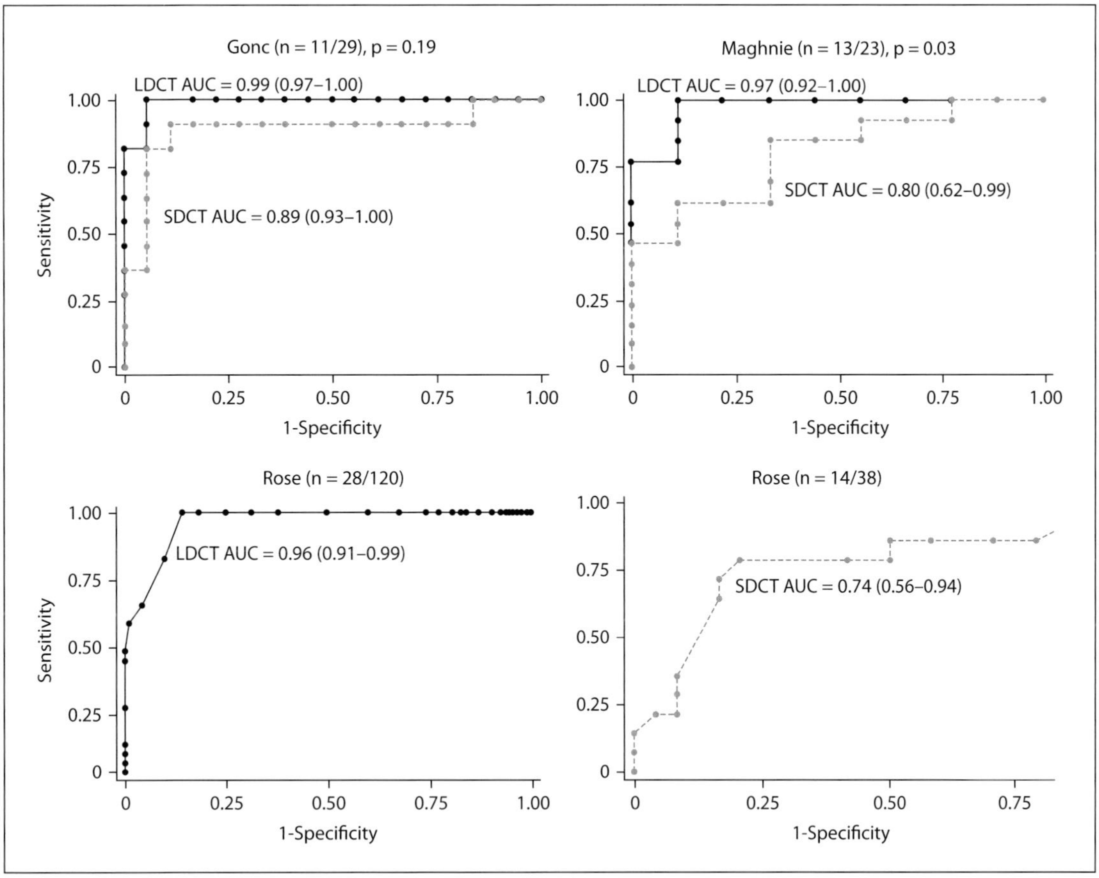

Fig. 1. ROC curves for LDCT (20- to 30-min cortisol levels; light lines) and SDCT (30-min cortisol levels; darker lines) diagnosing HPA insufficiency.

Statistical Analysis

We conducted data analysis using Stata statistical software, version 10.0 (StataCorp LP, College Station, Tex., USA).

To compare the performance of LDCT and SDCT, we used receiver-operator-characteristic (ROC) curve analysis. From each study's data, we calculated the area under the ROC curve (AUC) with 95% CIs (fig. 1). We categorized cortisol response into 3 intervals (high, indeterminate and low likelihood of CAI), which were defined by two thresholds. The first threshold was the cortisol value below which there was a high likelihood of CAI (likelihood ratio [LR] >9; rule-in threshold). The second threshold was the cortisol value above which there was a low likelihood of CAI (LR <0.15; rule-out threshold). Cortisol values between these thresholds (LR 0.15–9) defined the interval with indeterminate likelihood of CAI.

Likelihood ratios were calculated as the ratio of two probabilities: the probability of the test result among patients with CAI, divided by the probability of the same test result among patients without CAI.

Table 1. Study characteristics

Study	Basal cortisol (early morning)			Standard-dose stimulated cortisol (30 min/peak)			Low-dose stimulated cortisol (20–30 min)		
	n HPAI/ n total	HPAI† µg/dl*	no HPAI‡ µg/dl*	n HPAI/ n total	HPAI† µg/dl*	no HPAI‡ µg/dl*	n HPAI/ n total	HPAI† µg/dl*	no HPAI‡ µg/dl*
Studies with paired data									
Gonc et al. [7]	11/29	≤6	≥9	11/29	≤16	≥36	11/29	≤16	≥19
Maghnie et al. [8]	14/24	≤9	**≥15**	13/23	≤20	≥33	14/24	≤20	**≥22**
Study with unpaired data									
Rose et al. [6]‖	42/158	**≤3**	≥13	14/38	**≤16**	**≥39**	28/120	≤17	≥20
Adult mean§ (95% CI)	**33%** 210/635	**≤5**§ (4.7–5.3)	**≥13**§ (12.9–13.6)	**40%** 140/346	**≤16**§ (15.2–16.4)	**≥30**§ (29.9–32.3)	**33%** 193/586	**≤16**§ (15.2–16.0)	**≥22**§ (20.9–21.9)

HPAI = Hypothalamic-pituitary adrenal insufficiency.
Suggested pediatric and adult thresholds are in bold.
* Serum cortisol in µg/dl, to convert to nmol/l multiply by 27.56.
† Threshold below which cortisol values had a LR >9 (rule-in threshold).
‡ Threshold above which cortisol values had a LR <0.15 (rule-out threshold).
§ Mean, weighted by size of the studies.
‖ SDCT and LDCT were performed on different subsets of patients (no paired data).

Results

We were able to analyze pediatric patient-level data from 3 published studies, with 2 studies having paired data comparing results of the low-dose and standard-dose corticotropin stimulation tests on the same patients (table 1). The prevalence of CAI in the study samples ranged from 27% to 58%, with a mean of 33% (table 1). The age of the children varied from 1 to 18 years [6], 5 to 20 years [7], and 4 to 20 years [8].

Cortisol Testing

Cortisol testing methods varied from individual radioimmunoassay kits [6, 8] to immunometric test kits [7]. The lack of a standard cortisol assay method [9–11] explains some of the variability in diagnostic cortisol thresholds reported across studies.

Basal Cortisol

According to pediatric data from 3 studies (211 children), the lowest basal cortisol threshold was ≤3 µg/dl (88 nmol/l) to diagnose CAI and the highest basal threshold was ≥15 µg/dl (415 nmol/l) to exclude CAI. For comparison, in a meta-analysis of 12 studies of adults (635 subjects), a basal cortisol less than 5 µg/dl (138 nmol/l) best predicted CAI, while values greater than 13 µg/dl (365 nmol/l) best predicted a normal HPA axis.

Standard-Dose Corticotropin-Stimulated Cortisol Test

After standard-dose corticotropin stimulation, there was variability across studies in the optimal timing for measuring cortisol response; however, in no study was there a statistically significant difference in diagnostic discrimination at 30 min, 60 min, or at peak response.

A 30-min cortisol value of less than 16 µg/dl (440 nmol/l) was highly predictive of CAI. Values greater than 39 µg/dl (1,076 nmol/l) virtually exclude CAI in children (ruling out CAI). (For comparison, adults with a stimulated cortisol greater than 30 µg/dl (833 nmol/l) rules out CAI.)

Intermediate values – 16–39 µg/dl – should be considered diagnostically indeterminate in children. The area under the ROC curve for these test results is depicted in figure 1.

Low-Dose Corticotropin-Stimulated Cortisol Test

After low-dose corticotropin stimulation, 30-min cortisol measurements in 2 studies had superior test characteristics compared to measurements at other times [7, 8]. In our analyses of low-dose corticotropin stimulation, we used 30-min cortisol values, or, if not available, then the 20-min value [6].

A 20- to 30-min cortisol value of less than 16 µg/dl (440 nmol/l) was highly predictive of CAI. Values greater than 22 µg/dl (600 nmol/l) virtually exclude CAI in children (ruling out CAI). The area under the ROC curve using these diagnostic thresholds was 0.99 (95% CI 0.98–1.00). Given the a small number of pediatric studies and to achieve higher fidelity diagnosing or excluding CAI, the 'rule in' threshold value was selected as the lowest cortisol threshold to predict CAI (whereas weighted mean was 17 µg/dl or 470 nmol/l), the 'rule out' threshold value was selected as the highest cortisol threshold to exclude CAI (whereas weighted mean was 20 µg/dl or 550 nmol/l), and were reasonably close to match LDCT thresholds in adults. Using weighted mean thresholds did not significantly change the results.

For comparison, our meta-analysis of 11 studies using the low-dose stimulation test (589 subjects, primarily adults) found that values less than 16 µg/dl (440 nmol/l) best predicted CAI, while values greater than 22 μg/dl (600 nmol/l) were best for ruling out CAI. The area under the ROC curve using these diagnostic thresholds was 0.94 (95% CI: 0.90–0.94).

Comparison of Low-Dose and Standard-Dose Stimulation Tests

In the 2 studies with paired 30-min cortisol data for both tests (53 children) and one study with unpaired data (158 children), the low-dose test had a larger area under the ROC curve compared to the standard-dose test (see fig. 1 for area under the ROC curve). In the two studies that used either 1 μg or 1 μg/m^2 of the corticotropin analog, the low-dose test was statistical superior to the standard-dose test in area under the ROC curve.

Optimal Testing Strategy Algorithm in Children

We applied the previously published testing algorithm [4] to the data on children (fig. 2). The basal cortisol and LDCT thresholds described in figure 2 were based on the mean cortisol values weighted by study sample size (last row of table 1). The thresholds for the two sequential tests defined 5 subgroups: (1) low basal cortisol; (2) high basal cortisol; (3) indeterminate basal cortisol and low stimulated cortisol; (4) indeterminate cortisol and indeterminate stimulated cortisol, and (5) indeterminate basal cortisol and high stimulated cortisol. We calculated the expected probability of CAI, with 95% CIs, within each of the 5 subgroups.

We found that overall LDCT thresholds for evaluation of CAI performed well in children. However, basal cortisol thresholds, particularly the one to rule in CAI (<5 μg/dl) was not reliable.

Discussion

Our analysis suggests that the low-dose corticotropin stimulation test is superior to the standard-dose test in diagnosing central adrenal insufficiency in children, similar to findings in adults. Because all study subjects were ambulatory and presumably had normal sleep-wake cycles, these findings may not generalize to hospital settings or patients with acute illnesses. Nevertheless, there may be clinical settings where standard-dose testing is more appropriate to diagnose CAI, especially if the quality of the low-dose testing protocol cannot be assured.

The 3-step approach for evaluating patients with possible hypothalamic-pituitary adrenal insufficiency [4] may be used in children (fig. 2). However, in the first step of measuring a morning basal cortisol, one may consider using lower threshold (3

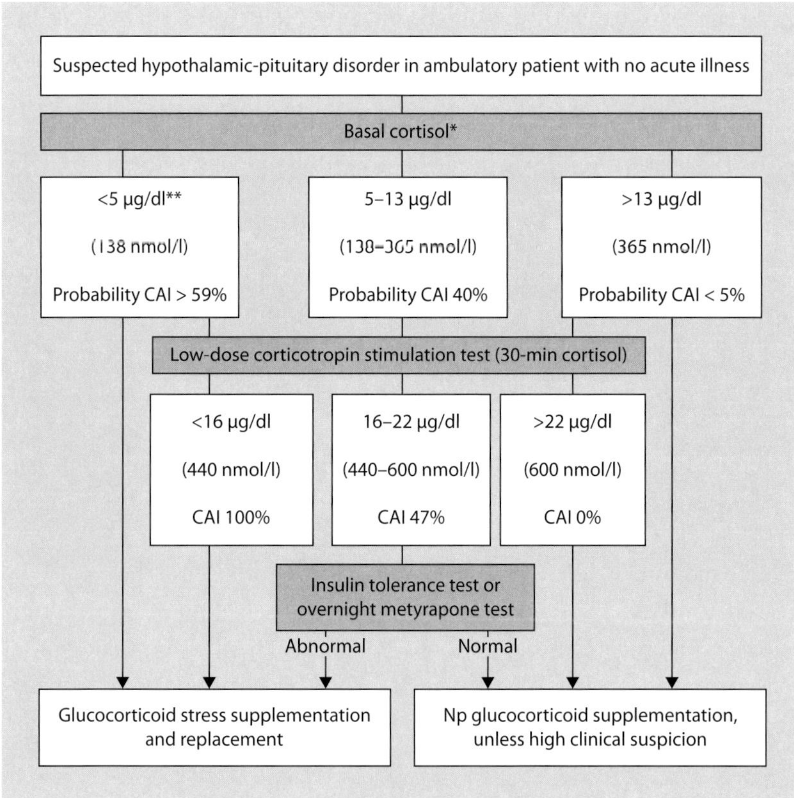

Fig. 2. Performance of adult optimal testing strategy for evaluating children with possible CAI. * A normal DHEA-S blood level makes CAI highly unlikely [17] and therefore supports the finding of a normal basal cortisol level. ** At <3 µg/dl (88 nmol/l) threshold probability CAI 100% (95% CI 99–100).

µg/dl or 88 nmol/l) to achieve higher fidelity in the diagnosis of adrenal insufficiency. The second step, a low-dose corticotropin stimulation test, performs well in children diagnosing or excluding adrenal insufficiency. If this test is indeterminate and there are no contraindications to integrated HPA axis testing, we suggest the third step of an insulin hypoglycemia test or metyrapone test. Although this three-step approach will accurately diagnose the majority of children, because it is not perfect, there will still be an important role for clinical judgment, especially regarding use of glucocorticoid supplementation during extreme stress. For convenience, in appropriate clinical circumstances, the first and second steps (basal and LDCT or SDCT) can be done at the same clinical visit to reduce the number of visits for testing.

Due to the lack of cortisol assay standardization and other reasons for measurement variability, the error in measuring cortisol can be up to 6 µg/dl (165 nmol/l), thus caution is advised when making clinical decisions based on cortisol values close to threshold values. In addition to high variability in the cortisol diagnostic thresholds, especially one to exclude CAI, a low likelihood of CAI does not exclude the possibility of future CAI, especially after progression of hypothalamic-pituitary disease or radiation therapy. Therefore, longitudinal assessments may be necessary.

The low-dose corticotropin stimulation test has not been validated in patients with acute illnesses, abnormal sleep-wake cycles, or acute hypothalamic-pituitary disorders (e.g. within 1 month of pituitary surgery). In addition, all studies of the low-dose test that we were able to analyze were conducted in the morning with the patients fasting. Afternoon cortisol values tend to be lower by 1–1.5 μg/dl (28–58 nmol/l) [12, 13], and the effect of eating or drinking is uncertain. We also have no information on how the low-dose corticotropin stimulation test would perform among patients with low serum protein levels, as cortisol in the circulation is highly protein bound.

There are several technical details to performing a low-dose test that must be rigorously addressed to avoid false-positive test results (falsely low 30-min stimulated cortisol value). Currently, there are two acceptable corticotropin analogs that can be used – cosyntropin (Cortrosyn, Amphastar Pharmaceuticals) or tetracosactrin (Synacthen, Novartis Pharma) – supplied in vials containing 250 μg of powder. Preparing the 1-μg dose requires a several-step process of first reconstituting with 250 ml of normal saline and then using a 1-ml aliquot (1 μg) for intravenous injection. There are additional steps for minimizing adherence of the medication to plastic tubing [14]. In addition, the timing of cortisol sampling after low-dose corticotropin administration is very important (we recommend collecting the blood sample 20–30 min after corticotropin analog administration), as later sampling may result in a false-positive result [15]. Thus, low-dose testing should be performed only by personnel knowledgeable of the multiple steps required for preparation and administration. If the quality of administering a 1-μg dose is suspect, then we recommend using the standard dose of 250 μg (reconstituted with 1 ml of sterile diluent) and measuring serum cortisol 30 min after intravenous injection. A result less than 16 μg/dl (440 nmol/l) – which is the same threshold used for low-dose testing – strongly suggests hypothalamic-pituitary AI. However, with standard-dose testing, the 30-min cortisol value must be greater than 30 μg/dl (833 nmol/l) to be reasonably confident in ruling out adrenal insufficiency.

In the two studies that used 1-μg corticotropin analog testing (Maghnie and Rose studies in fig. 1), the low-dose tests perform better than standard-dose test – the area under the ROC curve is better for the low-dose test. Although we do not have a head-to-head comparison of the 1-μg or 1-μg/m^2 and 0.5-μg/m^2 corticotropin testing, the latter dose appears to be inferior (the discriminatory capacity of 0.5 μg/m^2 LDCT is similar to SDCT). Therefore, the 1-μg corticotropin analog testing is preferable. None of the studies were designed to validate a dose adjustment for body surface for the 1-μg corticotropin stimulation test. Similar to adults, children with a mature hypothalamic-pituitary axis (typically older than 3 years) [16] may achieve the maximal total daily ACTH production rates which can reach 250 μg. Therefore, using corticotropin analog in a 1-μg dose without body surface adjustment is logical and feasible [8], given the precision due to technical difficulties diluting and administering available corticotropin formulations in doses even lower than 1 μg.

It is worth mentioning that low-dose corticotropin analog testing in children younger than age 3 years has not been well studied.

Research suggests [17, 18] that dehydroepiandrosterone sulphate (DHEA-S) blood levels might also help with assessing the hypothalamic-pituitary-adrenal axis, particularly when the results of the low-dose stimulation test are close to either of the two threshold values.

We found no studies testing the performance of the low-dose corticotropin analog test against a reference standard (insulin hypoglycemia test or metyrapone test) in the diagnosis of glucocorticoid-induced adrenal insufficiency. The diagnosis of asthmatic children using inhaled synthetic glucocorticoids is challenging for several reasons. First, the basal cortisol levels in children have a relatively low discriminatory capacity diagnosing central adrenal insufficiency, and synthetic glucocorticoid absorbed into the systemic circulation may affect basal cortisol levels (certain synthetic glucocorticoids may partially cross-react in cortisol assay). Second, the performance of the low-dose corticotropin analog test in patients has not been well validated against a reference standard. The washout period of the synthetic glucocorticoids and their metabolites (3–5 elimination half-times) may require prolonged discontinuation of inhaled glucocorticoid in order to obtain valid results of insulin hypoglycemia or overnight metyrapone test. Finally, the diagnostic thresholds used in the low-dose corticotropin test may prove to be different (dependent on the degree of cortisol suppression and on partial cross-reactivity of synthetic glucocorticoid in cortisol assay) in patients who have synthetic glucocorticoids in their circulation.

Establishing the diagnosis of hypothalamic-pituitary adrenal insufficiency, the accepted reference standard is an abnormal insulin tolerance test or metyrapone test. Both tests, however, can be unreliable. The average intra-subject variability in peak cortisol response to insulin-induced hypoglycemia is 8 to 12 percent [19], but in males with hypopituitarism it can vary by 42 percent [20]. Healthy control subjects have been known to 'fail' this test. Neither of these reference tests has been validated by assessing predictive accuracy, that is, the ability to predict adrenal crisis.

A limitation of our analysis is that we were unable to include data of one study that had published paired results of LDCT and SDCT, because we were unable to obtain the patient-level data [21]; however, spectrum bias in this study limits the value of its use for the purpose of our analysis, as the children were selected for Weintrob et al.

[21] study either due to unequivocal adrenal insufficiency or unequivocally normal HPA axis.

In summary, the performance of the three step algorithm, including low-dose corticotropin stimulation test for diagnosis of central adrenal insufficiency is valid in children older than age 3 years. The low-dose corticotropin stimulation test appears to be superior to the high-dose test for evaluating hypothalamic-pituitary adrenal insufficiency. However, it must be used by personnel, knowledgeable of the multiple steps required for preparation and administration.

References

1 Grinspoon SK, Biller BM: Clinical review 62: laboratory assessment of adrenal insufficiency. J Clin Endocrinol Metab 1994;79:923–931.

2 Hartzband PI, Van Herle AJ, Sorger L, Cope D: Assessment of hypothalamic-pituitary-adrenal (HPA) axis dysfunction: comparison of ACTH stimulation, insulin-hypoglycemia and metyrapone. J Endocrinol Invest 1988;11:769–776.

3 Wood JB, Frankland AW, James VH, Landon J: A rapid test of adrenocortical function. Lancet 1965; 191:243–245.

4 Kazlauskaite R, Evans AT, Villabona CV, Abdu TA, Ambrosi B, Atkinson AB, Choi CH, Clayton RN, Courtney CH, Gonc EN, Maghnie M, Rose SR, Soule SG, Tordjman K: Corticotropin tests for hypothalamic-pituitary adrenal insufficiency: a meta-analysis. J Clin Endocrinol Metab 2008;93: 4245–4253.

5 Ransohoff DF, Feinstein AR: Problems of spectrum and bias in evaluating the efficacy of diagnostic tests. N Engl J Med 1978;299:926–930.

6 Rose SR, Lustig RH, Burstein S, Pitukcheewanont P, Broome DC, Burghen GA: Diagnosis of ACTH deficiency: comparison of overnight metyrapone test to either low-dose or high-dose ACTH test. Horm Res 1999;52:73–79.

7 Gonc EN, Kandemir N, Kinik ST: Significance of low-dose and standard-dose ACTH tests compared to overnight metyrapone test in the diagnosis of adrenal insufficiency in childhood. Horm Res 2003; 60:191–197.

8 Maghnie M, Uga E, Temporini F, Di Iorgi N, Secco A, Tinelli C, Papalia A, Casini MR, Loche S: Evaluation of adrenal function in patients with growth hormone deficiency and hypothalamic-pituitary disorders: comparison between insulin-induced hypoglycemia, low-dose ACTH, standard ACTH and CRH stimulation tests. Eur J Endocrinol 2005;152:735–741.

9 Nye EJ, Grice JE, Hockings GI, Strakosch CR, Crosbie GV, Walters MM, Jackson RV: Comparison of adrenocorticotropin (ACTH) stimulation tests and insulin hypoglycemia in normal humans: low dose, standard high dose, and 8-hour ACTH-(1–24) infusion tests. J Clin Endocrinol Metab 1999;84: 3648–3655.

10 Odagiri E, Naruse M, Terasaki K, Yamaguchi N, Jibiki K, Takagi S, Tanabe M, Takano K: The diagnostic standard of preclinical Cushing's syndrome: evaluation of the dexamethasone suppression test using various cortisol kits. Endocr J 2004;51:295–302.

11 Clark PM, Neylon I, Raggatt PR, Sheppard MC, Stewart PM: Defining the normal cortisol response to the short Synacthen test: implications for the investigation of hypothalamic-pituitary disorders. Clin Endocrinol (Oxf) 1998;49:287–292.

12 Dickstein G, Shechner C, Nicholson WE, Rosner I, Shen-Orr Z, Adawi F, Lahav M: Adrenocorticotropin stimulation test: effects of basal cortisol level, time of day, and suggested new sensitive low dose test. J Clin Endocrinol Metab 1991;72:773–778.

13 Park YJ, Park KS, Kim JH, Shin CS, Kim SY, Lee HK: Reproducibility of the cortisol response to stimulation with the low dose (1 microg) of ACTH. Clin Endocrinol (Oxf) 1999;51:153–158.

14 Murphy H, Livesey J, Espiner EA, Donald RA: The low dose ACTH test: a further word of caution. J Clin Endocrinol Metab 1998;83:712–713.

15 Oelkers W: The role of high- and low-dose corticotropin tests in the diagnosis of secondary adrenal insufficiency. Eur J Endocrinol 1998;139: 567–570.

16 Miller WA: Adrenal cortex; in Sperling MA (ed): Pediatric Endocrinology. Philadelphia, Saunders, 2008, p 461.

17 Nasrallah MP, Arafah BM: The value of dehydroepiandrosterone sulfate measurements in the assessment of adrenal function. J Clin Endocrinol Metab, 2003;88:5293–5298.

18 Fischli S, Jenni S, Allemann S, Zwahlen M, Diem P, Christ ER, Stettler C: Dehydroepiandrosterone sulfate in the assessment of the hypothalamic-pituitary-adrenal axis. J Clin Endocrinol Metab 2008;93:539–542.

19 Vestergaard P, Hoeck HC, Jakobsen PE, Laurberg P: Reproducibility of growth hormone and cortisol responses to the insulin tolerance test and the short ACTH test in normal adults. Horm Metab Res 1997;29:106–110.

20 Pfeifer M, Kanc K, Verhovec R, Kocijancic A: Reproducibility of the insulin tolerance test (ITT) for assessment of growth hormone and cortisol secretion in normal and hypopituitary adult men. Clin Endocrinol (Oxf) 2001;54:17–22.

21 Weintrob N, Sprecher E, Josefsberg Z, Weininger C, Aurbach-Klipper Y, Lazard D, Karp M, Pertzelan A: Standard and low-dose short adrenocorticotropin test compared with insulin-induced hypoglycemia for assessment of the hypothalamic-pituitary-adrenal axis in children with idiopathic multiple pituitary hormone deficiencies. J Clin Endocrinol Metab 1998;83:88–92.

Rasa Kazlauskaite, MD
Department of Preventive Medicine, Rush University Medical Center
1700 W. Van Buren St, Ste 470
Chicago, IL–60612 (USA)
Tel. +1 312 942 3133, E-Mail Rasa_Kazlauskaite@rush.edu

Loche S, Cappa M, Ghizzoni L, Maghnie M, Savage MO (eds): Pediatric Neuroendocrinology.
Endocr Dev. Basel, Karger, 2010, vol 17, pp 108–120

Central Nervous System-Acting Drugs Influencing Hypothalamic-Pituitary-Adrenal Axis Function

Vittorio Locatelli · Elena Bresciani · Laura Tamiazzo · Antonio Torsello

Department of Experimental Medicine, and Interdepartmental Center for Bioinformatics and Proteomics
University of Milano-Bicocca, Monza, Italy

Abstract

The hypothalamic-pituitary-adrenal (HPA) axis is a major integrated system that maintains body homeostasis by regulating the neuroendocrine and sympathetic nervous systems and modulating immune function. It is well established that the central nervous system (CNS) integrates responses to different stimuli secreting a specific corticotropin-releasing hormone (CRH) and vasopressin (AVP). In turn, they stimulate the release of ACTH, which induces steroidogenesis in the adrenal gland. The HPA axis is regulated by diurnal rhythms and negative feedback by corticosteroids. Many neurotransmitters and neuropeptides are responsible for the modulation of CRH and AVP neurons. In addition to synthetic glucocorticoids that inhibit the HPA axis, GABA agonists, opioid peptides and endocannabinoids can inhibit cortisol secretion. On the contrary, serotonin, norepinephrine, dopamine, acetylcholine, ghrelin, angiotensin II and different cytokines can stimulate it. It follows that a number of neuroactive drugs, acting as agonists or antagonists on several brain neurotransmitter or neuropeptide receptors, can influence ACTH/cortisol secretion thereby interfering with clinical testing of the functionality of the HPA axis.

The hypothalamic-pituitary-adrenal (HPA) axis is a major system maintaining body homeostasis by regulating the neuroendocrine and sympathetic nervous systems and modulating immune function. The CNS integrates a number of different positive and negative influences that ultimately affect ACTH release. These signals converge on the CRH neurons, which are clustered largely in the parvocellular region of the paraventricular hypothalamic nucleus and make axonal connections to the median eminence of the hypothalamus. Following release into the hypothalamic-hypophysial portal system, CRH binds to specific receptors present on the membranes of corticotrope cells. Binding of CRH to its receptors activates adenylyl cyclase, thereby increasing both the biosynthesis and the release of ACTH [1]. Arginine vasopressin (AVP), that is co-expressed in some CRH neurons, also behaves as an ACTH secretagogue.

Table 1. Effect of neurotransmitters and other neuromediators on CRH/ACTH secretion

Excitatory
Epinephrine
Norepinephrine (α1)
Dopamine
Serototin
Acetylcholine
Histamine (H1)

Neuropeptide Y
Cholecystokinin
Angiotensin II
Calcitonin
Ghrelin
VIP
Glutamate
IL-1, IL-2, IL-6, TNF
Prostaglandins (E2)

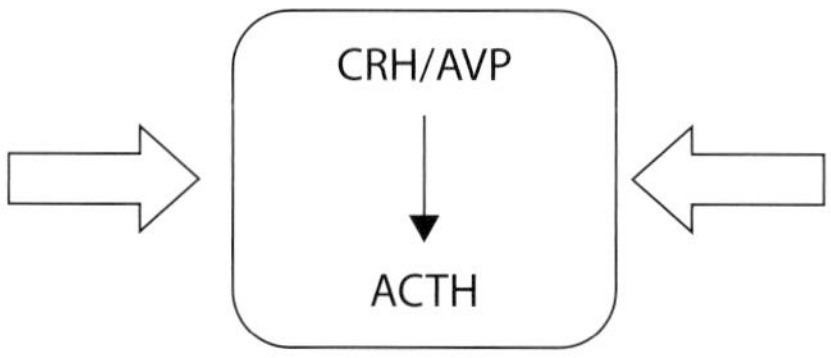

Inhibitory
GABA
Epinephrine
Norepinephrine (β)
Opiates and opioid peptides
Endocannabinoids (CB1)
NO
Leptin

AVP is endowed with little releasing activity by itself; however, it is a potent synergistic releaser in combination with CRH. This potentiation might play a physiologically relevant role in the stress response [2]. CRH and AVP are secreted into the hypophyseal-portal circulation in a pulsatile manner. The ultradian rhythms of CRH and AVP secretion are responsible for the ultradian rhythms of ACTH release. Similarly, circadian ACTH rhythms are induced by rhythmic hypothalamic activity. Important excitatory inputs originate from the suprachiasmatic nucleus, amygdala and raphe nuclei, which are sites of origin of the serotonergic projections and the locus coeruleus of the brain stem, where ascending noradrenergic fibers originate. As reported in table 1, the most important influences are cholinergic, serotonergic, adrenergic, and neuropeptide Y-ergic. CRH neurons are also activated by the immune system through the mediation of prostaglandin E_2 and several cytokines, reportedly IL-1, IL-2, IL-6 and TNF [3]. Inhibitory inputs on CRH secretion arise in the hippocampus and in the locus coeruleus of the midbrain [4]. The primary inhibitory influences are mediated by GABA and NO [5]. ACTH released from the pituitary is transported through the general circulation to the adrenal gland where it increases the steroidogenic activity. The highly integrated activity of the adrenal cortex, anterior pituitary and hypothalamus gives rise to the HPA axis, a system that maintains appropriate levels of glucocorticoids (GCs). The HPA axis integrates the diurnal rhythm in basal steroidogenesis, negative feedback by adrenal corticosteroids and steroidogenesis increases in response to stress. The feedback system is very important for limiting the duration of the tissue exposure to GCs, thus minimizing the catabolic, lipogenic, anti-reproductive, and immunosuppressive effects of these hormones. GCs easily cross the blood-brain barrier and enter into the brain. These steroids act on both the pituitary corticotropes and the hypothalamic neurons that secrete CRH and AVP. A still higher level of feedback control is acted in the hippocampus, an area that has been proposed to play important negative feedback inhibition by GCs-responsive neurons [6]. Hippocampal neurons project to the hypothalamus and affect the activity of CRH hypophysiotropic neurons and in turn determine the set point of pituitary responsiveness to GCs [6]. GCs bind two distinct intracellular receptors and the steroid-receptor complex binds to regulator sequences in the genome. Type I receptors are saturated by basal levels of GCs, whereas type II receptors approach saturation only in condition of elevated secretion, i.e. in peak phases of the circadian rhythm and during stress [7]. These differences as well as differences in regional distribution within the brain suggest that type I receptors determine basal activity of the hypothalamic-pituitary axis and type II mediate stress responses. GCs feedback takes place at different levels: in the pituitary, in the hypothalamus, and at the level of the hippocampus, which contains the highest concentration of GCs receptors. GCs can inhibit the release and synthesis of CRH and AVP in the PVN. They can inhibit POMC transcription and the release of ACTH stimulated by CRH and AVP. GCs may also induce fast feedback effects acting directly on neuronal cell membranes to change corticotropin secretion by non-genomic inhibition. Several studies have indicated that estradiol enhances responsiveness of the HPA axis to stressors which may be due in part to impairment of GCs-negative feedback [8]. Recent data indicate that the dysregulation of the HPA axis in the presence of estradiol occurs specifically via estrogen receptor alpha at the level of the PVN [9]. More recently the participation of transcriptional coregulators in the regulation of the *crh* gene in response to chronic stress and GCs has been emphasized [10].

This paper will briefly summarize the most cogent evidences of the role played by classical brain neurotransmitters on CRH/ACTH release as an introduction to understand how commonly used drugs can interfere with endocrine testing of the functionality of the HPA axis. Even if a huge body of studies has focused on the neurotransmitter systems that influence central regulation of the HPA axis some uncertainties are still present about the physiological relevance of some of these interactions.

Catecholamines

The adrenergic system and in particular norepinephrine (NE) has long been regarded as an inhibitor of the HPA axis in experimental animals, as demonstrated by the remarkable corticosterone surge measured after pharmacological blockade of the catecholaminergic neurotransmission. Further studies revealed, however, that catecholamines are endowed with stimulatory influences also. In fact, the intravenous infusion of the alpha1-agonist phenylephrine was shown to stimulate ACTH secretion [12]. In humans, the body of available data indicates the presence of both inhibitory and stimulatory influences on ACTH secretion. The stimulatory action would be exerted through the alpha1-receptors whereas inhibitory effects would be mediated by beta-receptors. Phentolamine, an alpha1-antagonist, antagonizes ACTH release induced by amphetamine. Similarly, propranolol, a nonselective beta-antagonist, can enhance the response of the HPA axis to the hypoglycemic stress [13].

Nonunivocal results have been obtained for dopamine, both in experimental animals and healthy humans. Instead, very cogent results have been obtained in Cushing patients, in whom a prolonged treatment with dopaminergic agonists can decrease cortisol secretion in 30% of subjects. However, in this instance the mechanism may involve a direct action on pituitary ACTH cells.

Serotonin

A stimulatory role of serotonin (5-HT) on the HPA axis is well established. Administration of 5-HT precursors, releasers, uptake inhibitors, or receptor agonists increase plasma ACTH and GCs levels [14]. 5-HT seems to play a role in the diurnal secretion of GCs as suggested by the suppression of the diurnal secretion rhythm after inhibition of 5-HT synthesis or 5-HT receptor antagonism by methysergide. The 5-HT antagonist cyproheptadine blunts the cortisol response to hypoglycemia, and the increase of 5-HT neurotransmission by fenfluramine, a 5-HT uptake inhibitor, stimulates ACTH secretion [15]. Knowledge of the stimulatory role of 5-HT in ACTH secretion has prompted the use of antiserotonergic drugs to block excessive ACTH secretion in Cushing patients.

Although clearly implicated in the stimulation of the HPA axis, the exact sites and mechanisms of action of 5-HT are not completely defined. The ambiguity is at least in part due to the existence of a large number of 5-HT receptor subtypes and to the existence of marked regional differences in the regulatory mechanisms. Fourteen of the 15 cloned serotonin receptors are expressed in the brain, often in overlapping areas, and it is likely that multiple receptors subtypes with similar or opposing actions are expressed in individual neurons, leading to a tremendous diversity of actions [16]. Recent studies by Heisler et al. [17], using different techniques, have shown that in the parvocellular zone of the PVN 5-HT2C receptors are the most abundant among all 5-HT receptor subtypes expressed, indicating that 5-HT2C receptors may play a key role in the regulation of the HPA axis. However, this conclusion cannot rule out the intervention of other 5-HT receptor subtypes located on cells in the proximity of CRH-containing neurons or on 5-HT terminals in the PVN.

Acetylcholine

Several lines of experimental evidence suggest that acetylcholine (ACh) has a stimulatory role on the HPA axis. ACh was shown to stimulate hypothalamic CRH secretion in a dose-dependent fashion. Further evidence for the cholinergic regulation of the CRH neurons was provided by the findings that both carbachol, a muscarinic receptor agonist, and nicotine, dose-dependently stimulated CRH secretion. These effects were antagonized by atropine and hexamethonium, respectively, suggesting that both muscarinic and nicotinic receptors are involved in the process [18]. The lack of subtype-selective muscarinic agonists and antagonists has made the functional roles of individual receptor subtypes difficult to determine. In studies with M2 receptors KO mice have demonstrated that M2 receptors may play a role in modulating muscarinic receptor-dependent stimulation of the pituitary-adrenal axis in response to cholinergic stimulation or in response to mild stress [19]. The acetylcholinesterase inhibitor, physostigmine, has been shown also to stimulate HPA activity in humans with a greater degree in young adult males than females [20].

GABA

GABA inhibits the HPA function and can antagonize the stress-induced activation of the HPA axis. Neuroanatomical and neuropharmacological studies have established that GABA inhibits the HPA axis at the level of the PVN. Among the diverse arrays of afferents impinging on the hypophysiotropic CRH neurons, more than a third contain the inhibitory neurotransmitter GABA [21]. These data highlight the importance of GABAergic neural circuits in the regulation of the neuroendocrine stress response [22]. However, published evidence indicates that the role played by GABA is not simply inhibiting the HPA axis. The neurotransmitter may play instead a complex modulatory role on the stress response [22]. It has been shown that sodium valproate, a GABA mimetic, and diazepam, a benzodiazepine, inhibit stress-induced beta-endorphin, beta-lipotropin and cortisol secretions, suggesting that also in humans endogenous GABA and benzodiazepine receptors participate in physiological mechanisms regulating the activity of the HPA axis [23].

Histamine

Systemic as well as central infusion of histamine (H) stimulate the release of ACTH and GCs in experimental animals. It is likely that histaminergic neurons are involved in the mediation of the insulin/hypoglycemia-induced release of ACTH and beta-endorphin and that this effect is mediated via activation of primarily postsynaptic H1-receptors and, to a lesser extent, via H2-receptors [24]. A stimulatory effect of H has been reported also in humans. Administration of meclastine, a specific antagonist of the H1 receptors, reduces both the ACTH response to insulin hypoglycemia and metopirone test [25].

Neuropeptides

Many neuropeptides can influence the activity of the HPA axis and among them angiotensin II can stimulate the release of ACTH from pituitary cell cultures [36]. In addition to stimulating receptors located in the pituitary, the existence of a hypothalamic site of action for angiotensin II through receptors located on vasopressin neurons is conceivable, as indicated by the concomitant release of AVP and ACTH after peripheral angiotensin II administration [26].

Vasoactive intestinal peptide (VIP), pituitary adenylate cyclase-activating polypeptide (PACAP) and related peptides have been shown to activate the HPA axis through a central mechanism of action [27].

Leptin has inhibitory effects on the HPA axis reducing the release of CRH from isolated hypothalami, and both the secretion and synthesis of cortisol are directly blocked by leptin in adrenocortical cells [28].

In contrast, ghrelin and synthetic GH secretagogues have a clear stimulatory effect on ACTH release [29].

Also opioid peptides can influence ACTH secretion by modifying the release of CRH at the hypothalamic level. Beta-endorphin or met-enkephalin infusions in humans reduce the circulating levels of ACTH and cortisol. Conversely, administration of the receptor antagonist naloxone induces an increase of circulating levels of ACTH and cortisol [30].

Endocannabinoids negatively regulate HPA axis with a primary action on the hypothalamus, but there is also some evidence of possible direct CB1 receptor-mediated modulation of the HPA axis at the anterior pituitary [31].

Excitatory amino acids are also involved in the stimulatory control of ACTH release. Glutamate might play a role in the stress response [32].

Data reported on the neurotransmitter control of ACTH secretion strongly suggest that a relevant number of neuroactive drugs, acting as agonists or antagonists on brain receptors for neurotransmitter or neuropeptides could influence ACTH/cortisol secretion thereby interfering with clinical testing of the functionality of the HPA axis. Due to space limitation only synthetic GCs and serotonergic drugs will be briefly summarized.

Synthetic GCs

GCs are compounds of very common use for the treatment of inflammatory, autoimmune, and neoplastic disorders. GCs exert rapid and delayed feedback inhibition on ACTH secretion. In experimental animals, the fast feedback effect is proportional to the rate of increase in GC concentrations. Delayed feedback is correlated to the dose and potency of the compound and duration of administration. Initially, they inhibit secretion of ACTH and CRH, later they decrease also POMC and CRH gene transcription decreasing hormone synthesis. In humans, any GC can suppress ACTH secretion, but the degree of suppression depends on the dose, potency, and duration of action of the steroid and the length of time of its administration. The longer the duration of action and the larger the dose administered, the longer the duration of suppression. Significant is also the timing of administration, the shorter the interval before the early morning peak of ACTH secretion the greater the suppressive effect of the steroid [33].

After withdrawal of chronic administration of pharmacologic doses of GCs, the HPA axis may remain suppressed for a long time. The duration of the suppression is, however, highly variable among patients with respect to the degree and duration of adrenal suppression following GC therapy, and it is therefore difficult to establish the relative risk in any given patient [34].

The most severe complication of steroid withdrawal after prolonged therapy is acute adrenal failure, whereas continued use of supraphysiological doses of GCs induce iatrogenic Cushing's syndrome. More than 99% of cases of Cushing's syndrome are due to administration of excessive amounts of GCs. With the exception of abnormal growth, the signs of hypercortisolism are frequently subtler in pediatric patients than in adults. In children, the most commonly observed features include an increase in body weight due in part to appetite increase, and a decrease in linear growth.

Although the use of topical, intra-articular, or aerosol therapy has the advantage of allowing more targeted therapy and therefore theoretically fewer systemic adverse effects, every route of exogenous GCs delivery has the potential to disturb the activity of the HPA axis [35]. Although most common with oral therapy, it is clear that also local delivery of steroids (e.g. cutaneous, intra-articular and inhaled therapy) can subtly provoke possible adverse effects. The most striking biochemical finding is suppressed endogenous cortisol levels, that can be masked because of the cross-reaction interference of many synthetic GCs with standard cortisol assays. Moreover, not all cases of exogenous Cushing's syndrome come from prescribed or therapeutic use of GCs. It is important to be aware that numerous cases of factitious Cushing's syndrome resulting from surreptitious use of steroids have been reported [35]. Patients can also receive GCs therapy unconsciously. This can occur in the form of alternative remedies which, upon inspection, contain GCs. A case of Cushing's syndrome caused by an herbal remedy containing betamethasone was described [36]. But also, OTC drugs and traditional curatives may also contain potent GCs. In another case, a neonate became cushingoid after continuation for 2 months of betamethasone drops that were prescribed for an upper respiratory infection [37]. In other cases, the use of megestrol acetate, a progestational agent used in the management of AIDS cachexia and in the treatment of breast, uterine, and prostate cancers, commonly considered not having glucocorticoid activity, was found responsible for the development of several cases of Cushing's syndrome, adrenal insufficiency, and hyperglycemia [38]. Excessive GC levels can also be reached in patients because of drug interactions. A 14-year-old female with perinatally acquired HIV in treatment with protease inhibitor therapy developed cushingoid features, with excessive weight gain and moon facies, within

2 weeks of receiving inhaled fluticasone/salmeterol for asthma treatment. Soon after discontinuing protease inhibitors and inhaled steroid, she required hospitalization for dyspnea, headache, muscle weakness, and extreme fatigue requiring hydrocortisone replacement therapy for presumed adrenal insufficiency. Cushing's syndrome and adrenal suppression were very likely caused by elevated steroid systemic concentrations resulting from the cytochrome P450 3A4 interaction between protease inhibitors and fluticasone [see ref. 57]. Health care professionals should be conscious of this important drug interaction in HIV-infected children and adolescents and be aware that rapid onset of hypercortisolism and adrenal suppression are possible.

Other drugs can inhibit cytochrome P450 3A4 enzyme system, and one of these is itroconazole, a triazole antifungal agent, that can result in increased fluticasone systemic effects when the inhaled fluticasone is added. Caution is recommended, and long-term treatment with such drugs should be avoided if possible [39].

In a survey on the safety of long-term treatment of inhaled steroids in asthmatic children, it was found that most patients show an improvement of their HPA axis during conventional dose of inhaled steroids as a probable result of the reduced chronic effect of many cytokines. However, some patients might experience further deterioration of the adrenal function during therapy, a phenomenon that might be constitutionally or genetically determined [40]. The clinical presentation of the adrenal insufficiency varies with the degree and rate of loss of adrenal function, as well as with the degree of stress the child is exposed to. The potential pitfalls and the most appropriate test for diagnosing HPA suppression have been reviewed by Zöllner [41].

Serotonergic Drugs

Serotonergic drugs are also widely prescribed drugs for the treatment of many diffused pathologies, comprising depression, panic disorders, and obesity. Many drugs commonly used as appetite suppressants such as fenfluramine, or agonists of the 5-HT1A receptors, used to treat generalized anxiety disorder as azapirones, and antidepressants of the selective serotonin reuptake inhibitor (SSRI) class are effective to stimulate ACTH and cortisol secretion [42]. All these drugs can, to a certain degree, stimulate the HPA axis; however, the careful examination of their pharmacological profile indicates that their mechanisms of action may implicate also non 5-HT-mediated actions. For example, it has been shown that the *l*-isomer of fenfluramine, that is more effective than the racemic *d,l*-fenfluramine on ACTH and cortisol secretion, is endowed with clear anti-dopaminergic effects [43]. On the opposite, the *d*-isomer is more potent on 5-HT release and uptake inhibition than the *l*-isomer, and it is ineffective on HPA axis. The azapirone compounds, acting as partial agonists at the 5-HT1A receptor are relatively more selective than fenfluramine. Ipsaperone and buspirone administration caused clear and significant elevations in ACTH/cortisol in healthy men and depressed subjects [44].

The compound m-chlorophenylpiperazine (m-CPP), a 5-HT agonist with some selectivity for the 5-HT2C receptor subtype, which is widely used to examine 5-HT receptor function in human subjects, has been found to induce a clear and dose-dependent ACTH/cortisol response in healthy subjects [45]. Neuroendocrine challenge studies in healthy male subjects suggest that antidepressant drugs, with different effects on the central neurotransmitter systems, can be characterized by different endocrine profiles after acute administration. Serotonin as well as NE reuptake-inhibiting antidepressants acutely stimulate cortisol/ACTH secretion in healthy volunteers and depressed patients, whereas mirtazapine, an antidepressant which does not inhibit the reuptake of NE or 5-HT, acutely inhibits the ACTH/cortisol release, probably due to blocking effects at the central 5-HT2 and/or H1 receptors [46]. Similar effects have been reported for trazodone, an antidepressant drug with alpha-adrenolytic activity that significantly decreased plasma cortisol concentrations [47], confirming that in humans alpha1-adrenergic mechanisms stimulate the basal secretion of cortisol. The different impact of single administration of these antidepressants on cortisol/ACTH secretion in healthy subjects and depressed patients is also reflected by a different time-course in the down-regulation of HPA axis hyperactivity in depression, as measured by serial DEX/CRH tests during short-term daily therapy. Reuptake-inhibiting antidepressants gradually normalize HPA axis hyperactivity in depressed patients during several weeks of daily treatment, whereas mirtazapine markedly reduces HPA axis activity within 1 week, followed by a partial re-enhancement of HPA function after several weeks of therapy. Flesinoxan has been investigated for its antidepressant properties and found very effective with few side effects against treatment-resistant patients and major depression [48]. In contrast to some 5-HT1A partial agonists such as buspirone, flesinoxan has been reported to aggravate the condition of panic patients [49]. Flesinoxan acts as a high-affinity selective 5-HT1A full agonist and therefore appears to be a potentially interesting neuroendocrine serotonergic probe. Its administration induced a significant and dose-dependent increase in ACTH, cortisol, prolactin, growth hormone and a decrease in body temperature in normal volunteers [50]. Citalopram is a highly selective SSRI available in well-tolerated intravenous form. These features have favored the use of citalopram as a specific neuropharmacologic challenge probe in assessing central 5-HT activity and function in vivo. Citalopram produced a dose-dependent increase in cortisol and prolactin in healthy subjects [51]. Fluoxetine, a selective SSRI antidepressant, when administered as a single 80-mg dose, induced only a slight increase in cortisol secretion when compared to placebo in an acute endocrine challenge test. Pretreatment with 80 mg fluoxetine did not change the ACTH release following blockade of the feedback regulation of peripheral corticosteroids on ACTH secretion by metyrapone [52]. In spite of the scarce effects on ACTH and cortisol secretion, a 4-week fluoxetine administration significantly blunted ACTH/cortisol release as well as the hypothermic response to acute ipsapirone. These data indicate that both postsynaptic hypothalamic 5-HT1A receptors, which mediate hormone responses

Table 2. Effect of acute administration of antidepressants on cortisol secretion

5-HT	NE	Drug	Cortisol
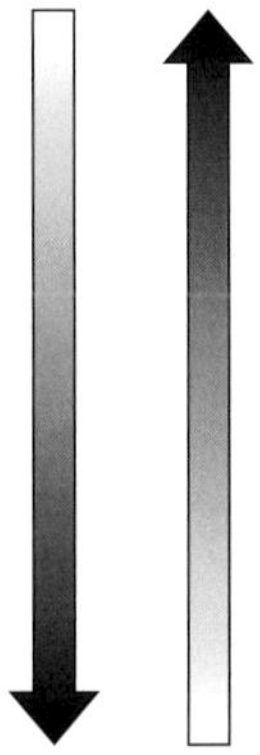		D-Oxaprotiline	+ (stimulation)
		Mianserine	+
		Desipramine	+
		Mirtazapine	– (inhibition)
		Atomoxetine	+
		Doxepine	+
		Amitryptiline	+
		Trazodone	–
		Venlafaxine	+
		Clormipramine	+
		Fluoxetine	+
		Fluvoxamine	+
		Citalopram	+

to 5-HT1A agonists and pre-synaptic 5-HT1A receptors which possibly mediate the hypothermic response, are rendered subsensitive by chronic SSRI administration [53]. Similarly, in healthy subjects there was a subsensitivity to an acute challenge with ipsapirone after a 20-day treatment with controlled-release ipsapirone preparations. The subsensitivity of postsynaptic 5-HT1A-receptors regained normal activity after 2 weeks of placebo administration [54].

Although implicated in the regulation of a number of physiological processes and their malfunction, the exact sites and modes of action of 5-HT often remain nondefined and elusive. The ambiguity is at least in part due to the existence of a large number of 5-HT receptor subtypes and to the marked regional differences in the regulatory mechanisms. An example is the reported differential control of the transcription of the encoding genes from one cell type to another in the rat brain during long term stimulation with antidepressant drugs [55]. But also the reported significant interindividual differences in the 5-HT system and responsiveness to serotonergic medications may play a relevant role [56] (table 2).

Conclusions

From this tracking shot, it appears that many drugs of common use can alter the normal functional activity of the HPA axis or can mask its real functional status. It is therefore mandatory to carry out an accurate investigation of the drug case history to seek out all prescription and nonprescription drugs taken by the subjects under consideration. Indeed, nonprescription drugs will become a more frequent clinical problem because of the increasing demand of the so-called natural therapies, further increasing the need of an accurate drug case history to avoid misdiagnosis, and most importantly to avoid inappropriate treatments of patients.

References

1 Antoni FA: Hypothalamic control of adrenocorticotropin secretion: advances since the discovery of 41-residue corticotropin-releasing factor. Endocr Rev 1986;7:351.

2 Gaillard RC, Al-Damluji S: Stress and the pituitary-adrenal axis. Baillieres Clin Endocrinol Metab 1987; 1:319.

3 Dunn AJ: Effects of cytokines and infections on brain neurochemistry. Clin Neurosci Res 2006;6:52.

4 Calogero AE: Neurotransmitter regulation of the hypothalamic corticotropin-releasing hormone neuron. Ann NY Acad Sci 1995;771:31.

5 Givalois L, Li S, Pelletier G: Central nitric oxide regulation of the hypothalamic-pituitary-adrenocortical axis in adult male rats. Brain Res Mol Brain Res 2002;102:1.

6 Jacobson L, Sapolsky R: The role of the hippocampus in feedback regulation of the hypothalamic-pituitary-adrenocortical axis. Endocr Rev 1991;12: 118.

7 Reul JM, de Kloet ER: Two receptor systems for corticosterone in rat brain: microdistribution and differential occupation. Endocrinology 1985;117:2505.

8 Ferrini M, Lima A, De Nicola AF: Estradiol abolishes autologous downregulation of glucocorticoid receptors in brain. Life Sci 1995;57:2403.

9 Weiser MJ, Handa RJ: Estrogen impairs glucocorticoid dependent negative feedback on the hypothalamic-pituitary-adrenal axis via estrogen receptor alpha within the hypothalamus. Neuroscience 2009; 159:883.

10 Lachize S, Apostolakis EM, van der Laan S, Tijssen AM, Xu J, de Kloet ER, Meijer OC: Steroid receptor coactivator-1 is necessary for regulation of corticotropin-releasing hormone by chronic stress and glucocorticoids. Proc Natl Acad Sci USA 2009;106: 8038–8042.

11 Weiner RI, Ganong WF: Role of brain monoamines and histamine in regulation of anterior pituitary secretion. Physiol Rev 1978;58:905.

12 Labrie F, Gagné B, Lefèvre G, Meunier H: CRF stimulates adenylate cyclase activity in the intermediate lobe of the pituitary gland. Mol Cell Endocrinol 1983;30:347.

13 Plotsky PM, Bruhn TO, Vale W: Hypophysiotropic regulation of adrenocorticotropin secretion in response to insulin-induced hypoglycemia. Endocrinology 1985;117:323.

14 Fuller RW: The involvement of serotonin in regulation of pituitary-adrenocortical function. Front Neuroendocrinol 1992;13:250.

15 Cavagnini F, Panerai AE, Valentini F, Bulgheroni P, Peracchi M, Pinto M: Inhibition of ACTH response to oral and intravenous metyrapone by antiserotoninergic treatment in man. J Clin Endocrinol Metab 1975;41:143.

16 Palacios JM, Waeber C, Hoyer D, Mengod G: Distribution of serotonin receptors. Ann NY Acad Sci 1990;600:36.

17 Heisler LK, Pronchuk N, Nonogaki K, Zhou L, Raber J, Tung L, Yeo GS, O'Rahilly S, Colmers WF, Elmquist JK, Tecott LH: Serotonin activates the hypothalamic-pituitary-adrenal axis via serotonin 2C receptor stimulation. J Neurosci 2007;27:6956.

18 Calogero AE, Gallucci WT, Bernardini R, Saoutis C, Gold PW, Chrousos GP: Effect of cholinergic agonists and antagonists on rat hypothalamic corticotropin-releasing hormone secretion in vitro. Neuroendocrinology 1988;47:303.

19 Rhodes ME, Billings TE, Czambel RK, Rubin RT: Pituitary-adrenal responses to cholinergic stimulation and acute mild stress are differentially elevated in male and female M[2] muscarinic receptor knockout mice. J Neuroendocrinol 2005;17:817.

20 Rubin RT, Sekula LK, O'Toole S, Rhodes ME, Czambel RK: Pituitary-adrenal cortical responses to low-dose physostigmine and arginine vasopressin administration in normal women and men. Neuropsychopharmacology 1999;20:434.

21 Miklós IH, Kovács KJ: GABAergic innervation of corticotropin-releasing hormone [CRH]-secreting parvocellular neurons and its plasticity as demonstrated by quantitative immunoelectron microscopy. Neuroscience 2002;113:581.

22 Cullinan WE, Ziegler DR, Herman JP: Functional role of local GABAergic influences on the HPA axis. Brain Struct Funct 2008;213:63.

23 Petraglia F, Bakalakis S, Facchinetti F, Volpe A, Muller EE, Genazzani AR: Effects of sodium valproate and diazepam on beta-endorphin, beta-lipotropin and cortisol secretion induced by hypoglycemic stress in humans. Neuroendocrinology 1986;44:320.

24 Kjaer A, Knigge U, Madsen EL, Søe-Jensen P, Bach FW, Warberg J: Insulin/hypoglycemia-induced adrenocorticotropin and beta-endorphin release: involvement of hypothalamic histaminergic neurons. Endocrinology 1993;132:2213.
25 Allolio B, Deuss U, Kaulen D, Winkelmann W: Effect of meclastine, a selective H1 receptor antagonist, upon ACTH release. Clin Endocrinol [Oxf] 1983;19:239.
26 Sumitomo T, Suda T, Nakano Y, Tozawa F, Yamada M, Demura H: Angiotensin II increases the corticotropin-releasing factor messenger ribonucleic acid level in the rat hypothalamus. Endocrinology 1991;128:2248.
27 Nussdorfer GG, Malendowicz LK: Role of VIP, PACAP, and related peptides in the regulation of the hypothalamo-pituitary-adrenal axis. Peptides 1998; 19:1443.
28 Ahima RS, Prabakaran D, Mantzoros C, Qu D, Lowell B, Maratos-Flier E, Flier JS: Role of leptin in the neuroendocrine response to fasting. Nature 1996;382:250.
29 Giordano R, Pellegrino M, Picu A, Bonelli L, Balbo M, Berardelli R, Lanfranco F, Ghigo E, Arvat E: Neuroregulation of the hypothalamus-pituitary-adrenal [HPA] axis in humans: effects of GABA-, mineralocorticoid-, and GH-secretagogue-receptor modulation. Scientif World J 2006;6:1.
30 Iyengar S, Kim HS, Wood PL: Mu-, delta-, kappa- and epsilon-opioid receptor modulation of the hypothalamic-pituitary-adrenocortical [HPA] axis: subchronic tolerance studies of endogenous opioid peptides. Brain Res 1987;435:220.
31 Malcher-Lopes R, Franco A, Tasker JG: Glucocorticoids shift arachidonic acid metabolism toward endocannabinoid synthesis: a non-genomic anti-inflammatory switch. Eur J Pharmacol 2008;583: 322.
32 Jezova D: Control of ACTH secretion by excitatory amino acids: functional significance and clinical implications. Endocrine 2005;28:287.
33 Orth DN, Kovacs WJ: The adrenal cortex; in Wilson JD (ed): Williams Textbook of Endocrinology, ed 9. Philadelphia, Saunders,1998, pp 605–610.
34 Henzen C, Suter A, Lerch E, Urbinelli R, Schorno XH, Briner VA: Suppression and recovery of adrenal response after short-term, high-dose glucocorticoid treatment. Lancet 2000;355:542.
35 Hopkins RL, Leinung MC: Exogenous Cushing's syndrome and glucocorticoid withdrawal. Endocrinol Metab Clin North Am 2005;34:371.
36 Krapf R: Development of Cushing's syndrome after use of a herbal remedy. Lancet 2002;360:1884.
37 Agadi S: Iatrogenic Cushing's syndrome: a different story. Lancet 2003;361:1059.
38 Mann M, Koller E, Murgo A, Malozowski S, Bacsanyi J, Leinung M: Glucocorticoid like activity of megestrol: a summary of Food and Drug Administration experience and a review of the literature. Arch Intern Med 1997;157:1651.
39 Naef R, Schmid C, Hofer M, Minder S, Speich R, Boehler A: Itraconazole comedication increases systemic levels of inhaled fluticasone in lung transplant recipients. Respiration 2007;74:418.
40 Priftis KN, Papadimitriou A, Nicolaidou P, Chrousos GP: The hypothalamic-pituitary-adrenal axis in asthmatic children. Trends Endocrinol Metab 2008; 19:32.
41 Zöllner EW: Hypothalamic-pituitary-adrenal axis suppression in asthmatic children on inhaled corticosteroids. 2. The risk as determined by gold standard adrenal function tests: a systematic review. Pediatr Allergy Immunol 2007;18:469.
42 Ambrogio AG, Pecori Giraldi F, Cavagnini F: Drugs and HPA axis. Pituitary 2008;11:219.
43 Garattini S, Mennini T: Critical notes on the specificity of drugs in the study of metabolism and functions of brain monoamines. Int Rev Neurobiol 1988;29:259.
44 Meltzer HY, Maes M: Effects of buspirone on plasma prolactin and cortisol levels in major depressed and normal subjects. Biol Psychiatry 1994;35:316.
45 Bagdy G, Arato M: Gender-dependent dissociation between oxytocin but not ACTH, cortisol or TSH responses to m-chlorophenylpiperazine in healthy subjects. Psychopharmacology (Berl) 1998;136:342.
46 Laakmann G, Schüle C, Baghai T, Waldvogel E: Effects of mirtazapine on growth hormone, prolactin, and cortisol secretion in healthy male subjects. Psychoneuroendocrinology 1999;24:769.
47 Monteleone P: Effects of trazodone on plasma cortisol in normal subjects: a study with drug plasma levels. Neuropsychopharmacology 1991;5:61.
48 Ansseau M, von Frenckell R, Franck G, Geenen V, Legros JJ: Dexamethasone suppression test and MMPI scales. Neuropsychobiology 1986;16:68.
49 Jenck F, Martin JR, Moreau JL: The 5-HT1A receptor agonist flesinoxan increases aversion in a model of panic-like anxiety in rats. J Psychopharmacol 1999;13:166.
50 Pitchot W, Wauthy J, Hansenne M, Pinto E, Fuchs S, Reggers J, Legros JJ, Ansseau M: Hormonal and temperature responses to the 5-HT1A receptor agonist flesinoxan in normal volunteers. Psychopharmacology (Berl) 2002;164:27.
51 Lotrich FE, Pollock BG: Candidate genes for antidepressant response to selective serotonin reuptake inhibitors. Neuropsychiatr Dis Treat 2005;1:17.

52 von Bardeleben U, Holsboer F, Gerken A, Benkert O: Mood elevating effect of fluoxetine in a diagnostically homogeneous inpatient population with major depressive disorder. Int Clin Psychopharmacol 1989;4(suppl 1):31.
53 Lerer B, Gelfin Y, Gorfine M, Allolio B, Lesch KP, Newman ME: 5-HT1A receptor function in normal subjects on clinical doses of fluoxetine: blunted temperature and hormone responses to ipsapirone challenge. Neuropsychopharmacology 1999;20:628.
54 Berlin I, Warot D, Legout V, Guillemant S, Schöllnhammer G, Puech AJ: Blunted 5-HT1A-receptor agonist-induced corticotropin and cortisol responses after long-term ipsapirone and fluoxetine administration to healthy subjects. Clin Pharmacol Ther 1998;63:428.
55 Lanfumey L, Mongeau R, Cohen-Salmon C, Hamon M: Corticosteroid-serotonin interactions in the neurobiological mechanisms of stress-related disorders. Neurosci Biobehav Rev 2008;32:1174.
56 Yatham LN, Steiner M: Neuroendocrine probes of serotonergic function: a critical review. Life Sci 1993; 53:447.
57 St Germain RM, Yigit S, Wells L, Girotto JE, Salazar JC: Cushing syndrome and severe adrenal suppression caused by fluticasone and protease inhibitor combination in an HIV-infected adolescent. AIDS Patient Care STDS 2007;21:373.

Vittorio Locatelli
Department of Experimental Medicine
University of Milano-Bicocca
Via Cadore, 48, IT–20052 Monza (Italy)
Tel. +39 0264488201, Fax +39 0264488068, E-Mail vittorio.locatelli@unimib.it

Loche S, Cappa M, Ghizzoni L, Maghnie M, Savage MO (eds): Pediatric Neuroendocrinology.
Endocr Dev. Basel, Karger, 2010, vol 17, pp 121–133

Genetic Factors in the Development of Pituitary Adenomas

Silvia Vandeva · Maria A. Tichomirowa · Sabina Zacharieva · Adrian F. Daly · Albert Beckers

Department of Endocrinology, University of Liège, Domaine Universitaire du Sart-Tilman, Liège, Belgium

Abstract

Pituitary adenomas are one of the most frequent intracranial tumors. Usually, they are benign but are of great clinical significance because of tumor compression syndrome and hormone overproduction. The interest in this pathology is increasing, particularly after some recent reports on their prevalence that proved to be 3–5 times more than previously estimated. Pituitary tumors arise in a sporadic setting and rarely as part of hereditary genetic syndromes. Such rare hereditary conditions like MEN1, Carney complex and McCune-Albright syndrome give significant insight into pituitary tumorigenesis. Newer genes associated pituitary tumor development include CDKN1B (MEN4) and *AIP*, the latter of which is involved in the pathophysiology of 15% of FIPA kindreds. The number of genes involved in pituitary tumorigenesis is progressively increasing and the possible mechanisms of action include signal transduction pathways, cell cycle regulators, growth factors, chromosome instability and others. Nevertheless, in the majority of sporadic adenomas, the primary genetic defect remains unknown. Furthermore, there is not a well established relationship between the genotype and its influence on the protein expression, ligand-receptor interaction, tumor growth or hormone hyperproduction. Further studies should evaluate the clinical significance of genetic alterations and their implications for existing and new therapeutic options.

The interest and significance of understanding pituitary tumorigenesis is increasing, particularly after some recent reports on the prevalence of clinically apparent pituitary adenomas. There has been a discrepancy in tumor prevalence based on radiological (22.5%) or autopsy (14.4%) series on the one hand [1] and epidemiological studies based on cancer registers on the other, with the latter showing a relatively rare frequency 190–280 cases/million (1:3,571 to 1:5,263 individuals) [2]. A recent cross-sectional study in the province of Liège, Belgium, showed that the actual prevalence of clinically apparent pituitary adenomas is 3–5 times more than previously thought (1:1,064 individuals) [3].

The majority of pituitary tumors are benign but they are clinically significant because of tumor compression syndrome and hormone overproduction. They are usually monoclonal and on a functional basis they can be classified as hormone-producing or nonfunctional pituitary adenomas [4]. About 5% of pituitary adenomas could occur in a familial setting, like multiple endocrine neoplasia type 1 (MEN1), Carney complex syndrome (CNC) and newly described familial isolated pituitary adenomas (FIPA) [5]. McCune-Albright syndrome (MAS) could theoretically lead to pituitary adenomas in a hereditary setting, but none has been reported to date [6]. The largest proportion of pituitary adenomas, however, occur sporadically.

Recently, mutations in the aryl hydrocarbon receptor-interacting protein gene (*AIP*/*Ara9*), a tumor suppressor gene, were discovered [7] which were subsequently noted to occur in about 15% of all FIPA families [8]. It is estimated that this condition contributes equally with MEN1 to the total percentage of pituitary tumors occurring in a familial setting. More than 70% of cases with clinical characteristics of MEN1, familial or sporadic, are found to have mutations in *MEN1,* a tumor suppressor gene [9]. A recently described mutation of the *CDKN1B* gene (coding cyclin-dependent kinase inhibitor $p27^{kip1}$), found in 2 patients with MEN-4 syndrome, explains a very limited number of cases in patients negative for *MEN1* genetic alterations [10, 11]. CNC in more that 60% of cases is caused by mutations in the protein kinase A 1α regulatory subunit gene (*PRKAR1A*), also a tumor suppressor gene [12]. Several mechanisms of tumor suppressor gene inactivation have been described, heterozygous or homozygous loss of the alleles encoding the gene and methylation of promoter regions [13]. McCune-Albright syndrome is due to a mutation in the *gsp* gene, coding the α-unit of the Gs protein, and similarly is involved in up to 40% of the sporadic GH-producing tumors [6].

However, for the most part, the genetic alterations giving rise to pituitary adenomas are still not known. A number of studies on sporadic pituitary adenomas give insight on the possible mechanisms of tumorigenesis. Apart from tumor suppression genes, genetic defects or changes in protein expression have been shown in signal transduction pathways (PKA, PKC, PI3K), cell cycle regulation (cyclin D), growth factors and their receptors (FGF, FGFR), chromosomal aneuploidity (PTTG), oncogene activation (Ras) and some other factors [13].

This review summarizes many of the genetic defects implicated in pituitary tumorigenesis described to date. It emphasizes on pituitary adenomas occurring in a familial setting, especially in the setting of familial isolated pituitary adenomas (FIPA).

Familial Isolated Pituitary Adenomas

FIPA is a new clinical entity, the idea of which arose in the late 1990s, when it became evident that pituitary adenomas could exist in a familial setting not related to MEN1 and CNC. FIPA kindreds are characterized by the absence of *MEN1* and *PRKAR1* mutations [14]. There have been single reports of familial pituitary adenomas and IFS (isolated familial somatotropinoma) which was already known as a clinical entity [14, 15].

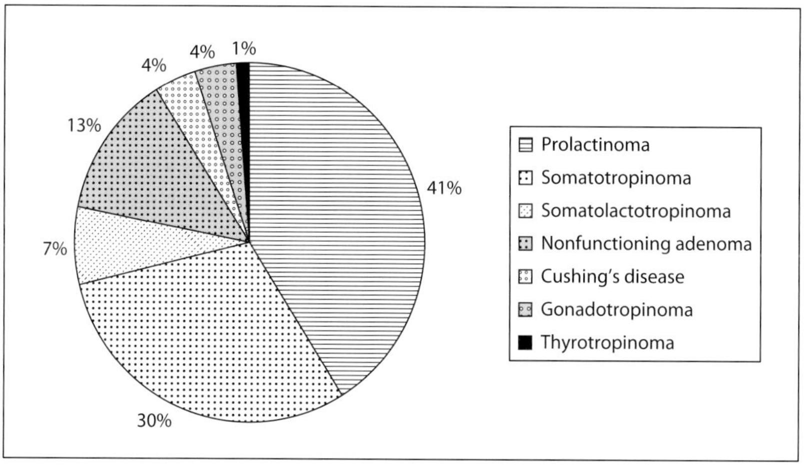

Fig. 1. Distribution of pituitary adenomas by tumor type in FIPA.

In 2000, the first organized efforts to collect and classify such familial kindreds were made, and the results of this program were published in 2006. Patients within the same family could present either the same or different pituitary adenoma type which led to the classification of FIPA kindreds as homogeneous or heterogeneous, respectively [16]. In the homogeneous group prolactinomas and somatotropinomas prevail. In the heterogeneous group there was at least one prolactinoma or somatotropinoma in combination with any other kind of pituitary tumor. To date more than 120 FIPA families have been described. On this basis, it was estimated that they comprise about 2.5% of the total pituitary adenoma patient population [14].

Pituitary tumors in the FIPA setting show some clinical differences compared to sporadic adenomas. Patients are about 4 years younger at diagnosis in the FIPA cohort and the youngest generations are diagnosed significantly earlier compared to their ancestors. Prolactinomas comprise about 40% of all tumors (fig. 1), virtually all males with prolactinomas presented with macroprolactinomas, characterized by a greater aggressiveness. Familial somatotropinomas comprise about 30% of cases, while another 7% are somatomamotropinomas. There is a 10-year difference between the age of diagnosis of patients with homogeneous acromegaly and those with acromegaly in the heterogeneous FIPA kindreds (and as compared with sporadic adenomas) and they are more frequently disposed to invasion. Nonsecreting adenomas, accounting for about 13%, are diagnosed about 8 years earlier and show more aggressive behavior compared to the sporadic cases [5].

There are some differences compared to MEN1 pituitary tumors as well. FIPA patients with homogeneous acromegaly and Cushing's disease were diagnosed earlier than in MEN1. The proportion of prolactinomas is greater in MEN1 compared to FIPA (63 vs. 40%). On the contrary, somatotropinomas are more frequent in FIPA than in MEN1 (34 vs. 8.8%) [17].

Searching for genetic abnormalities in the familial settings of pituitary adenomas unrelated to MEN1 and CNC started with familial acromegaly and over the years a site of a possible mutation was defined by linkage analysis between microsatellite markers D11S956 and D11S527 on chromosome 11q13.1–q.13.3 [18]. In a key study, Vierimaa et al. [7] performed a detailed genomewide screen and DNA mapping for potential genes involved in the pathogenesis of familial pituitary tumor kindreds. Inactivation mutations in the gene encoding *AIP* on chromosome 11q13.3 were found. Furthermore, tumor samples from affected individuals showed loss of heterozygosity at the *AIP* locus, meaning that tumors were null for *AIP*. Combinations of somatotropinomas and prolactinomas were observed in these families. In this Finnish cohort two mutations were identified, Q14X both in familial and sporadic pituitary adenoma cases, and IVS3–1G>A mutation in exon 4 in a sporadic case. Another mutation, R304X, was found in an Italian sibling pair with acromegaly. Interestingly, the relatively frequent Q14X Finnish mutation was not found in any other FIPA family in Europe, Japan and the USA and is thought to be a founder mutation [7, 8].

The biggest cohort of 73 FIPA families (156 patients) was studied in an international cooperative project involving nine countries [8]. Ten *AIP* mutations, nine of which were novel, were found in 15% of the FIPA families. The already described R304X mutation was found in another (apparently unrelated) Italian FIPA family. In the homogeneous acromegaly cohort only 50% demonstrated AIP mutations. In the last 3 years many more mutations have been identified both in FIPA kindreds and more rarely in sporadic pituitary tumors (fig. 2) [19].

The significance of the different *AIP* mutations on pituitary function, tumor formation, protein expression or ligand-receptor interaction is not clear, but some studies on *AIP* structure throw light on the subject. AIP is an immunophilin protein of 330 amino acids which contains several conserved regions, three tetratricopeptide repeat (TPR) domains and one domain characteristic of the immunophilin proteins – FK506 binding protein-type peptidyl-prolyl *cis-trans*-isomerase (FKBP-PPI) [20]. The third TPR seems to play a key role in the function of AIP as it is responsible for the interaction with the aryl hydrocarbon receptor (AHR) and with a dimer of heat shock protein 90 (hsp90). In murine models mutation of this domain prevents or decreases coimmunoprecipitation with hsp90, AHR, or both. Removal of the final carboxy-terminal amino acids or alanine replacement of any of the four last amino acids interrupts interaction with AhR only. Less is known about the N-terminal end of AIP, although it shows a highly conserved amino acid sequence across species [15]. In FIPA kindreds several mutations that lead to stop codons have been identified which would result in errors in encoding the third TPR domain, the carboxy-terminus or both: Q142X, Q217X, Q239X and R304X [8]. Two frameshift mutation, Q285fs and E174fs, also cause stop codons resulting in loss of the sequences coding for the hsp90- and AhR-binding sites. A G47-R54del mutation, responsible for amino acid deletion, was found in the FKBP-PPI region and potentially could cause interference

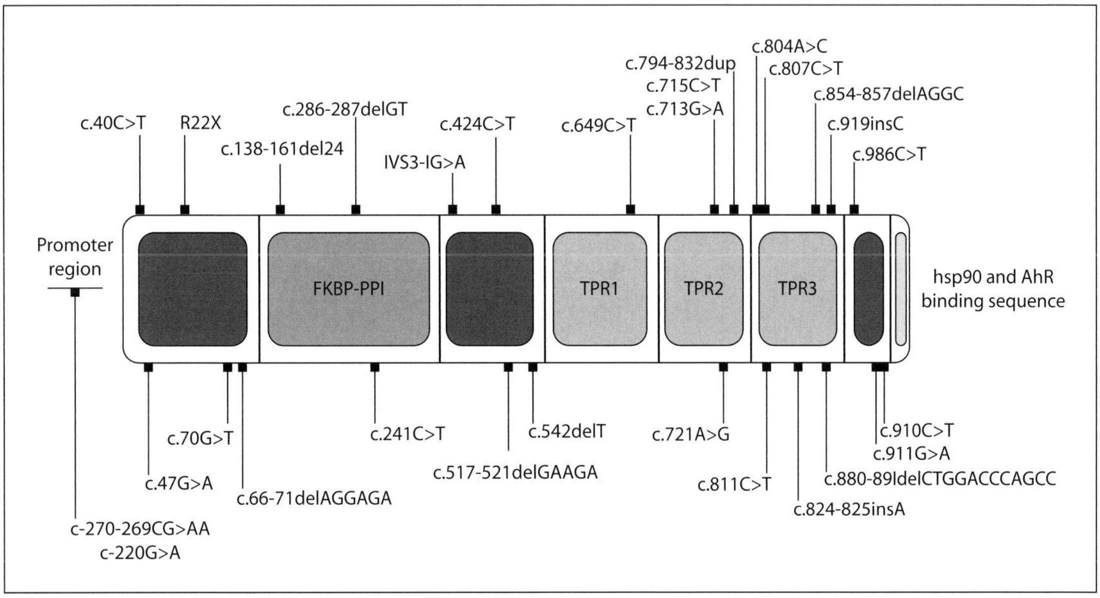

Fig. 2. Mutations in the *aryl hydrocarbon receptor interacting protein gene (AIP)* found in FIPA and sporadic adenomas. FKBP-PPI – FK506-binding protein-type peptidyl-propyl *cis-trans*-isomerase. TPR = Tetratricopeptide repeat domain; hsp 90 = heat shock protein 90; AhR = aryl hydrocarbon receptor.

in the function of the region. The functional effect of some missense mutations, like R271W, K241E and R16H remains to be determined. R271W is in the highly conserved third TPR domain. Interestingly, the R16H mutation for example, situated in the highly conserved N-terminal end has been described not only in sporadic and FIPA cases but also in two patients with colorectal carcinoma and family history of colorectal, carcinoid and other tumors [8, 15, 21].

From clinical point of view, the bearers of the mutation were quite heterogeneous in characteristics: GH-secreting tumors predominate and they were pure somatotropinomas (62%) or somatolactotropinomas (33%) but on immunohistochemistry mixed staining for GH and FSH was also found. There was also one hetereogeneous family with nonfunctional adenoma and prolactinoma. It has been shown that the same *AIP* mutation could result in a different phenotype in different families. However, the most important clinical conclusions were that patients harboring the mutation were significantly younger at diagnosis and the maximum tumor diameter was significantly larger [8].

Studies regarding the function of *AIP* could help in understanding the association of mutations with pituitary adenoma formation. AIP is shown to play an important role in modulation of AhR levels. By interacting with phosphodiesterase PDE2A it may suppresses dioxin- and cAMP-related AhR nuclear translocation and gene transcription. AhR on the other hand influences number of cellular signaling cascades such as dioxin-mediated responses and induction of hepatic cytochrome P450 subtype 1A1 expression. On a transcriptional level it is involved in a complex cross-talk with hypoxia inducible factor-1α (HIF-1α), aryl hydrocarbon nuclear translocator (ARNT), and may interact with nuclear factor-κB, retinoblastoma protein, and estrogen receptor- α. AhR interacts with p27, inducing its expression and with cyclin E, reducing its expression, both of which are related to suppression of cycin-dependent kinase 2 (CDK2) activity and in turn cell cycle progression [22]. Recently, it has also been shown that AIP inhibits cell proliferation and phosphodiesterase PDE4A5. PDE4A5 is a c-AMP-specific phosphodiesterase which has the property to hydrolyze cAMP and thus could control cAMP levels and activity of cAMP signaling pathway. Altogether this suggests complex mechanisms of action of AIP, however the exact mechanisms related to pituitary tumorigenesis remain to be determined [15, 22].

MEN1

Multiple endocrine neoplasia syndrome type 1 is an autosomal-dominant disease caused by mutation in the *MEN1* gene located on chromosome 11q13, clinically characterized by a great variety of hormone-producing or nonfunctioning tumors, mostly involving the parathyroid, pituitary and pancreas. The *MEN1* gene is a tumor suppressor gene, it has 10 exons and encodes a 610-amino acid protein, menin [23]. The exact mechanisms of menin-related tumorigenesis remain unclear, although the most likely pathways involve cell cycle control and proliferation. It is known that menin has at least three nuclear localization signals at its C-terminal, most probably responsible for DNA interaction and controlling of gene transcription [24]. Studies investigating menin's tumor suppression properties show that it acts as a repressor of telomerase activity via hTERT (a protein component of telomerase) [24]. On the whole, work to date reveals a great variety of potential menin-related molecular mechanisms of action. It takes part in transcriptional regulation through activating protein-1 (AP-1), transcription factor JunD, members of the nuclear factor-κB (NF-kB) and Smad family; regulation of histone methylation as in the case with CDKN1B and CDKN2A, genome stability, and cell cycle control [9].

Up to now hundreds of different mutations in *menin* have been described, most of them leading to premature stop codons and no genotype-phenotype relation has been noted, except for the preponderance of pituitary adenomas which were more common in familial MEN1 compared to sporadic MEN1 [25]. In patients that are bearers of a *MEN1* mutation, pituitary adenomas are found in about 40% of the cases; prolactinomas predominate and there are some differences compared to sporadic pituitary tumors [17]. Prolactinomas were found to be larger in MEN1 and macroprolactinomas twice as frequent (85 vs. 42%) than in the sporadic pituitary tumor cases. MEN1 prolactinomas were relatively more resistant to dopamine agonist therapy.

Furthermore, increased female-male ratio was observed concerning development of pituitary adenoma and acromegaly in MEN1 patients [17].

In about 20% of MEN1 cases mutations of *menin* are absent which could be explained by the involvement of other genes in the syndrome. Recently, one of the possible culprits was found, a germline nonsense mutation (TGG>TAG at codon 76) in the *CDKN1B* gene. *CDKN1B* consists of 3 exons and encodes the cyclin-dependent kinase inhibitor $p27^{Kip1}$. This syndrome was initially found as occurring spontaneously in the rat and subsequently in a human kindred presenting a MEN1-like syndrome. In the human, it was characterized by acromegaly, primary hyperparathyroidism, renal angiomyolipoma and testicular cancer among the various members of one family [10]. Soon after that a sporadic case was described involving a female patient with small-cell neuroendocrine cervical carcinoma, Cushing's disease and hyperparathyroidism. Loss of heterozygosity (LOH) of the *CDKN1B* locus and lack of p27 was observed [11]. This MEN-like syndrome is now designated MEN4.

Carney Complex

Carney complex (CNC) is a rare autosomal-dominant disease, described in about 500 patients to date and characterized by cutaneous pigmentation, atrial and other myxomas, adrenal hyperplasia, Schwann cell tumors and pituitary disorders. In about 60% of the cases, it is caused by mutation in the protein kinase A 1α regulatory subunit gene *PRKAR1A*. *PRKAR1A* is a tumor suppressor gene which consists of 11 exons. In pituitary tumors that occur in this familial setting losses of its normal allele at chromosomal region 17q22–24 are found [26]. Another locus at 2p16, still uncharacterized, is thought to be involved in some families [27]. More than 40 mutations in *PRKAR1A* have been described, most of them leading to premature stop codons and absence of mutated protein, although several missense mutations allowing synthesis of a mutated PRKAR1A have also been found. Data from all these studies show that either loss or alteration of protein function could be related to increased PKA activity and hence tumorigenesis [28]. Up to 75% of CNC cases exhibit hypersecretion of prolactin, growth hormone (GH) and/or insulin-like growth factor-I (IGF-I). Nevertheless, clinically apparent acromegaly develops only in occasional cases. The disease is slowly progressing and the mean age of diagnosis is at about 35.8 years. Another characteristic of CNC is that, unlike in MEN1, pituitary tumors are characterized by a somatomammotropic cell multifocal hyperplasia, against a background of normal pituitary [9].

McCune-Albright Syndrome

McCune-Albright syndrome (MAS) is characterized by polyostotic fibrous dysplasia, cutaneous hyperpigmentation and endocrine hyperactivity including precocious puberty, Cushing's syndrome, thyrotoxicosis and gigantism. It is caused by mosaicism for a mutation in the *GNAS* (guanine nucleotide-activating α-subunit) gene, located on the 20q13, encoding the stimulatory Gsα-subunit of the heterotrimeric G protein [6]. The same mutation was first detected in sporadic adenomas [29]. Like in CNC, it affects the cAMP-dependent protein kinase signaling pathway which most probably reflects some similarities in the clinical characteristics of both syndromes. GH hypersecretion is observed in about 20% of the cases, although tumor development is uncommon and histopathology shows somatotrope and lactotrope hyperplasia. Somatotropinomas in MAS could be often resistant to cabergoline and long-acting octreotide [6]. The familial occurrence of pituitary adenomas in MAS has not been reported but remains theoretically possible.

Sporadic Tumors

Signal Transduction Pathways

Two syndromes related to mutations in cAMP-dependent protein kinase signaling pathways have already been described, CNC and MAS. The *GNAS* mutation is also found in up to 40% of sporadic pituitary adenomas. The most common defect leads to amino acid substitution of highly conserved Arg 201 and rarely Gln227 in the Gsα protein [6]. When bound to GTP, Gsα unit dissociates from the βγ complex which leads to adenylate-cyclase activation and cAMP production. The switch-off mechanism is GTP hydrolysation and precisely this is disrupted as a result of the mutations, leading to excessive signaling downstream, with GH-transcriptional activation and somatotrope proliferation [6]. Furthermore, recent studies report *GNAS* mother imprinting in sporadic pituitary adenomas. Thus, sporadic tumors without *GNAS* mutation could be due to a partial loss of this imprinting [30]. Apart from somatotrope adenomas and nonfunctioning adenomas, *GNAS* mutations have been identified in one case with an ACTH-secreting pituitary adenoma. The *GNAS* mutation positive adenomas have a better prognosis, as they are smaller, characterized by lower levels of GH and show a blunted response to GHRH [31].

Efforts in searching for additional alterations in the other participants of the signal transduction pathway led to the discovery of an inactivating mutation in the α-subunit of GIP2, a protein coupled to the inhibitory G-protein Gi2α. No mutations were found in either of the other G protein subunits, PKA subunits or *PRKAR1A* in sporadic adenomas. On the other hand, the PKA pathway could interact with PKC pathway on several levels, having the same end result – increased CREB activation. In the PKC pathway, increased expression of PKCα subunit was found in aggressive pituitary adenomas and subsequently a somatic mutation (Gly294Asp) at the calcium-binding site was identified in some of these tumors [32]. Another gene involved in tumorigenesis, and especially in invasive growth is the phosphoinositide 3-kinase *gene PIK3CA*, with somatic mutations in exons 9 and 20 and gene amplification recently being demonstrated [33].

Cell Cycle Regulators and Associated Genetic Alterations

One of the chief regulators of the cell cycle are the cyclin D proteins (cyclins 1, 2 and 3). The cell-cycle nuclear D1 gene (*CCND1*) is found with allelic imbalance in about 25% of sporadic pituitary adenomas. Nevertheless, as there is no change of the proteins expression, the significance of the mutation remains to be determined [34].

The retinoblastoma gene (*RB1*) is a tumor-suppressor gene, located on 13q14.2 and encodes the Rb protein that takes a vital part in cell-cycle transition from G1 to S phase. In murine knock-out models almost all develop pituitary adnomas by the age of 12 months. In human sporadic tumors there seem to be no somatic mutations, nor LOH, except for aggressive tumors. Another possible explanation for protein deactivation is methylation of the *RB1* promotor or deletion of the regions encoding the protein-binding pocket domain [35].

Cyclin-dependent kinase nuclear 2A protein (CDKN2A, p16) is a cyclin-dependent kinase inhibitor which participates in the Rb1 pathway. The *CDKN2A* gene is located on chromosome 9p. It has been found that LOH or homozygous loss of the gene is uncommon in pituitary tumors but one-third of the nonfunctioning tumors showed LOH of two regions, telomeric and centromeric to *CDKN2A*, which suggests participation of other genes in this region in tumorigenesis. Other studies show that pituitary tumors with low p16 expression are associated with methylation of exon 1, which was subsequently confirmed in 70% of nonfunctioning tumors and 9.5% of GH-producing tumors [13].

Ras protein participates in the signal transduction of the mitogen-activated phosphokinase (MAPK) pathway. Mutations of *ras* proto-oncogenes are common in a number of solid tumors, like colorectal and thyroid cancer. In pituitary tumors *RAS* mutations are related to invasive behavior [33].

Another possible participant in the pituitary tumor pathogenesis is the growth arrest and DNA-damage-inducible gene-45 *(GADD-45)*. GADD-45 negatively regulates cell cycle and its expression was found to be significantly lower in GH and prolactin-producing pituitary adenomas. The possible mechanism is supposed to be *GADD-45* promoter methylation [36].

ZAC, a tumor suppressor gene, is located on chromosome 6q24–25 and it encodes a zinc finger transcription factor, inducing apoptosis and cell cycle arrest. In a healthy pituitary it is highly expressed, while the majority of the pituitary adenomas show a significant downregulation [37]. No mutations were found and the discovery of a second promoter of ZAC and epigenetic alterations could probably explain the changes of protein expression [38].

Other Factors

There is evidence that growth factor signaling could be implicated in pituitary tumorigenesis, as for example fibroblast growth factors and their receptors. An N-terminally truncated isoform of pituitary tumor-derived FGFR4 (ptd FGFR4) was found to be overexpressed in pituitary adenomas and its tumorogenetic role was demonstrated in transgenic mice. The cause of this is alternative transcription initiation from a cryptic intronic promoter and the possible mechanism is loss of affinity for extracellular matrix which predisposes to aggressive tumor growth. Another member of this family, *FGFR2* was found epigenetically silenced, a condition associated with hypomethylation and overexpression of melanoma associated antigen (MAGE-A) in pituitary tumors [39].

The pituitary tumor-transforming gene (PTTG) belongs to the securin family, it was first found to inhibit chromatide separation during mitosis in rat pituitary GH- and prolactin-secreting cells. The possible mechanisms of this oncogene's action are not only restricted to chromosomal aneuploidy, it was shown that PTTG stimulates basic fibroblast growth factor (bFGF)-mediated angiogenesis and thus tumor growth. PTTG overexpression is associated with invasion not only in pituitary tumors, but in colorectal and breast neoplasms. Nevertheless, until now no genetic alterations are found to explain expression changes [40]. Maternally expressed 3, *MEG3*, first discovered as the human homolog of the murine *Gtl2* gene, is thought to be involved in growth control during early development. It was shown that an alternatively spliced isoform of MEG3, called MEG3a is highly expressed in normal pituitary cells but not at all in nonfunctioning and GH-secreting pituitary adenomas. Possible explanation of this loss of expression is the recent finding of hypermethylation in exon 1 in tumors without *MEG3* expression [41]. Additionally there is evidence for the involvement in pituitary tumorigenesis of some other factors like hypoxia inducible factor (HIF)-1α, matrix metaloproteinases, bone morphogenic protein, Wnt and others [13, 39].

Conclusion

In this review, many of the genetic defects implicated in pituitary tumorigenesis have been highlighted (table 1) with an accent on familial settings, especially FIPA. Although there have been great advances in the identification of new genetic alterations, the causes of pituitary adenoma formation remains unclear in the majority of the pituitary tumors. Furthermore, the association of these known genetic alterations with protein expression, tumor growth and clinical manifestation is still to be determined in many cases. A number of proteins are shown to interact in a complex crosstalk in mitogenic and angiogenic signal pathways. Future studies will need to elucidate the exact molecular mechanisms and their potential use in the development of new therapeutic approaches.

Table 1. Genetic alterations in pituitary adenomas

Gene	Molecular defect	Pituitary tumor
MEN1	inactivating mutations decreased menin expression	all pituitary adenoma types
CDKN1B	germline nonsense mutation lack of p27 staining in tumors	MEN1-like syndrome
AIP	germline mutations and LOH decreased mRNA and AIP in some tumors	15% of FIPA and rare in sporadic adenomas, more aggressive behavior
Gsp	somatic inactivating mutations, mother imprinting constant Gsa activation	40% GH tumors, mosaicism in MAS, Non-secreting adenomas
PRKAR1	truncation mutation, decreased protein expression	somatolactotrope hyperplasia and adenomas in CNC
Cyclin D (CCND1)	allelic imbalance, overexpression, unknown effect on protein level	somatotropinomas, nonsecreting adenomas
Cyclin D3 (CCND3)	increased expression	pituitary adenomas all
Cyclin E (CCNE)	increased expression	corticotropinomas
Cyclin A (CCNA1)	increased expression	pituitary adenomas
Pdt-FGFR4	alternative transcription initiation	pituitary adenomas, invasive growth
FGFR2	decreased expression	different pituitary adenomas
PTTG	increased expression	pituitary adenomas all types, invasive growth
BMP-4	diminished expression	prolactinoma
GADD45G	promoter methylation, protein underexpression	prolactinomas, somatotropinomas, nonsecreting adenomas
MEG3a	promoter methylation	NF adenomas
PKC	point mutation, increased protein expression	prolactinoma, invasive growth
RB1	promoter methylation, loss of 13q14, decreased Rb expression	pituitary adenomas, invasive growth
ZAC	promoter methylation	nonsecreting adenomas
CDKN2A	promoter methylation, decreased expression	pituitary adenomas, nonfunctioning, macroadenomas

Table 1. Continued

Gene	Molecular defect	Pituitary tumor
CDKN1A	decreased expression, increased expression	nonsecreting adenomas, hormone-producing adenomas
CDKN2B	promoter methylation	pituitary adenomas
CDKN2C	decreased expression	corticotropinomas
H-ras	point mutation, amplification	metastatic mituitary carcinoma
PI3CA	somatic mutations, gene amplification	pituitary tumors, invasive growth

References

1 Ezzat S, Asa SL, Couldwell WT, Barr CE, Dodge WE, Vance ML, McCutcheon IE: The prevalence of pituitary adenomas: a systematic review. Cancer 2004;101:613–619.

2 Davis JR, Farrell WE, Clayton RN: Pituitary tumours. Reproduction 2001;121:363–371.

3 Daly AF, Rixhon M, Adam C, Dempegioti A, Tichomirowa MA, Beckers A: High prevalence of pituitary adenomas: a cross-sectional study in the province of Liege, Belgium. J Clin Endocrinol Metab 2006;91:4769–4775.

4 Melmed S: Mechanisms for pituitary tumorigenesis: the plastic pituitary. J Clin Invest 2003;112:1603–1618.

5 Daly AF, Jaffrain-Rea ML, Ciccarelli A, et al: Clinical characterization of familial isolated pituitary adenomas. J Clin Endocrinol Metab 2006;91:3316–3323.

6 Levine MA: Clinical implications of genetic defects in G proteins: oncogenic mutations in G alpha s as the molecular basis for the McCune-Albright syndrome. Arch Med Res 1999;30:522–531.

7 Vierimaa O, Georgitsi M, Lehtonen R, Vahteristo P, Kokko A, Raitila A, Tuppurainen K, Ebeling TM, Salmela PI, Paschke R, Gundogdu S, De Menis E, Makinen MJ, Launonen V, Karhu A, Aaltonen LA: Pituitary adenoma predisposition caused by germline mutations in the AIP gene. Science 2006;312: 1228–1230.

8 Daly AF, Vanbellinghen JF, Khoo SK, et al: Aryl hydrocarbon receptor interacting protein gene mutations in familial isolated pituitary adenomas: analysis in 73 families. J Clin Endocrinol Metab 2007;92: 1891–1896.

9 Horvath A, Stratakis CA: Clinical and molecular genetics of acromegaly: MEN1, Carney complex, McCune-Albright syndrome, familial acromegaly and genetic defects in sporadic tumors. Rev Endocr Metab Disord 2008;9:1–11.

10 Pellegata NS, Quintanilla-Martinez L, Siggelkow H, et al: Germ-line mutations in p27Kip1 cause a multiple endocrine neoplasia syndrome in rats and humans. Proc Natl Acad Sci USA 2006;103:15558–15563.

11 Georgitsi M, Raitila A, Karhu A, et al: Germline CDKN1B/p27kip1 mutation in multiple endocrine neoplasia. J Clin Endocrinol Metab 2007;92:3321–3325.

12 Kirschner LS, Carney JA, Pack SD, et al: Mutations of the gene encoding the protein kinase A type I-alpha regulatory subunit in patients with the Carney complex. Nat Genet 2000;26:89–92.

13 Heaney AP: Pituitary tumour pathogenesis. Br Med Bull 2006;75–76:81–97.

14 Beckers A, Daly A: The clinical, pathological, and genetic features of familial isolated pituitary adenomas. Eur J Endocrinol 2007;157:371–382.

15 Verloes A, Stevenaert A, Teh BT, Petrossians P, Beckers A: Familial acromegaly: case report and review of the literature. Pituitary 1999;1:273–277.

16 Valdes-Socin H, Poncin J, Stevens V, Stevenaert A, Beckers A: Adenomes hypophysaires familiaux isolés non liés avec la mutation somatique NEM-1: suivi de 27 patients. Ann Endocrinol 2000;61:301.

17 Verge's B, Boureille F, Goudet P, Murat A, Beckers A, Sassolas G, Cougard P, Chambe B, Montvernay C, Calender A: Pituitary disease in MEN type 1 (MEN1): data from the France-Belgium MEN1 multicenter study. J Clin Endocrinol Metab 2002; 87:457–465.

18 Luccio-Camelo DC, Une KN, Ferreira RE, Khoo SK, Nickolov R, Bronstein MD, Vaisman M, Teh BT, Frohman LA, Mendonca BB, Gadelha MR: A meiotic recombination in a new isolated familial somatotropinoma kindred. Eur J Endocrinol 2004;150: 643–648.
19 Daly AF, Tichomirowa MA, Beckers A: Update on familial pituitary tumors: from multiple endocrine neoplasia type 1 to familial isolated pituitary adenoma. Horm Res 2009;71(suppl 1):105–111.
20 Carver LA, Bradfield CA: Ligand-dependent interaction of the aryl hydrocarbon receptor with a novel immunophilin homolog in vivo. J Biol Chem 1997; 272:11452–11456.
21 Georgitsi M, Karhu A, Winqvist R, Visakorpi T, Waltering K, Vahteristo P, Launonen V, Aaltonen LA: Mutation analysis of aryl hydrocarbon receptor interacting protein (AIP) gene in colorectal, breast, and prostate cancers. Br J Cancer 2007;96:352–356.
22 Huang G, Elferink CJ: Multiple mechanisms are involved in Ah receptor-mediated cell cycle arrest. Mol Pharmacol 2005;67:88–96.
23 Chandrasekharappa SC, Guru SC, Manickam P, et al: Positional cloning of the gene for multiple endocrine neoplasia-type 1. Science 1997;276:404–407.
24 La P, Desmond A, Hou Z, Silva AC, Schnepp RW, Hua X: Tumor suppressor menin: the essential role of nuclear localization signal domains in coordinating gene expression. Oncogene 2006;25:3537–3546.
25 Lemos MC, Thakker RV: Multiple endocrine neoplasia type 1 (MEN1): analysis of 1336 mutations reported in the first decade following identification of the gene. Hum Mutat 2008;29:22–32.
26 Kirschner LS, Carney JA, Pack SD, et al: Mutations of the gene encoding the protein kinase A type I-alpha regulatory subunit in patients with the Carney complex. Nat Genet 2000;26:89–92.
27 Stratakis CA, Carney JA, Lin JP, et al: Carney complex, a familial multiple neoplasia and lentiginosis syndrome: analysis of 11 kindreds and linkage to the short arm of chromosome 2. J Clin Invest 1996; 97:699–705.
28 Boikos SA, Stratakis CA: Carney complex: the first 20 years. Curr Opin Oncol 2007;19:24–29.
29 Landis CA, Masters SB, Spada A, Pace AM, Bourne HR, Vallar L: GTPase inhibiting mutations activate the α chain of Gs and stimulate adenylyl cyclase in human pituitary tumours. Nature 1989;340:692–696.
30 Mantovani G, Ballare E, Giammona E, Beck-Peccoz P, Spada A: The *gsalpha* gene: predominant maternal origin of transcription in human thyroid gland and gonads. J Clin Endocrinol Metab 2002;87:4736–4740.
31 Riminucci M, Collins MT, Lala R, et al: An R201H activating mutation of the GNAS1 (Gsalpha) gene in a corticotroph pituitary adenoma. Mol Pathol 2002;55:58–60.
32 Boikos SA, Stratakis CA: Molecular genetics of the cAMP-dependent protein kinase pathway and of sporadic pituitary tumorogenesis. Hum Mol Genet 2007;16:R80–R87.
33 Lin Y, Jiang X, Shen Y, Li M, Ma H, Xing M, Lu Y: Frequent mutations and amplifications of the PIK3CA gene in pituitary tumors. Endocr Relat Cancer 2009;16:301–310.
34 Hibberts NA, Simpson DJ, Bicknell JE, et al: Analysis of cyclin D1 (CCND1) allelic imbalance and overexpression in sporadic pituitary tumors. Clin Cancer Res 1999;5:2133–2139.
35 Quereda V, Malumbres M: Cell cycle control of pituitary development and disease. J Mol Endocrinol 2009;42:75–86.
36 Zhang X, Sun H, Danila DC, et al: Loss of expression of GADD45 gamma, a growth inhibitory gene, in human pituitary adenomas: implications for tumorigenesis. J Clin Endocrinol Metab 2002;87:1262–1267.
37 Pagotto U, Arzberger T, Theodoropoulou M, et al: The expression of the antiproliferative gene ZAC is lost or highly reduced in nonfunctioning pituitary adenomas. Cancer Res 2000;60:6794–6799.
38 Valleley EM, Cordery SF, Bonthron DT: Tissue-specific imprinting of the ZAC/PALGL 1 tumour suppressor gene results from variable utilization of monoallelic and biallelic promoters. Hum Mol Genet. 2007;16:972–981.
39 Ezzat S: Epigenetic control in pituitary tumors. Endocr J 2008;55:951–957.
40 Yu R, Melmed S: Pituitary tumor transforming gene: an update. Front Horm Res 2004;32:175–185.
41 Gejman R, Batista SL, Zhong Y, Zhou Y, Zhang X, Swearingen B, Stratakis CA, Hedley-Whyte ET, Klibanski A: Selective loss of MEG3 expression and intergenic differentially methylated region hypermethylation in the MEG3/DLK1 locus in human clinically non-functioning pituitary adenomas. J Clin Endocrinol Metab 2008;93:4119–4125.

Prof. Albert Beckers, MD, PhD
Department of Endocrinology, CHU de Liège
Domaine Universitaire du Sart Tilman
BE–4000 Liège (Belgium)
Tel. +32 4 3668223, Fax +32 4 3667261, E-Mail albert.beckers@chu.ulg.ac.be

Loche S, Cappa M, Ghizzoni L, Maghnie M, Savage MO (eds): Pediatric Neuroendocrinology.
Endocr Dev. Basel, Karger, 2010, vol 17, pp 134–145

Diagnosis and Treatment of Cushing's Disease in Children

Martin O. Savage[a] · Renuka P. Dias[a] · Li F. Chan[a] · Farhad Afshar[b] · Nicolas P. Plowman[c] · Matthew Matson[d] · Ashley B. Grossman[a] · Helen L. Storr[a]

[a]Department of Endocrinology, William Harvey Research Institute, Barts and the London School of Medicine and Dentistry, Departments of [b]Neurosurgery, [c]Radiotherapy and [d]Radiology, Barts and the Royal London NHS Trust, London, UK

Abstract

Cushing's disease (CD) is rare in the paediatric age range, but presents a diagnostic and therapeutic challenge. Most paediatric endocrinologists have limited experience managing children or adolescents with CD and thus benefit from close consultation with adult colleagues. A diagnostic protocol for investigation is required which broadly follows the model for adult patients. Treatment strategies for CD are described and critically appraised. The management of paediatric CD patients after cure also presents challenges for optimizing growth, bone health, reproduction and body composition from childhood into and during adult life.

Cushing's disease (CD) in childhood and adolescence is very rare, compared to the more common endocrine pathologies such as disorders of growth, puberty and thyroid which make up the major part of paediatric endocrine practice. CD is caused by an ACTH-secreting pituitary adenoma and is the commonest cause of Cushing's syndrome (CS) in children over 5 years of age [1–3].

Some aspects of paediatric CD differ from those present in adults. Examples are the increased frequency in prepubertal males compared to females, the frequent absence of radiological evidence of a corticotrope adenoma on pituitary radiological imaging, the more exuberant cortisol response to bolus IV CRH and the more rapid response to external beam pituitary radiotherapy. These features will be discussed together with other diagnostic and therapeutic aspects of paediatric CD.

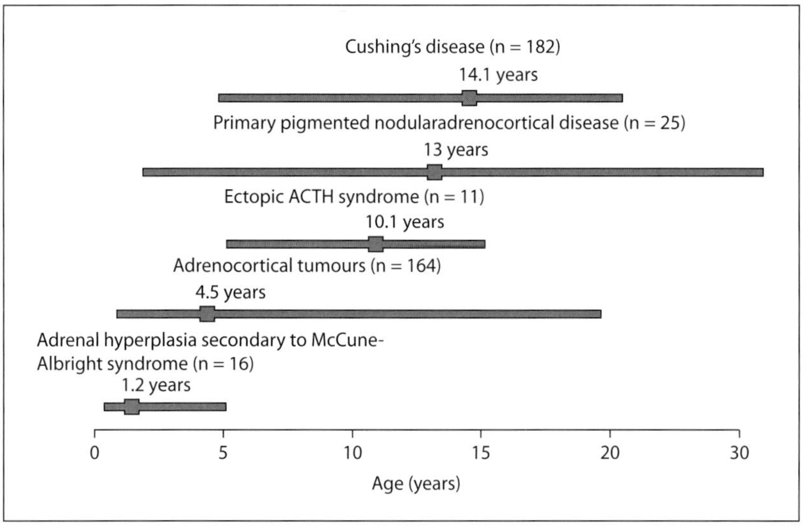

Fig. 1. Different aetiologies of paediatric CS from the literature (n = 398 cases) shown at ages of peak incidence (boxes) [2].

Diagnosis of Paediatric Cushing's Disease

Epidemiology

The peak incidence of paediatric CD occurs during the adolescent or preadolescent years with median age of presentation in 141 cases taken from the literature being 14.1 years [2]. The youngest child in our own series of 37 cases was aged 5.8 years at diagnosis. The ages of peak incidence of different causes of CS in childhood and adolescence are shown in figure 1.

Whereas in adults, CD comprises 49–71% of CS cases, in the paediatric population it accounts for 75–80% of cases [2]. Paediatric CD is almost always caused by a pituitary microadenoma [4]. We have seen only one macroadenoma in 37 paediatric cases [2]. However, very rarely this has been reported and has been described as an early manifestation of MEN1 [5]. In adults, CD has a female preponderance [6]. Until recently, no comment had been made about sex distribution in children with CD. We analysed sex at diagnosis in fifty CD patients aged from 6 to 30 years and found a significant predominance of males in the prepubertal patients [7]. There were similar incidences of males and females during puberty and an increasing predominance of females in the post-pubertal patients. In our current series of 37 CD cases aged from 5.8 to 17.8 years there are 24 males and 13 females. Our report was the first to describe this male predominance in young patients, however examination of cases in the large series from the NIH [3] reveals the same phenomenon. No clear explanation for this exists, although it is tempting to suggest that the oestrogenic milieu during

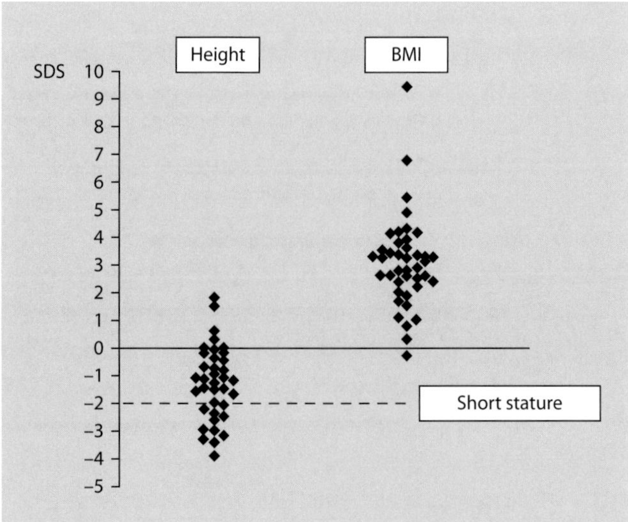

Fig. 2. Height and body mass index (BMI) SDS values in 42 paediatric patients with CS: CD (n = 35), and primary nodular adrenal hyperplasia (n = 7). The dotted line indicates the SDS value below which patients are significantly shorter than average.

female puberty may be related to the relative increase in females with CD during and following adolescence.

Clinical Presentation

The recognition of features which might alert the clinician to the diagnosis of CD is of crucial importance in effective diagnosis and treatment. Most children and adolescents have a typical Cushingoid appearance. A subtle or sub-clinical presentation or even cyclical features are uncommon. However, parents and general practitioners frequently fail to recognise the pathological nature of the change of the child's appearance. The mean length of symptoms prior to diagnosis in our 37 patients was 2.5 ± 1.7 years (range 0.3–6.6 years).

Facial appearance was always changed and 100% of our patients complained of weight gain. Striae were present in 50% of patients, being more frequent in the older patients. It was not unusual for a young child with CD to present with obesity and poor growth, but without the classical features of plethora, hirsutism, acne and striae. Additional features were virilisation, hypertension, emotional lability and fatigue. Muscle weakness and easy bruising were rare.

Characteristics of Growth

Short stature (height less than –2.0 SD) was present in 43% of our patients and growth velocity when available was subnormal. One of the most striking features was the contrast between height SDS, being almost always below the mean, and BMI SDS being consistently above it (fig. 2), as has been previously reported [1, 3]. We recently compared height and BMI SDS values in 29 patients with CD and 44 age-matched patients with simple obesity. There was a significant difference in the ratio of these two variables between the two groups [8], height being increased in simple obesity and relatively decreased in CD. Bone age (BA) at diagnosis in 17 patients was delayed in 15 (mean delay 2.0 'years'; range –0.5 to 4.1 'years') and correlated negatively with height SDS ($r = -0.70$; $p < 0.01$), duration of symptoms ($r = 0.48$; $p = 0.05$) and age at diagnosis ($r = 0.48$; $p = 0.05$) [9].

Puberty Development

There are few reports of pubertal development in CD, although it is recognised that virilisation with pseudo-precocious puberty are common features [1, 3]. Pubertal development was analysed in 27 patients at diagnosis and abnormal virilisation, defined as unusual advance of Tanner pubic hair stage compared to testicular volume or breast development was identified in 12 [10]. In these patients the SDS values of serum androstenedione, DHEAS, as previously reported [11] and testosterone were higher ($p = 0.03$, 0.008, 0.03 respectively) than in subjects without abnormal virilisation and SHBG SDS values were lower ($p = 0.006$). Gonadotropin levels were subnormal in the patients who had commenced true puberty suggesting a suppressive effect of chronic hypercortisolaemia.

Investigations

The investigation of patients with suspected Cushing's syndrome has been extensively reviewed [12, 13]. Guidelines for the diagnosis of paediatric CD have also been published [1, 2]. We will therefore highlight some aspects which we have found helpful during the management of CD in children and adolescents over the past 27 years. The scheme of investigations in children should be based on those performed in adults [12] and consists initially of confirmation or exclusion of the diagnosis of CS followed by investigations to confirm aetiology of CD. This scheme is shown in table 1.

Confirmation or Exclusion of Cushing's Syndrome

Initially, we perform three consecutive 24 h urine collections for urinary free cortisol (UFC). If there is doubt about the interpretation of these values we proceed to admit the child for measurement of serum cortisol at 3 time-points (09.00 h, 18.00 h and midnight [sleeping]) to assess circadian rhythm. Determination of midnight cortisol

Table 1. Scheme of investigation for patients with suspected CS

Confirmation or exclusion of CS
1. Urinary free cortisol excretion (24-hour urine collection) daily × 3
2. Serum cortisol circadian rhythm study (09.00 h, 18.00 h, midnight [sleeping])
3. Low-dose dexamethasone suppression test (LDDST) • Dose; 0.5 mg 6-hourly [09.00 h, 15.00 h, 21.00 h, 03.00 h] × 48 h • Dose for patients weighing <40 kg; 30 µg/kg/day • Serum cortisol measured at 0 and 48 h
Definition of aetiology of CS
1. Plasma ACTH (09.00 h)
2. CRH test (1.0 µg/kg i.v.)
3. Analysis of change in serum cortisol during LDDST
4. Adrenal or pituitary MRI scan
5. Bilateral inferior petrosal sinus sampling for ACTH (with CRH)

in the sleeping child gives the highest sensitivity for the diagnosis of Cushing's syndrome [14]. The value in normal subjects is <50 nmol/l, although some young children may reach their cortisol nadir earlier than midnight.

We then perform a low-dose dexamethasone suppression test (LDDST), using the adult dose regimen of 0.5 mg 6 hourly (at 09.00, 15.00, 21.00 and 03.00 h) for 48 h, unless the child weighs <40 kg – which is unusual – when we use the NIH-recommended dose of 30 µg/kg/day [3]. In the LDDST, blood is taken for serum cortisol at 0 and at 48 hrs, when it is normally undetectable (<50 nmol/l). These tests performed individually, and particularly in combination, have a high sensitivity for Cushing's syndrome and an even higher specificity for the exclusion of this diagnosis.

Confirmation of Cushing's Disease

Having confirmed the presence of CS, the priority is to establish that the patient has ACTH-dependent CS. This is most easily confirmed by determination of basal 09.00 h plasma ACTH. In all of our patients with CD, ACTH was detectable, ranging from 12 to 128 ng/l (NR 10–50) (fig. 3) [4].

We routinely perform a CRH test (1 µg/kg i.v.) and in 27 CD patients serum cortisol increased by >20% (range 106–554%) [15]. Although it is arguable that ectopic ACTH syndrome is so rare in children that the CRH test is not justified, we find an

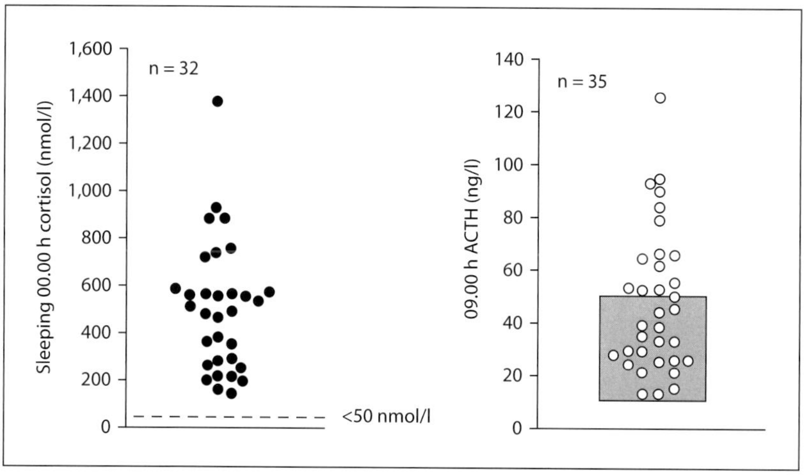

Fig. 3. Midnight serum cortisol and 09.00 h plasma ACTH values in children and adolescents with CD. Note loss of circadian variation with elevation of midnight cortisol and detectable ACTH values. Normal range of ACTH shown by the grey box.

increased cortisol response contributes to the diagnosis of CD. We no longer perform a routine high dose dexamethasone suppression test (HDDST). This recent decision follows an analysis of serum cortisol suppression during L and HDDSTs. In adult patients with ACTH-dependent CS, the change in cortisol during LDDST has been shown to distinguish between pituitary and ectopic ACTH secretion, questioning the value of the HDDST [16].

We have now reported similar findings in children [17]. In 24 patients with CD, mean baseline serum cortisol values of 590.7 ± 168.8 nmol/l decreased to 337.4 ± 104.0 nmol/l at 48 h during LDDST ($p < 0.05$; mean decrease, 45.1%) with 66% decreasing by >30%. Cortisol suppression during LDDST correlated with that during HDDST ($r = 0.45$, $p < 0.05$). Consequently, decrease of cortisol during the LDDST strongly supports the diagnosis of CD.

Radiological Investigations

Pituitary imaging using MRI is an important step towards the successful treatment of Cushing's disease by trans-sphenoidal surgery (TSS). As previously mentioned, most paediatric ACTH-secreting pituitary tumours are microadenomas with a diameter <5 mm [4]. The majority of these have a hypointense signal on MRI, which fails to enhance with gadolinium [3, 12]. In the large NIH series, approximately 50% of microadenomas were visible on pituitary MRI [3]. In our series pituitary imaging was relatively unhelpful, showing a normal appearance in over half of the patients, with a

Table 2. Paediatric Cushing's disease: pituitary imaging, surgical identification of adenoma and cure by TSS

Total number of patients	Adenoma CT/MRI image, n (%)	Concordance of image with surgery, n (%)	Cure by TSS, n (%)
36	19/36 (53)	10/36 (28)	24/36 (67)

n = Number of patients; MRI = magnetic resonance imaging; CT = computed tomography imaging; TSS = trans-sphenoidal selective adenomectomy.

low predictive value of the position of the adenoma, as identified at surgery (table 2) [18, 19]. In some cases, the distinction between CD and ectopic ACTH syndrome may be in doubt. Here, a CT scan of the chest using 0.5-cm cuts will usually exclude a bronchial carcinoid tumour [6].

Bilateral Inferior Petrosal Sinus Sampling for ACTH

The technique of bilateral inferior petrosal sinus sampling for ACTH (BIPSS) was developed mainly at the NIH during the 1980s [20] and has become routine in adult practice. It was hoped that BIPSS would distinguish CD from ectopic ACTH syndrome and also provide a method of identifying a lateral or central source of pituitary ACTH secretion [12]. In children, because of the extreme rarity of the ectopic ACTH syndrome, the aim of BIPSS is primarily to contribute to the localisation of the microadenoma by demonstrating lateral or midline ACTH secretion.

The first paediatric data were reported in the large NIH series where a predictive value of lateralization was 75–80% [1, 3]. We have been performing BIPSS in paediatric patients since 1986 and reported our experience, suggesting that ACTH sampling gave a better prediction of the site of the microadenoma than pituitary imaging [19].

BIPSS is a highly specialised technique and in our unit is performed by the same radiologist who regularly studies adult patients. We do not usually use general anaesthesia (GA) to avoid potential alteration of ACTH secretion. However, in 2 children aged 5.8 and 6.2 years GA was used. The youngest patient we studied without GA was aged 8.4 years. We have now performed BIPSS in 29 paediatric CD patients, without complications, The results are shown in table 3. A more recent study from the NIH described experience of BIPSS in 94 paediatric patients and reported that localisation of ACTH secretion concurred with the site of the adenoma at surgery in 58% of cases, concluding that the technique was not an essential part of a paediatric investigation protocol [21]. The percentage of lateralisation, however, increased to 70% (51/73) after exclusion of 18 centrally located and 4 bilateral lesions.

Table 3. BSIPSS results, surgical identification of adenoma and cure by TSS

Total number of patients	BSIPSS results		Concordance of BSIPSS result with surgery, n (%)	Cure by TSS, n (%)
	lateralisation, n (%)	non-lateralisation, n (%)		
29	23 (79)	6 (21)	24 (83)	22/29 (76)

n = Number of patients; BSIPSS = bilateral simultaneous inferior petrosal sinus sampling; TSS = trans-sphenoidal selective adenomectomy.

Treatment of Cushing's Disease

CD in childhood causes considerable morbidity and requires prompt and expert treatment, which should be curative. The approach to treatment has evolved over the years. Initially bilateral adrenalectomy was widely practised and while effective in lowering hypercortisolaemia, the pituitary adenoma remained in situ and there was an appreciable risk of post-adrenalectomy Nelson's syndrome [22]. In the management of 37 cases of CD, we have only performed adrenalectomy twice, when the patients were extremely unwell and not fit to undergo pituitary surgery. In one of these patients, the hypercortisolaemia was uncontrollable by oral metyrapone and treatment was given with IV etomidate which successfully controlled the cortisol levels prior to adrenalectomy [23]. Medical therapy to lower cortisol using metyrapone or ketoconazole is a short-term option but cannot be recommended as definitive therapy for CD.

Trans-Sphenoidal Surgery

The aim of trans-sphenoidal pituitary surgery (TSS) is the selective removal of the adenoma. This is now considered first-line therapy for paediatric CD [2]. It is important that normal pituitary tissue remains in situ for future growth and development. TSS is regarded as a safe and effective procedure in children [24–26]. Adult CD studies show variable surgical success rates depending on which definition of cure is adopted.

Selective microadenomectomy can be technically very difficult in children. As discussed above, the microadenomas may be very small and an appreciable rate of failure, i.e. lack of definite cure, exists even in the hands of the most experienced trans-sphenoidal surgeons [4]. We recently analysed our experience over the past 25 years and considered the factors which contributed to successful surgical therapy [19]. The overall cure rate from TSS in 33 paediatric patients with microadenomas treated by TSS from 1982 to 2008 was 61% and in 29 of these patients, treated since routine

BIPSS was introduced as pre-operative preparation, the cure rate was 76% (table 3). We therefore feel that the ability of BIPSS to correctly identify the lateral or central position of the adenoma has contributed to an increased rate of surgical success [19]. Other paediatric series report cure rates varying from 45 to 78% [24–29]. Our adult endocrine unit has traditionally used the definition of undetectable post-operative serum cortisol (<50 nmol/l) for successful treatment, i.e. cure [30]. We have used the same definition for paediatric cases.

Pituitary Radiotherapy

Pituitary radiotherapy (RT) has been considered a therapeutic option for paediatric CD for many years. Children with CD have been shown to respond more rapidly than adults [31]. In our centre, external beam RT is used as second-line therapy, following unsuccessful TSS. Our practice is to make a decision to proceed to RT, usually within 2–4 weeks of TSS, when it is clear from circulating cortisol levels that complete removal of the adenoma has not been achieved [32]. The RT protocol we follow consists of delivering 45 Gy in 25 fractions over 35 days [32]. We have treated 13 patients during the past 26 years with a successful cure rate of 85% which occurred at a mean interval of 0.8 years (range 0.3–2.9) following completion of therapy.

We recently analysed long-term pituitary function in 6 of these patients and have reported that although GH deficiency was frequent initially, some recovery may occur in adult life [33]. Gonadotropin secretion was generally preserved with normal, or early puberty, and TSH and ACTH deficiency was minimal [32]. We have not studied cognitive function following pituitary RT. However, we know of no data demonstrating a decrease in IQ related to targeted pituitary RT, as opposed to therapy using a broader field as for paediatric brain tumours.

Post-Cure Growth and Development and Pituitary Function

Most patients with paediatric CD have subnormal growth rates and short stature at diagnosis [1, 2]. The challenge is to reverse these problems so as to achieve acceptable adult height and body composition. Key articles from the NIH described the abnormalities of height and GH secretion together with a rather pessimistic view of post-treatment catch-up growth and adult height [34, 35]. We also reported disappointing post-cure catch-up, which we attributed to continuing GH deficiency, occurring either from TSS, pituitary RT or the long-standing effects of chronic hypercortisolaemia on pituitary and growth plate physiology [36].

Our approach now is to test for GH deficiency 3 months after TSS or completion of RT. If GH therapy is demonstrated, we start therapy in a standard GH dose of 0.025 mg/kg/day. GnRH analogue therapy may be added to delay puberty and epiphyseal closure. Results demonstrate that catch-up growth usually occurs and adult height within range of target height was achieved for the majority of patients [37]. GH deficiency may persist for many years [38] but in the adult follow-up patients was usually not severe enough to indicate GH replacement as recommended for the adult GH deficiency syndrome.

Normal body composition was more difficult to achieve. Many patients remained obese and BMI SDS was elevated ($p < 0.01$) at a mean interval of 3.9 years after cure in 14 patients [37]. A long-term follow-up study of childhood and adolescent CD showed that total body fat and the ratio of visceral to subcutaneous fat was abnormally high in the majority of patients studied 7 years after cure [39]. The implications of chronic excess visceral fat in terms of risk for adult metabolic syndrome deserve future study. Bone mineral density was closer to normal, a finding which we also reported, together with some patients having normal bone mineral density at diagnosis [40].

Conclusions

Paediatric CD contains a number of characteristic features. Early diagnosis remains a challenge because of the frequent lack of appreciation of the nature of the pathology by parents and general practitioners. Once suspected, the patient requires investigation using a formal protocol and the choice and interpretation of tests is most productively discussed with an adult specialist with experience of CD. Concerning effective and curative therapy, referral should be considered to a centre ideally combining paediatric and adult endocrinology, TSS and pituitary RT. The choice of neurosurgeon experienced in TSS in children is likely to significantly improve the chance of cure. Whereas the prognosis for cure is good in the majority of children and adolescents, post-treatment management presents challenges for optimization of growth, puberty and body composition.

References

1 Magiakou MA, Chrousos GP: Cushing's syndrome in children and adolescents: Current diagnostic and therapeutic strategies. J Endocrinol Invest 2002;25: 181–194.

2 Storr HL, Chan LF, Grossman AB, Savage MO: Paediatric Cushing's syndrome: epidemiology, investigation and therapeutic advances. Trends Endocrinol Metab 2006;18:167–174.

3 Magiakou MA, Mastorakos G, Oldfield EH, Gomes MT, Doppman JL, Cutler GB, Nieman LK, Chrousos GP: Cushing's syndrome in children and adolescents. Presentation, diagnosis and therapy. N Engl J Med 1994;331:629–636.

4 Fahlbusch R: Neurosurgical management of Cushing's disease in children; in Savage MO, Bourguignon JP, Grossman AB (eds): Frontiers of Paediatr Neuroendocrinol. Oxford, Blackwell Scientific Publications, 1994, pp 68–72.

5 Stratakis CA, Schussheim DH, Freedman SM, Keil MF, Pack SD, Agarwal SK, Skarulis MC, Weil RJ, Lubensky IA, Zhuang Z, Oldfield EH, Marx SJ: Pituitary macroadenoma in a 5-year-old: an early expression of multiple endocrine neoplasia type 1. J Clin Endocrinol Metab 2000;85:4776–4780.

6 Besser GM, Trainer PJ: Cushing's syndrome; in Besser GM, Thorner MO (eds): Comprehensive and Clinical Endocrinololg, ed 3. Edinburgh, Mosby, 2002, pp 193–202.
7 Storr HL, Isidori AM, Monson JP, Besser GM, Grossman AB, Savage MO: Pre-pubertal Cushing's is more common in males, but there is no increase in severity at diagnosis. J Clin Endocrinol Metab 2004;89:3818–3820.
8 Greening JE, Storr HL, Mckenzie SA, Davies KM, Martin L, Grossman AB, Savage MO: Linear growth and body mass index in paediatric patients with Cushing's disease or simple obesity. J Endocrinol Invest 2006;29:885–887.
9 Peters CJ, Ahmed ML, Storr HL, Davies KM, Martin LJ, Allgrove J, Grossman AB, Savage MO: Factors influencing skeletal maturation at diagnosis of paediatric Cushing's disease. Horm Res 2007;68:31–35.
10 Dupuis C, Storr HL, Perry LA, Ho JTF, Ahmed L, Ong KK, Dunger DB, Monson JP, Grossman AB, Besser GM, Savage MO: Abnormal puberty in paediatric Cushing's disease; relationships with adrenal androgens, sex hormone binding globulin and gonadotrophin concentrations. Clin Endocrinol 2007;66: 838–843.
11 Hauffa B, Kaplan SL, Grumbach MM: Dissociation between plasma adrenal androgens and cortisol in Cushing's disease and ectopic ACTH-producing tumour: relation to adrenarche. Lancet 1984;i:1373–1376.
12 Newell-Price J. Trainer P, Besser GM, Grossman AB: The diagnosis and differential diagnosis of Cushing's and pseudo-Cushing's syndrome. Endocr Rev 1998;19 647–672.
13 Nieman LK, Biller BM, Findling JW, Newell-Price J, Savage MO, Stewart PM, Montori V: The diagnosis of Cushing's syndrome: an Endocrine Society Clinical Practice Guideline. J Clin Endocrinol Metab 2008; 93:1526–1540.
14 Batista DL, Riar J, Keil M, Stratakis CA: Diagnostic tests for children who are referred for the investigation of Cushing's syndrome. Pediatrics 2007;120: 575–586.
15 Peters CJ, Storr HL, Grossman, AB, Savage MO: The role of corticotrophin-releasing hormone in the diagnosis of Cushing's syndrome. Eur J Endocrinol 2006;155:S93–S98.
16 Isidori A, Kaltsas GA, Mohammed S, Morris DG, Jenkins P, Chew SL, Monson JP, Besser GM, Grossman AB: Discriminatory value of the low-dose dexamethasone suppression test in establishing the diagnosis and differential diagnosis of Cushing's syndrome. J Clin Endocrinol Metab 2003;88:5299–5306.
17 Dias RP, Storr HL, Perry LA, Isidori AM, Grossman AB, Savage MO: The discriminatory value of the low-dose dexamethasone suppression test in the investigation of paediatric Cushing's syndrome. Horm Res 2006;65:159–162.
18 Lienhardt A, Grossman AB, Dacie JE, Evanson J, Huebner A, Afshar F, Plowman PN, Besser GM, Savage MO: Relative contributions of inferior petrosal sinus sampling and pituitary imaging in the investigation of children and adolescents with ACTH-dependent Cushing's syndrome. J Clin Endocrinol Metab 2001;86:5711–5714.
19 Storr HL, Afshar F, Matson M, Sabin I, Savage KM, Evanson J, Plowman PN, Besser GM, Monson JP, Grossman AB, Savage MO: Factors influencing cure by transsphenoidal selective adenomectomy in paediatric Cushing's disease. Eur J Endocrinol 2005; 152:825–833.
20 Oldfield EH, Doppman JL, Nieman LK, Chrousos GP, Miller DL, Katz DA, Cutler GB Jr, Loriaux DL: Petrosal sinus sampling with corticotropin-releasing hormone to distinguish Cushing's disease from pseudo-Cushing's states or normal physiology. N Engl J Med 1991;325:897–905.
21 Batista D, Gennari M, Riar J, Chang R, Keil MF, Oldfield EH, Stratakis CA: An assessment of petrosal sinus sampling for localisation of pituitary microadenomas in children with Cushing disease. J Clin Endocrinol Metab 2006;91:221–224.
22 Hopwood NJ, Kenny FM: Incidence of Nelson's syndrome after adrenalectomy for Cushing's disease in children: results of a nationwide survey. Am J Dis Child 1977;131:1353–1356.
23 Greening JE, Brain CE, Perry LA, Mushtaq I, Sales Marques J, Grossman AB, Savage MO: Efficient short-term control of hypercortisolaemia by low-dose etomidate in severe paediatric Cushing's syndrome. Horm Res 2005;64:140–143.
24 Massoud AF, Powell M, Williams RA, Hindmarsh PC, Brook CG: Transsphenphoidal surgery for pituitary tumours. Arch Dis Child 1997;76:398–404.
25 Knappe UJ, Ludecke DK: Transnasal microsurgery in children and adolescents with Cushing's disease. Neurosurgery 1996;39:484–493.
26 Kanter AS, Diallo AO, Jane JA Jr, Sheehan JP, Asthagiri AR, Oskouian RJ, Okonkwo DO, Sansur CA, Vance ML, Rogol AD, Laws ER Jr: Single-center experience with pediatric Cushing's disease. J Neurosurg 2005;103(5 suppl):413–420.
27 Joshi SM, Hewitt RJ, Storr HL, Rezajooi K, Ellamushi H, Grossman AB, Savage MO, Afshar F: Cushing's disease in children and adolescents: 20 years of experience in a single neurosurgical centre. Neurosurgery 2005;57:281–285.

28 Leinung MC, Kane LA, Scheithauer BW, Carpenter PC, Laws ER Jr, Zimmerman D: Long-term follow-up of transsphenoidal surgery for the treatment of Cushing's disease in childhood. J Clin Endocrinol Metab 1995;80:2475–2479.
29 Devoe DJ, Miller WL, Conte FA, Kaplan SL, Grumbach MM, Rosenthal SM, Wilson CB, Gitelman SE: Long term outcome in children and adolescents after trans-sphenoidal surgery for Cushing's disease. J Clin Endocrinol Metab 1997;82: 3196–3202.
30 Trainer PJ, Lawrie HS, Verhelst J, Howlett TA, Lowe DG, Grossman AB, Savage MO, Afshar F, Besser GM: Transsphenoidal resection in Cushing's disease: undetectable serum cortisol as the definition of successful treatment. Clin Endocrinol 1993;56:25–31.
31 Jennings AS, Liddle GW, Orth DN: Results of treating childhood Cushing's disease with pituitary irradiation. N Engl J Med 1977;297:957–962.
32 Storr HL, Plowman PN, Carroll PV, Francois I, Krassas G, Afshar F, Besser GM, Grossman AB, Savage MO: Clinical and endocrine responses to pituitary radiotherapy in paediatric Cushing's disease. J Clin Endocrinol Metab 2003;88:34–37.
33 Chan LF, Storr HL, Plowman PN, Perry LA, Besser GM, Grossman AB, Savage MO: Long-term anterior pituitary function in patients with paediatric Cushing's disease treated with pituitary radiotherapy. Eur J Endocrinol 2007;156:477–482.
34 Magiakou MA, Mastorakos G, Gomez MT, Rose SR, Chrousos GP: suppressed spontaneous and stimulated growth hormone secretion in patients with Cushing's disease before and after surgical cure. J Clin Endocrinol Metab 1994;78:131–137.
35 Magiakou MA, Mastorakos G, Chrousos GP: Final stature in patients with endogenous Cushing's syndrome. J Clin Endocrinol Metab 1994;79:1082–1085.
36 Lebrethon M-C, Grossman AB, Afshar F, Plowman PN, Besser GM, Savage MO: Linear growth and final height after treatment of Cushing's disease in childhood. J Clin Endocrinol Metab 2000;85:3262–3265.
37 Davies JH, JH, Storr HL, Davies K, Monson JP, Besser GM, Afshar F, Plowman PN, Grossman AB, Savage MO: Final adult height and body mass index after cure of paediatric Cushing's disease. Clin Endocrinol 2005;62:466–472.
38 Carroll PV, Monson JP, Grossman AB, Besser GM, Plowman PN, Afshar F, Savage MO: Successful treatment of childhood-onset Cushing's disease is associated with persistent reduction in growth hormone secretion. Clin Endocrinol 2005;60:169–174.
39 Leong GM, Abad V, Charmandari E, Reynolds JC, Hill S, Chrousos GP, Nieman LK: Effects of child- and adolescent-onset endogenous Cushing syndrome on bone mass, body composition and growth: a 7-year prospective study into young adulthood. J Bone Miner Res 2007;22:110–118.
40 Scommegna S, Greening JP, Storr HL, Davies KM, Shaw NJ, Monson JP, Grossman AB, Savage MO: Bone mineral density at diagnosis and following successful treatment of disease. J Endocrinol Invest 2005;28:231–235.

Prof. Martin Savage
Department of Endocrinology, Barts and the London School of Medicine and Dentistry
John Vane Science Centre, Charterhouse Square
London EC1M 6BQ (UK)
Tel. +44 20 7882 6233, Fax +44 7882 6234, E-Mail m.o.savage@qmul.ac.uk

Loche S, Cappa M, Ghizzoni L, Maghnie M, Savage MO (eds): Pediatric Neuroendocrinology.
Endocr Dev. Basel, Karger, 2010, vol 17, pp 146–159

Prolactinomas in Children and Adolescents

Annamaria Colao[a] · Sandro Loche[b]

[a]Department of Molecular and Clinical Endocrinology and Oncology, 'Federico II' University, Naples, Italy;
[b]Servizio di Endocrinologia Pediatrica, Ospedale Microcitemico ASL Cagliari, Cagliari, Italy

Abstract

Prolactinomas are the most common pituitary adenomas in children and adolescents followed by adrenocorticotropic hormone-secreting and growth hormone-secreting adenomas. Females are slightly more affected than males (who have macroadenomas more frequently). Compared with the adult setting, in children macroadenomas are more frequent than microadenomas. Diagnosis is generally based on clinical symptoms of primary or secondary gonadal failure, growth delay and/or tumor compressive symptoms. Treatment is based on medical therapy with dopamine agonists, to control prolactin levels and reduce tumor size. Surgery is indicated in patients with tumors resistant to dopamine agonists as well as in those showing severe neurological symptoms at diagnosis. Radiotherapy should be limited to the cases with aggressive tumors, nonresponsive to dopamine agonists, because of the risk of neurological damage and hypopituitarism later in the lives of these patients.

All histotypes of pituitary adenomas are less common in children than in adults, but their frequency increases during the adolescent years [1–3]. Their estimated incidence is still unknown but they constitute less than 3% (1.2% by Gold [4]) of supratentorial tumors in children [1–3], and 2.3–6% of all pituitary tumors treated surgically [3, 5–9]. Moreover, most published series included as pediatric patients those with onset of symptoms until the age of 20 years, so that the actual prevalence might be lower [10]. The average annual incidence of pituitary adenomas in childhood has been estimated to be 0.1/million children [11]. Pituitary carcinomas are rare in adults and extremely rare in children [12, 13].

There is the perception that pituitary adenomas in children are more aggressive and present greater invasiveness than in adults, but data on this aspect are not sufficiently clear. The prolactin (PRL)-secreting adenoma is the most frequent adenoma histotype in children, followed by the adrenocorticotropic hormone (ACTH)-secreting and the growth hormone (GH)-secreting adenomas [10]. There is a slightly greater prevalence in females [3, 9, 14]. However, since prolactinomas occur more frequently

Table 1. Prevalence of clinical symptoms and signs in children/adolescents with pituitary adenomas: data extracted from Colao [10]

Symptom	Frequency
Visual field defects	+++
Secondary hypopituitarism	+++
Galactorrhea	+++
Premature telarche	++
Primary amenorrhea	++
Headache	++
Menstrual irregularities	++
Delayed puberty	++
Gynecomastia	+
Osteoporosis	+
Weight increase	+
Delayed/arrest growth	-/+

–/+ = Rare; + = present; ++ = frequent; +++ = frequent in macroadenomas.

in females in the early post-pubertal years [15, 16], the gender distribution mainly reflects the relative contribution of the two main groups, PRL- and ACTH-secreting adenomas, which present a higher prevalence in the females. Macroadenomas on presentation are more likely in boys than in girls [3, 8, 17]. In our series [18], microprolactinomas were more frequent in females (10 of 17), while macroprolactinomas were slightly, but not significantly, more frequent in males (7 of 9). Nonfunctioning pituitary adenomas, TSH-secreting, and gonadotropin-secreting adenomas are extremely rare in children, accounting for only 3–6% of all pituitary tumors [4, 19, 20].

Clinical Presentation

PRL-secreting adenomas are usually diagnosed at the time of puberty or in the post-pubertal period [21]. Clinical manifestations vary in keeping with the age and sex of the child. Pre-pubertal children generally present with a combination of headache, visual disturbances, growth failure, and amenorrhea (table 1). However, growth failure, that is considered a prominent symptom [17–20, 22], was found rarely in two different retrospective studies [18, 23]. In fact, we found growth arrest only in one male patient with microprolactinoma (4%), while all the remaining 25 patients had normal heights, and pubertal development was appropriate for their age [18]. Cannavò et al. [23] reported short stature in 3 of 30 adolescents with either micro- or macroprolactinoma (10%). In a re-evaluation of the young/adolescent patients with hyperprolactinemia admitted

Table 2. Presentation of prolactinomas in children and adolescents, from 1995 to 2004 at the Department of Endocrinology and Oncology, University 'Federico II' of Naples

Case no.	Sex	Age at diagnosis	Height	Percentile	Weight	BMI	Basal PRL	Volume	Presenting symptoms	Associated deficiency
1	F	10.5	120	1	48.8	33.9	1,700	1,982.6	H, G	ACTH, TSH, GH
2	F	11	135	10	50	27.4	312	578.2	H, G	none
3	F	12	140	3	51.1	26.1	444	1,626.1	A1, G, VFD, H	TSH, GH
4	F	13	153.8	24	57.9	24.5	200	508.5	A1, G, VFD, H	ACTH
5	F	13	154.6	25	62.1	26.0	160	527.0	A2	none
6	F	13.3	160	50	60.3	23.6	90.1	198.9	A2	none
7	F	13.5	148	3	54.4	24.8	200	2,172.6	A1, G, VFD, H	ACTH
8	F	13.7	155	20	55.5	23.1	94	139.4	A2	none
9	F	14	155.5	10	54.9	22.7	160	821.4	A1, G, VFD, H	none
10	F	14	160	50	62.3	24.3	110	58.1	O	none
11	F	14.1	157	15	65	26.4	110	78.8	O	none
12	F	14.5	152	4	65	28.1	336	1,033.7	A1, G	none
13	F	14.5	161	51	60.3	23.3	93	52.2	O, G	none
14	F	14.5	165	65	52.9	19.4	94	119.6	A2	none
15	F	14.5	167.7	80	59.4	21.1	70	127.4	A2, G	none
16	F	14.8	163.9	51	64.9	24.2	105	104.6	O	none
17	F	15	160	28	60.1	23.5	94	115.8	A2	none
18	F	15.3	152.2	3	65.5	28.3	171	803.2	A1, G, H	none
19	F	15.3	160.1	26	62.5	24.4	71	69.5	O, G	none
20	F	15.5	158.9	26	66.6	26.4	500	123.6	A1	none
21	F	15.7	161.2	30	61.2	23.6	71	29.1	O, G	none
22	F	15.8	154.2	1	57.7	24.3	1,700	3,058.6	A1, H	ACTH, TSH, GH
23	F	16.3	160	25	58.8	23.0	259	327.8	A1	none
24	F	16.5	164.5	60	61.2	22.6	145	550.1	O, G, H	none
25	F	17	160.2	25	74.5	29.0	1,246	1,362.7	A2, G, H	none
26	F	17	161.1	25.5	70.3	27.1	171	60.5	A1, G, H	none
27	F	17.3	156.7	18	58.8	23.9	93	60.3	O, G	none
28	F	17.5	160	25	62.3	24.3	336	493.4	A1, G	none
29	F	17.8	155.5	10	61.1	25.3	145	82.0	O, G, H	none

Table 2. Continued

Case no.	Sex	Age at diagnosis	Height	Percentile	Weight	BMI	Basal PRL	Volume	Presenting symptoms	Associated deficiency
30	M	7	122.5	52	41.1	27.4	165	183.9	G, Gy, H	none
31	M	8.5	132.2	60	49.7	28.4	1,600	2,379.2	VFD	ACTH, ADH, TS
32	M	10	135	35	42	23.0	88	117.6	Gy	none
33	M	11.1	135	10	52.7	28.9	1,600	2,379.2	VFD	ACTH, ADH, TS
34	M	12	140	10	61	31.1	3,065	3,394.2	G, Gy, VFD, H	none
35	M	12.8	151.1	25.2	66.6	29.2	165	82.0	G, Gy, H	none
36	M	13.5	165	75	77.5	28.5	1,043	2,649.5	VFD, H	none
37	M	14	158.5	48	62.2	24.8	142	81.8	Gy, H, GI	none
38	M	14	160.2	50	68.8	26.8	640	1,446.2	Gy, H	none
39	M	14	166.8	75	80.3	28.9	720	1,311.9	G, Gy, VFD, H	none
40	M	14.8	166.4	25	81.1	29.3	1,850	1,419.7	H, VFD	ACTH, TSH, GH
41	M	15	158.8	5	59.5	23.6	1,600	2,459.7	VFD	ACTH, ADH, TS
42	M	15	165.5	30	71.1	26.0	142	152.4	Gy, GI	GH
43	M	15.2	160.1	7	68.8	26.8	1,048	1,750.3	VFD, H	ACTH, TSH
44	M	16	150	1	55.5	24.7	720	1,436.2	G, Gy, VFD, H	GH
45	M	16	165	7	70.3	25.8	3,300	4,578.9	H, VFD	FSH, LH, TSH, G
46	M	16.5	170	25	76.9	26.6	640	430.1	Gy, H	none
47	M	16.5	178.8	75	82.2	25.7	3,065	2,044.8	G, Gy, VFD, H	none
48	M	17	162.2	3	71.1	27.0	1,700	948.3	H	ACTH, TSH, GH
49	M	18	167.7	10	71.2	25.3	105	1,397.7	Gy, GI	none
50	M	18	172.2	27	68.8	23.2	3,300	3,835.6	H, VDF	FSH, LH, TSH, G

G = Galactorrhea; Gy = gynecomastia; H = headache; VFD = visual field defects; A1 = primary amenorrhea; A2 = secondary amenorrhea; O = oligomenorrhea.

to the University Federico II from January 1st 1995 to December 31st 2004, we found short stature in 7 of 50 patients (14%), 5 girls and 2 boys (table 2). Another 2 patients, 1 girl and 1 boy, had their height below or at the 5th percentile and another 8 (3 girls) had their height between the 5th and 10th percentiles (table 2). As expected, the percentiles of height in the patients with extrasellar/invasive macroprolactinomas were lower than in those bearing smaller tumors ($p = 0.015$ comparing microprolactinomas

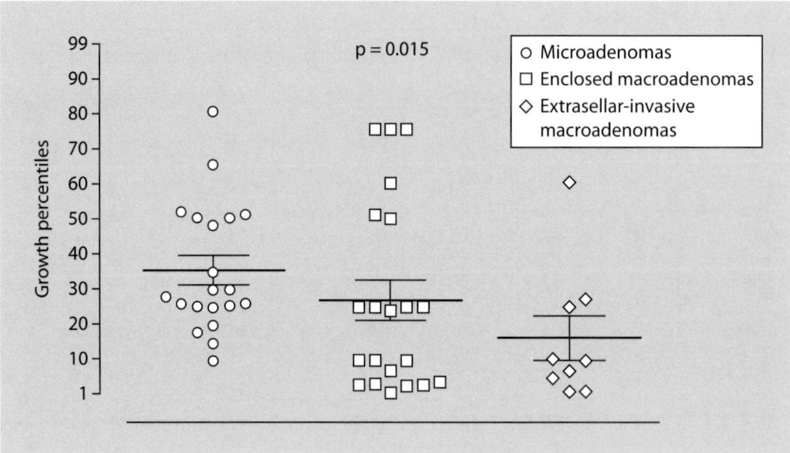

Fig. 1. Growth percentiles at diagnosis in 50 patients divided according to tumor dimensions.

vs. extrasellar tumors; fig. 1). We also found at diagnosis that macroadenomas were slightly more frequent in boys than in girls (76.2 vs. 48.3%, p = 0.09). This gender difference is similar to that observed in the adult population [24].

The most common symptoms of prolactinomas in peripubertal age are those associated with deficiency of the pituitary-gonadal axis (table 2). Menstrual irregularities in girls are common in all types of pituitary adenomas, except those causing Nelson's syndrome [10, 20]. As in the adults [24], the size of the prolactinoma is reported to correlate well with baseline PRL levels [17] and in our 50 patients, we found a high correlation between PRL levels and tumor volume (r = 0.84, p < 0.0001; fig. 2).

Weight gain has been reported to occur in patients with hyperprolactinemia [25–27] but never described in children. Indeed, among our 50 patients, 23 had a normal BMI (>25), 25 were overweight (BMI 25.1–30) and 2 were obese (BMI >30). In our series, PRL levels were also correlated with BMI (r = 0.48, p = 0.024; fig. 2).

Headache and/or visual field defects were common first symptoms in the majority of patients with macroadenomas [10, 18, 20]. This finding was confirmed in the re-evaluation of 50 patients (table 2): in 28 of 29 girls the first symptoms were amenorrhea, primary or secondary, or oligomenorrhea. In young patients, galactorrhea should be carefully investigated by expressing the breast, because teenagers may not spontaneously refer it as a symptom and frequently it is not spontaneous [14]. Cannavò et al. [23] also reported galactorrhea in 91% of their patients. In boys, the most common symptom was headache (15 of 21 patients) associated with gynecomastia (12 of 21 patients).

Impairment of other pituitary hormone secretion was reported to occur in a minority of patients at diagnosis [10, 18, 20, 23] and in some patients hypopituitarism

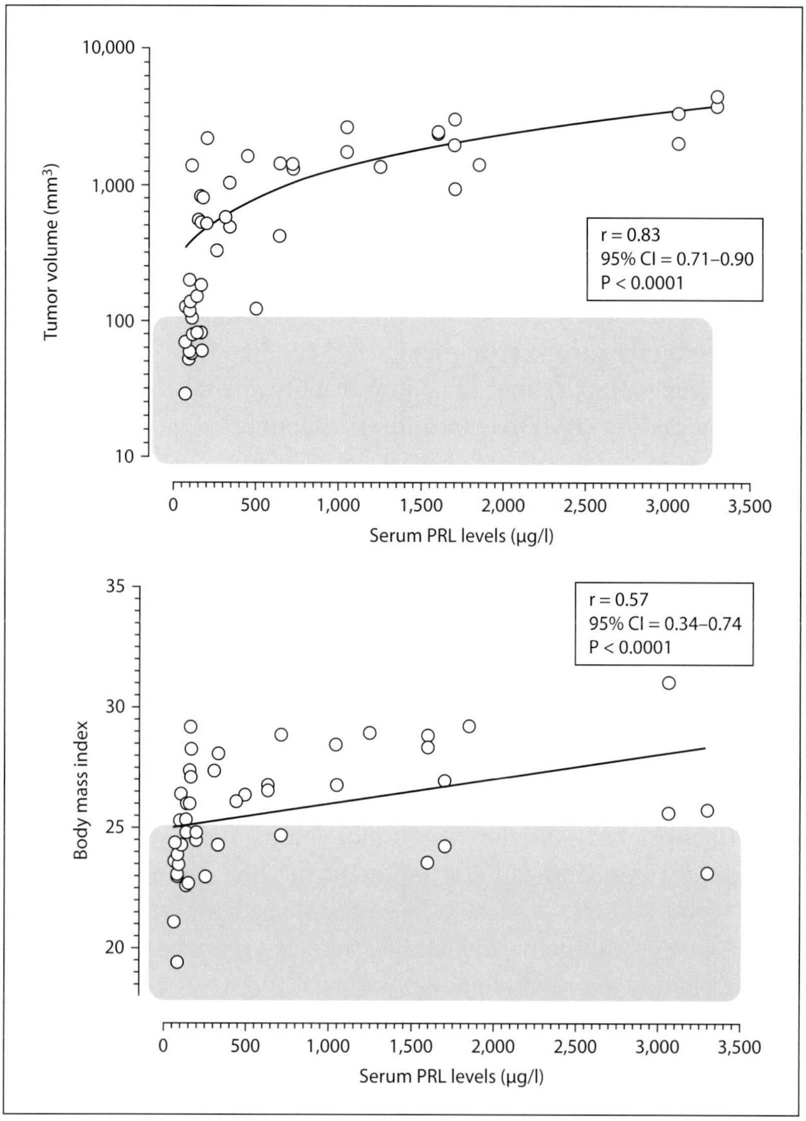

Fig. 2. Results of correlation analysis in the 50 children or adolescents with prolactinomas. Top: Correlation between serum PRL levels and tumor size. The PRL scale is logarithmic. The grey area corresponds to the median microadenoma volume. Bottom: Correlation between serum PRL levels and BMI. The PRL scale is logarithmic. The grey area corresponds to the normal body mass index.

developed after surgery. Indeed, pituitary deficiency in the context of a microprolactinoma is rare (4.7%), while one third of the patients with enclosed macroadenomas and 77.8% of those with extrasellar macroadenomas had some degree of pituitary deficiency (table 2). Deficiency of GH secretion was the most common (12/50 patients) followed by ACTH deficiency (10/50). While it is essential to immediately replace ACTH deficiency, mostly if the patients undergo neurosurgery, it is better to delay GH replacement by at least 6 months to verify if the control of hyperprolactinemia and the reduction of tumor volume after pharmacotherapy (see below) will produce the disappearance of the GH deficiency [28, 29]. This was nicely documented in a 13-year-old Japanese boy with pituitary prolactinoma and growth delay by >2 years treated with bromocriptine alone for 140 weeks [30]. Treatment normalized PRL levels and significantly reduced the tumor mass; his height improved (from –2.1 to –1.7 SDS). It has also been shown, however, that GH treatment associated with bromocriptine was useful to improve growth rate without inducing tumor growth but even without preventing tumor shrinkage in prepubertal children [31].

Lastly, the most frequent complications of hyperprolactinemia in adult patients is decreased bone mineral density (BMD), determining osteoporosis in some patients [32–34]. In a study focusing on the role of hyperprolactinemia in men, Di Somma et al. [35] reported a more severe impairment of BMD in young patients than in patients in whom hyperprolactinemia occurred at an older age. In 20 patients with diagnosis of hyperprolactinemia during adolescence, we found significantly lower BMD values in adolescents than in young adult patients with hyperprolactinemia [36]. This finding is confirmed in a large cohort of patients. In 26 patients all having a diagnosis of prolactinomas before the age of 18 years, the bone mineral density at the lumbar spine was significantly lower than in age-matched controls (–2.11 ± 0.74 vs. 0.06 ± 0.02, $p < 0.0001$). In the patients, the z-score at the lumbar spine ranged from –3.5 to 0.02. The z-score was significantly correlated with osteocalcin and Ntx levels (fig. 3) but not with gender (table 3), BMI, PRL levels or tumor volume (data not shown).

During childhood, prolactinomas can also represent the first tumor in multiple endocrine neoplasia type 1 (MEN1) syndrome. In 2 juvenile patients reported [37], a 14-year-old girl developed prolactinoma and manifested delayed puberty and growth arrest while a 16-year-old boy was asymptomatic.

Diagnosis

The differential diagnosis of hyperprolactinemia should consider any process interfering with dopamine (DA) synthesis, its transport to the pituitary gland or its action at lactotrope DA receptors. A single measurement of PRL levels is unreliable since PRL secretion is markedly influenced by physical and emotional stress. A complete revision of the diagnosis of hyperprolactinemia lies beyond the scope of this review.

Some peculiar conditions should, however, be reminded [38]. Serial serum PRL measurements at 0, 30 and 60 min after the needle was inserted into an antecubital vein is a valuable and simple measure to identify stress-related hyperprolactinemia in order to avoid diagnostic pitfalls and unnecessary treatments. It is important to exclude from the assay the monomeric PRL forms, *big-prolactin* (b-PRL) and big big-prolactin (bb-PRL); the latter may contain immunoglobulin (IgG) [39]. These

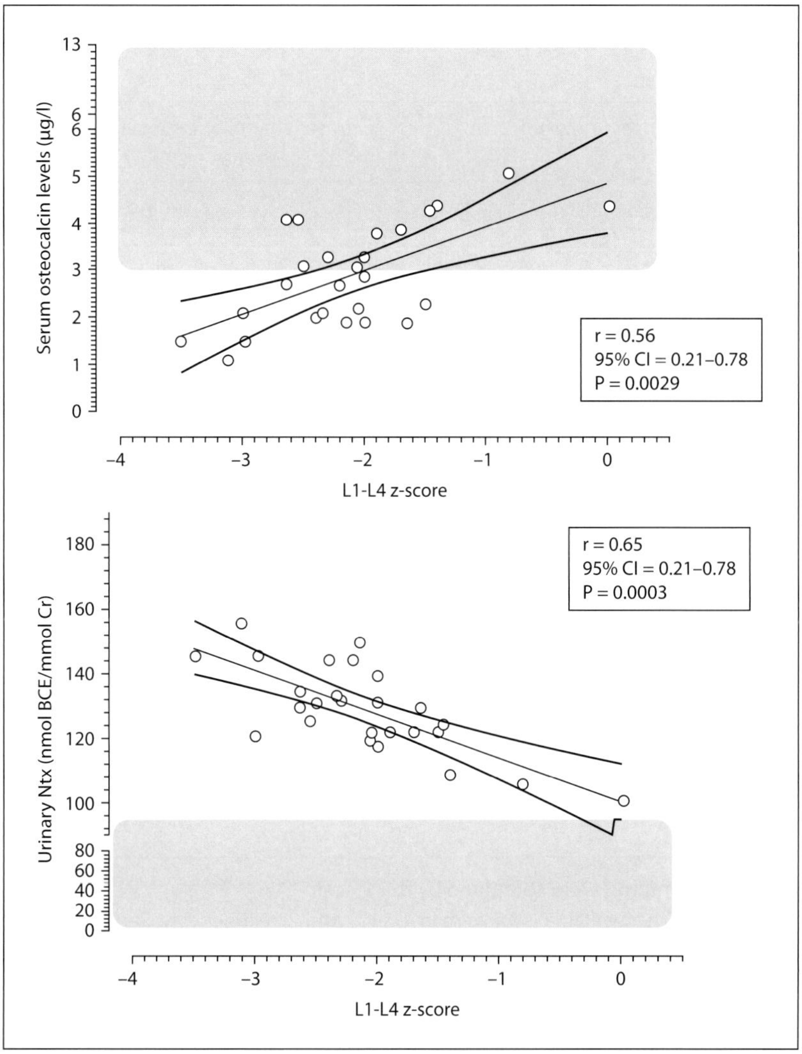

Fig. 3. Results of correlation analysis in the 26 children or adolescents with prolactinomas in which the bone mineral density analysis and bone markers were available. Correlation between z-SDS of BMD on L1-L4 and serum osteocalcin levels (top) and urinary cross-linked N-telopeptides of type I collagen (bottom). The grey areas correspond to the normal ranges of osteocalcin and cross-linked N-telopeptides of type I collagen.

molecular complexes are seldom active but may recorded by the PRL assay. The absence of a clinical syndrome of hyperprolactinemia will suggest the presence of macroprolactin. The 'high-dose hook effect' could be a serious problem in the differential diagnosis between prolactinomas and nonfunctioning adenomas (NFPA): it is mandatory, in these cases and in every patient with pituitary mass and hyperprolactinemia, to dilute PRL samples routinely (1:10 and 1:100 dilutions) or to use

Table 3. Presentation of prolactinomas in children and adolescents: the two-decade experience of the Department of Endocrinology and Oncology, University 'Federico II' of Naples (data are shown as mean ± SD or as prevalence shown as percentage of total number)

	Microadenomas and/or enclosed macroadenomas			Extrasellar and/or invasive macroadenomas		
	boys	girls	p	boys	girls	p
Number	8	24	<0.0001	13	5	0.020
Age at diagnosis, years	13.3±3.3	14.9±1.6	0.075	14.5±2.7	13.7±2.7	0.58
BMI	26.6±2.0	24.4±2.1	0.015	26.8±4.0	27.6±4.0	0.71
Basal PRL levels, μg/l	470.2±554.4	166.3±108.5	0.014	1,764.3±1092.8	1,058.0±702.3	0.20
Tumor volume on MRI, mm^3	414±466	294±294	0.39	2,398±1009	2,041±650	0.48
Pituitary deficiencies, %	25.0	4.2	0.29	100.0	100.0	1.0
z-score on L1-L4*	–2.65±0.60	–2.02±0.80	0.18	–1.85±0.65	–2.70±0.42	0.12
Osteocalcin levels, μg/l*	2.3±0.8	3.3±1.0	0.09	2.9±1.3	2.0±0.1	0.37
Urinary Ntx, nmol BCE/ mmol creatinine*	140.4±8.7	128.5±12.7	0.11	124.3±14.7	132.7±16.5	0.35

p values refer to the Mann-Whitney test. Percentages were compared by the χ^2 test.
* These data were not available in all patients. The available data were in 4, 11, 9 and 2, respectively. Serum PRL levels = 5–25 μg/l in females and 5–15 μg/l in males; Serum osteocalcin levels = 3.0–13.0 μg/l; urinary cross-linked N-telopeptides of type I collagen (Ntx): 13–96 nmol bone collagen equivalent (BCE)/mmol crea (creatinine) in females and 23–110 nmol BCE/mmol creatinine in males.

alterative methods to immunoradiometric assays. The difference between macroprolactinomas and 'pseudoprolactinomas' is essential to provide a correct treatment approach [40]. This problem is, however, of little value in children and adolescents as non functioning macroadenomas are very rare at this age.

Treatment Strategy

As for the adult patients [20], indications for therapy are: (1) to reduce tumor size, and (2) to control PRL excess. In adult asymptomatic patients with hyperprolactinemia there is no absolute requirement to treat as studies examining the natural history of untreated microprolactinomas demonstrated that significant growth of these tumors is uncommon [20]. However, in children prolactinomas are diagnosed in presence of symptoms so that treatment is always required. In the absence of complications needing immediate surgery, such as visual loss, hydrocephalus, or cerebrospinal fluid leak, pharmacotherapy with dopamine agonists should be considered the first treatment approach. to note, surgery is safe in children as in adults and the new technology of the minimally invasive surgery by the use of the endoscope is to be preferred [41, 42]. In children and adolescents, bromocriptine (BRC) has been used successfully by several investigators [10]. In our series, BRC at doses ranging from 2.5 to 20 mg/day orally induced restoration of normal PRL levels in 38.5% of the patients [18]. In the remaining 16 patients, 10 with macro- and 6 with microprolactinoma, PRL levels remained above the normal range despite a progressive increase of the dose of the drug. However, the possibility that some patients were indeed not taking BRC appropriately cannot be ruled out as poor compliance to any chronic treatment is a well-known phenomenon in children and adolescents. In addition, some patients required drug discontinuation for intolerable side effects overall regarding the gastrointestinal tract. Cabergoline, at doses ranging from 0.5 to 3.5 mg/week orally, is also effective in adolescent patients with large tumors and symptoms of tumor expansion. In our patients, cabergoline induced normalization of PRL levels in all but 3 cases, who, however, had a significant response in terms of decrease in PRL levels and tumor shrinkage. These data are in line with those obtained in the adult population [43–45]. None of the patients complained of severe side effects and none was withdrawn from treatment because of side effects. Cabergoline has been reported to be tolerated even at rather high doses [46]. Only one case of pituitary apoplexy following cabergoline treatment in a young patient has been reported so far [47]. Twelve of our 50 patients (one with enclosed macroprolactinoma and 11 with microprolactinoma) achieved disappearance of the tumor so that were withdrawn from treatment in accordance with our protocol [48]. In fact, the cure of a prolactinoma was generally defined as complete tumor removal at surgery but withdrawal from medical therapy has recently been reported to result in remission of hyperprolactinemia in a high percentage of patients. We first reported the persistence of normal PRL levels in more than 60% of the patients undergoing 5-year cabergoline withdrawal [48]. This finding was not related to the initial diagnosis but rather to the PRL suppression and/or tumor shrinkage during treatment [48].

The only relevant safety issue to be considered in patients treated with cabergoline is a recent alarm on a possible consequent cardiac valve derangement [49]. This phenomenon appears in patients with Parkinson's disease, who are older and require higher doses of the drug than the patients with prolactinomas [20]. Anyhow, this aspect deserves some attention and dedicated observational studies are ongoing.

Radiotherapy, is not a routine treatment option in prolactinomas even if when aggressive as in children. As reviewed by Gillam et al. [20], about 250 patients have been reported who have undergone treatment with conventional radiotherapy alone, or after failure of medical and/or surgical therapy. Normalization of PRL levels was infrequent, with an overall normalization rate for the entire series of 34.1%, and in most of these cases, only with an extended latency. A similar number of patients was reported after treatment with single-dose stereotactic radiotherapy alone, or after failure of medical and/or surgical therapy [20]. Normalization of PRL levels was infrequent, with an overall normalization rate for the entire series similar to that reported for conventional radiotherapy (31.4%). There is only one study reporting the outcome of single dose stereotactic radiotherapy as primary therapy for prolactinomas [20]. Seventy-seven patients underwent gamma knife radiosurgery as primary treatment of prolactinomas: in the absence of any dopamine agonist treatment, 2 years after radiosurgery normalization of PRL levels was attained in only 16 (20.8%).

Moreover, the effects of radiotherapy should be balanced against all complications deriving from the treatment itself. The risk of damage is dose dependent, with a 78% risk of optic neuropathy in patients receiving >15 Gy, and 27% risk for those receiving 10–15 Gy to the optic apparatus [50, 51]. Consequently, pituitary adenomas with significant suprasellar extension, or those with less than 5 mm clearance between the tumor margin and the optic apparatus are poor candidates for single-dose radiotherapy [52]. Tumors with cavernous sinus invasion might, alternatively, be good candidates for single-dose radiotherapy, as the cranial nerves in the cavernous sinus are relatively radioresistant [53]. The most frequent long-term morbidity of conventional radiotherapy is radiation-induced hypopituitarism, with a cumulative actuarial risk of approximately 50% at 10–20 years [54, 55]. The incidence of hypopituitarism following single-dose stereotactic radiotherapy is difficult to establish at present: it varies widely from 0 to 36%, but a long-term follow-up study with a mean follow-up of 17 years showed a relatively high cumulative incidence of hypopituitarism by 72% [20]. Additional complications that occur months to years after radiotherapy of pituitary adenomas include cerebrovascular accidents, optic nerve damage, neurologic dysfunction and soft tissue reactions [56]. Secondary radiation-induced intracranial malignancies were shown to have a cumulative risk of 2.0% at 10 years and a 2.4% risk at 20 years [57, 58]. The risk of damage to the optic apparatus is approximately 1%, cranial neuropathies involving nerves that traverse the cavernous sinus (III, IV, V, VI) are less common, and often transient [52, 58, 59]. Radiation necrosis of surrounding brain tissue occurs in approximately 0.2–0.8% of cases [20]. To date, no case of secondary intracranial malignancies has been reported after single-dose radiotherapy but in children and adolescents the long-term life expectancy might be a factor to consider in limiting radiotherapy only to those tumors with proven aggressiveness and nonresponding to medical therapy.

Conclusion

Prolactinomas are the most common pituitary adenomas in children and adolescents and are generally of large dimensions. They are diagnosed because of gonadal and growth arrest and/or tumor compressive symptoms. Once the prolactinoma is diagnosed, medical therapy with dopamine agonists is indicated in order to control PRL levels and reduce tumor size. Some results suggest that responsive patients can be withdrawn from dopamine agonists (especially cabergoline) therapy after a period of treatment longer than 3 years, provided that some criteria are applied. In patients with tumors resistant to dopamine agonists as well as in those showing severe neurological symptoms at diagnosis surgery is indicated. Radiotherapy should be limited to the cases with aggressive tumors, nonresponsive to dopamine agonists, because of the risk of neurological damage and hypopituitarism later in the lives of these patients.

References

1 Odom GL, Davis CH, Woodhall B: Brain tumors in children: clinical analysis in 164 cases. Pediatrics 1956;18:856–869.

2 Sano K: Problems in the treatment of children with brain tumors. Prog Exp Tumor Res 1987;30:1–9.

3 Mindermann T, Wilson CB: Pediatric pituitary adenomas. Neurosurgery 1995;36:259–269.

4 Gold EB: Epidemiology of pituitary adenomas. Epidemiol Rev 1981;3:163–183.

5 Abe T, Lüdecke DK, Saeger W: Clinically nonsecreting pituitary adenomas in childhood and adolescence. Neurosurgery 1998;42:744–751.

6 Abe T, Tara LA, Lüdecke DK: Growth hormone-secreting pituitary adenomas in childhood and adolescence: features and results of transnasal surgery. Neurosurgery 1999;45:1–10.

7 Boop FA, Teo C, Pihoker K: Pediatric pituitary tumors; in Krisht AF, Tindall GT (eds): Comprehensive Management of Pituitary Disorders. Hagerstown, Lippincott Williams & Wilkins, 1999, pp 315–326.

8 Partington MD, Dudley HD, Laws ER, Scheithauer BW: Pituitary adenomas in childhood and adolescence: results of transsphenoidal surgery. J Neurosurg 1994;80:209–216.

9 Laws ER, Scheithauer BW, Groover RV: Pituitary adenomas in childhood and adolescence. Prog Exp Tumor Res 1987;30:359–361.

10 Colao A: Pituitary tumors in childhood; in New MI (eds): Pediatric Endocrinology. Endotext. www.endotext.org

11 Ludecke DK, Herrmann HD, Schulte FJ: Special problems with neurosurgical treatment of hormone-secreting pituitary adenomas in children. Prog Exp Tumor Res 1987;30:362–370.

12 Haddad SF, VanGilder JC, Menezes AH: Pediatric pituitary tumors. Neurosurgery 1991;29:509–514.

13 Colao A, Ochoa AS, Auriemma RS, Faggiano A, Pivonello R, Lombardi G: Pituitary carcinomas; in Guitelman M, Bronstein M, Arzt E (eds): Pituitary Today. II. Molecular, Physiological and Clinical Aspects. Front Horm Res. Basel, Karger, 2009, in press.

14 Lafferty AR, Chrousos GP: Pituitary tumors in children and adolescents. J Clin Endocrinol Metab 1999;84:4317–4323.

15 Colao A, Lombardi G: GH and PRL excess. Lancet 1998;352:1455–1461.

16 Dissaneevate P, Warne GL: Hyperprolactinaemia and pituitary adenomas in adolescence. J Pediatr Endocrinol Metab 1998;11:531–541.

17 Tyson D, Reggiardo D, Sklar C, David R: Prolactin-secreting macroadenomas in adolescents. Response to bromocriptine therapy. Am J Dis Child 1993;147:1057–1061.

18 Colao A, Loche S, Cappa M, et al: Prolactinomas in children and adolescents. Clinical presentation and long term follow-up. J Clin Endocrinol Metab 1998;83:2777–2780.

19 Kane LA, Leinung MC, Scheithauer BW, et al: Pituitary adenomas in childhood and adolescence. J Clin Endocrinol Metab 1994;79:1135–1140.

20 Artese R, D'Osvaldo DH, Molocznik I, et al: Pituitary tumors in adolescent patients. Neurol Res 1998;20:415–417.

21 Gillam MP, Molitch ME, Lombardi G, Colao A: Advances in the treatment of prolactinomas. Endocr Rev 2006;27:485–534.

22 Duntas LH: Prolactinomas in children and adolescents: consequences in adult life. J Pediatr Endocrinol Metab 2001;14:1227–1232.

23 Cannavò S, Venturino M, Curto L, De Menis E, D'Arrigo C, Tita P, Billeci D, Trimarchi F: Clinical presentation and outcome of pituitary adenomas in teenagers. Clin Endocrinol (Oxf) 2003;58:519–527.

24 Colao A, Di Sarno A, Cappabianca P, Briganti F, Pivonello R, Di Somma C, Faggiano A, Biondi B, Lombardi G: Gender differences in the prevalence, clinical features and response to cabergoline in hyperprolactinemia. Eur J Endocrinol 2003;148:325–331.
25 Creemers LB, Zelissen PMJ, van't Verlaat JW, Koppeschaar HPF: Prolactinoma and body weight: a retrospective study. Acta Endocrinol Scand 1991; 125:392–396.
26 Delgrange, Donkier J, Maiter D: Hyperprolactinemia as a reversible cause of weight gain in male patients? Clin Endocrinol (Oxf) 1999;50:271–272.
27 Greenman Y, Torjman K, Stern N: Increased body weight associated with prolactin secreting pituitary adenomas: weight loss with normalization of prolactin levels. Clin Endocrinol (Oxf) 1998;48:547–553.
28 George LD, Nicolau N, Scanlon MF, Davies JS: Recovery of growth hormone secretion following cabergoline treatment of macroprolactinomas. Clin Endocrinol (Oxf) 2000;53:595–599.
29 Colao A, Vitale G, Cappabianca P, Briganti F, Ciccarelli A, De Rosa M, Zarrilli S, Lombardi G: Outcome of cabergoline treatment in men with prolactinoma: effects of a 24-month treatment on prolactin levels, tumor mass, recovery of pituitary function, and semen analysis. J Clin Endocrinol Metab 2004;89:1704–1711.
30 Sakazume S, Obata K, Takahashi E, Yoshino A, Murakami N, Sakuta R, Murai T, Nagai T: Bromocriptine treatment of prolactinoma restores growth hormone secretion and causes catch-up growth in a prepubertal child. Eur J Pediatr 2004; 163:472–474.
31 Oberfield SE, Nino M, Riddick L, et al: Combined bromocriptine and growth hormone (GH) treatment in GH-deficient children with macroprolactinoma in situ. J Clin Endocrinol Metab 1992;75: 87–90.
32 Klibanski A, Neer RM, Beitins IZ, Ridgway C, Zarvas NT, Mc Arthur JW: Decreased bone density in amenorrheic women. N Engl J Med 1980;303: 1511–1514.
33 Schlechte J, El-Khoury G, Kathol M, Walkner L: Forearm and vertebral bone mineral in treated and untreated hyperprolactinemic amenorrhea. J Clin Endocrinol Metab 1987;64:1021–1026.
34 Biller BMK, Baum HBA, Rosenthal DI, Saxe VC, Charpie PM, Klibanski A: Progressive trabecular osteopenia in women with hyperprolactinemic amenorrhea. J Clin Endocrinol Metab 1992;75:692–697.
35 Di Somma C, Colao A, Di Sarno A, et al: Bone marker and bone density responses to dopamine agonist therapy in hyperprolactinemic males. J Clin Endocrinol Metab 1998;83:807–813.
36 Colao A, Di Somma C, Loche S, et al: Prolactinomas in children and adolescents: persistent bone loss after 2 years of prolactin normalization. Clin Endocrinol 2000;52:319–328.
37 Oiwa A, Sakurai A, Sato Y, Sakuma T, Yamashita K, Katai M, Aizawa T, Hashizume K: Pituitary adenomas in adolescent patients with multiple endocrine neoplasia type 1. Endocr J 2002;49:635–640.
38 Di Sarno A, Rota F, Auriemma R, De Martino MC, Lombardi G, Colao A: An evaluation of patients with hyperprolactinemia: have dynamic tests had their day? J Endocrinol Invest 2003;26(7 suppl):39–47.
39 Cavaco B, Leite V, Santos MA, et al: Some forms of big big prolactin behave as a complex of monomeric with an immunoglobulin G in patients with macroprolactinoma or prolactinomas. J Clin Endocrinol Metab 1995;80:3507–3512.
40 Colao A, Di Somma C, Pivonello R, Faggiano A, Lombardi G, Savastano S: Medical therapy for clinically non-functioning pituitary adenomas. Endocr Relat Cancer 2008;15:905–915.
41 Abe T, Ludecke DK: Transnasal surgery for prolactin-secreting pituitary adenomas in childhood and adolescence. Surg Neurol 2002;57:369–378; discussion 378–379.
42 Cappabianca P, Cavallo LM, de Divitiis E: Endoscopic endonasal transsphenoidal surgery. Neurosurgery 2004;55:933–940; discussion 940–941.
43 Colao A, Di Sarno A, Sarnacchiaro F, et al: Prolactinomas resistant to standard dopamine agonists respond to chronic cabergoline treatment. J Clin Endocrinol Metab 1997;82:876–883.
44 Colao A, Di Sarno A, Landi ML, et al: Macroprolactinoma shrinkage during cabergoline treatment is greater in naive patients than in patients pretreated with other dopamine agonists: a prospective study in 110 patients. J Clin Endocrinol Metab 2000;85:2247–2252.
45 Di Sarno A, Landi ML, Marzullo P, et al: The effect of quinagolide and cabergoline, two selective dopamine receptor type 2 agonists, in the treatment of prolactinomas. Clin Endocrinol (Oxf) 2000;53:53–60.
46 Howell DL, Wasilewski K, Mazewski CM, Hudgins RJ, Meacham LR: The use of high-dose daily cabergoline in an adolescent patient with macroprolactinoma. J Pediatr Hematol Oncol 2005;27:326–329.
47 Knoepfelmacher M, Gomes MC, Melo ME, Mendonca BB: Pituitary apoplexy during therapy with cabergoline in an adolescent male with prolactin-secreting macroadenoma. Pituitary 2004;7:83–87.

48 Colao A, Di Sarno A, Cappabianca P, Di Somma C, Pivonello R, Lombardi G: Withdrawal of long-term cabergoline therapy for tumoral and nontumoral hyperprolactinemia. N Engl J Med 2003;349:2023–2033.
49 Colao A, Galderisi M, Di Sarno A, et al: Increased prevalence of tricuspid regurgitation in patients with prolactinomas chronically treated with cabergoline. J Clin Endocrinol Metab 2008;93:3777–3784.
50 Leber KA, Bergloff J, Pendl G: Dose-response tolerance of the visual pathways and cranial nerves of the cavernous sinus to stereotactic radiosurgery. J Neurosurg 1998;88:43–50.
51 Tishler RB, Loeffler JS, Lunsford LD, et al: Tolerance of cranial nerves of the cavernous sinus to radiosurgery. Int J Radiat Oncol Biol Phys 1993;27:215–221.
52 Brada M, Ajithkumar TV, Minniti G: Radiosurgery for pituitary adenomas. Clin Endocrinol (Oxf) 2004;61:531–534.
53 Chen JC, Giannotta SL, Yu C, Petrovich Z, Levy ML, Apuzzo ML: Radiosurgical management of benign cavernous sinus tumors: dose profiles and acute complications. Neurosurgery 2001;48:1022–1030; discussion 1030–1032.
54 Snyder PJ, Fowble BF, Schatz NJ, Savino PJ, Gennarelli TA: Hypopituitarism following radiation therapy of pituitary adenomas. Am J Med 1986; 81:457–462.
55 Littley MD, Shalet SM, Beardwell CG, Ahmed SR, Applegate G, Sutton ML: Hypopituitarism following external radiotherapy for pituitary tumors in adults. Q J Med 1989;70:145–160.
56 Erfurth EM, Bulow B, Mikoczy Z, Svahn-Tapper G, Hagmar L: Is there an increase in second brain tumors after surgery and irradiation for a pituitary tumor? Clin Endocrinol (Oxf) 2001;55:613–616.
57 Minniti G, Traish D, Ashley S, Gonsalves A, Brada M: Risk of second brain tumor after conservative surgery and radiotherapy for pituitary adenoma: update after an additional 10 years. J Clin Endocrinol Metab 2005;90:800–804.
58 Witt TC: Stereotactic radiosurgery for pituitary tumors. Neurosurg Focus 2003;14:e10.
59 Sheehan JP, Niranjan A, Sheehan JM, et al: Stereotactic radiosurgery for pituitary adenomas: an intermediate review of its safety, efficacy, and role in the neurosurgical treatment armamentarium. J Neurosurg 2005;102:678–691.

Annamaria Colao, MD, PhD
Department of Molecular and Clinical Endocrinology and Oncology
'Federico II' University
via S. Pansini 5, IT–80131 Napoli (Italy)
Tel. +39 81 7462132, Fax +39 81 7463668, E-Mail colao@unina.it

Loche S, Cappa M, Ghizzoni L, Maghnie M, Savage MO (eds): Pediatric Neuroendocrinology.
Endocr Dev. Basel, Karger, 2010, vol 17, pp 160–174

Pituitary Tumors: Advances in Neuroimaging

G. Morana[a] · M. Maghnie[b] · A. Rossi[a]

Departments of [a]Pediatric Neuroradiology and [b]Pediatrics, IRCCS 'G. Gaslini', University of Genoa, Genoa, Italy

Abstract

Pediatric pituitary tumors, albeit relatively infrequent, can significantly alter the quality of life of affected children. Accurate diagnostic differentiation is essential for both safe and effective disease management. Recent advances in neuroimaging have enabled the neuroradiologist to study the pituitary region in greater detail than ever before. Magnetic resonance imaging (MRI) represents the examination method of choice for evaluating hypothalamic-pituitary-related endocrine diseases due to its ability to provide strongly contrasted high-resolution, multiplanar and spatial images. Specifically, MRI allows the detection of the pituitary lesions responsible of the clinical picture and offers useful information about the relationship with adjacent anatomical structures in order to plan the medical or surgical strategy. A rigorous imaging exam technique is necessary in order to obtain images of high diagnostic quality. Advanced MR techniques, including diffusion-weighted imaging and MR spectroscopy, may be helpful in particular cases. Computerized tomography (CT) has a complementary role in the identification of intralesional calcifications or to better evaluate bone structures prior to trans-sphenoidal surgery. The aim of this work is to provide an overview of the most relevant neuroradiological features of pituitary region tumors and to propose an appropriate and accurate differential diagnosis.

Modern neuroimaging techniques represent an essential tool in the evaluation of pituitary tumors, and the advent of MRI has remarkably improved overall diagnostic accuracy. This article begins with some background information regarding imaging techniques and normal evolution of the pituitary gland appearance on MRI. Then, the most relevant neuroradiological characteristics of pituitary region tumors are described, with emphasis on pituitary adenomas and their main differential diagnosis. Finally, a brief discussion about incidentalomas is provided.

Background

Imaging Techniques

MRI is the imaging modality of choice for evaluating the sellar region because of its superior tissue contrast differentiation and lack of invasiveness. The most relevant information is provided by T_1- and T_2-weighted images obtained on sagittal and coronal planes. For T_1-weighted imaging, conventional spin-echo techniques are usually employed. Typically, these will yield optimal results at 3-mm slice thickness. Spoiled gradient-echo (SPGR) three-dimensional sequences are an excellent alternative to obtain very thin slice (i.e. 1.5 mm or less) T_1-weighted images that can be reconstructed in any plane [1]. Regarding T_2-weighted imaging, fast (i.e. turbo) spin-echo sequences are preferable over conventional spin-echo ones. Contrast material administration is a mainstay in the evaluation of pituitary tumors; thin slice (3 mm) contrast-enhanced T_1-weighted sequences should be obtained on sagittal and coronal planes. If necessary, transverse T_1-weighted sequences (5 mm) can be performed for the evaluation of the whole brain. Dynamic T_1-weighted spin-echo acquisition within 1–2 min after i.v. contrast medium may slightly improve the sensitivity of MR for the detection of small pituitary adenomas [2]. Advanced MR techniques, including diffusion-weighted imaging and MR spectroscopy, may be helpful in particular cases.

CT currently has a complementary role in the identification of intralesional calcifications or to better evaluate bone structures (e.g. in the study of the skull base before trans-sphenoidal surgery). For these purposes, a spiral acquisition covering the anatomic region of interest is sufficient. Radioprotection remains a significant issue especially in infants and children which requires careful consideration.

Normal Evolution and MRI Appearance

The pituitary gland undergoes dynamic changes [3, 4] in size and shape throughout life, depending on age and sex.

In newborns, the gland is typically convex, sometimes pear-shaped, with very high signal intensity on T_1-weighted images (fig. 1). This appearance persists for the first month and gradually changes during the second month (fig. 1), until the adult appearance, with a flat superior surface and isointensity of the anterior lobe to the white matter on T_1- and T_2-weighted images, is achieved. These changes correlate with the intense endocrine activity, lactotrope hyperplasia, and protein synthesis known to occur in the gland during the neonatal period [5]. By the second month of life, the posterior neural lobe of the gland becomes progressively recognizable next to the dorsum sellae as the 'bright spot', because of its marked hyperintensity on T_1-weighted images. This finding has been demonstrated to

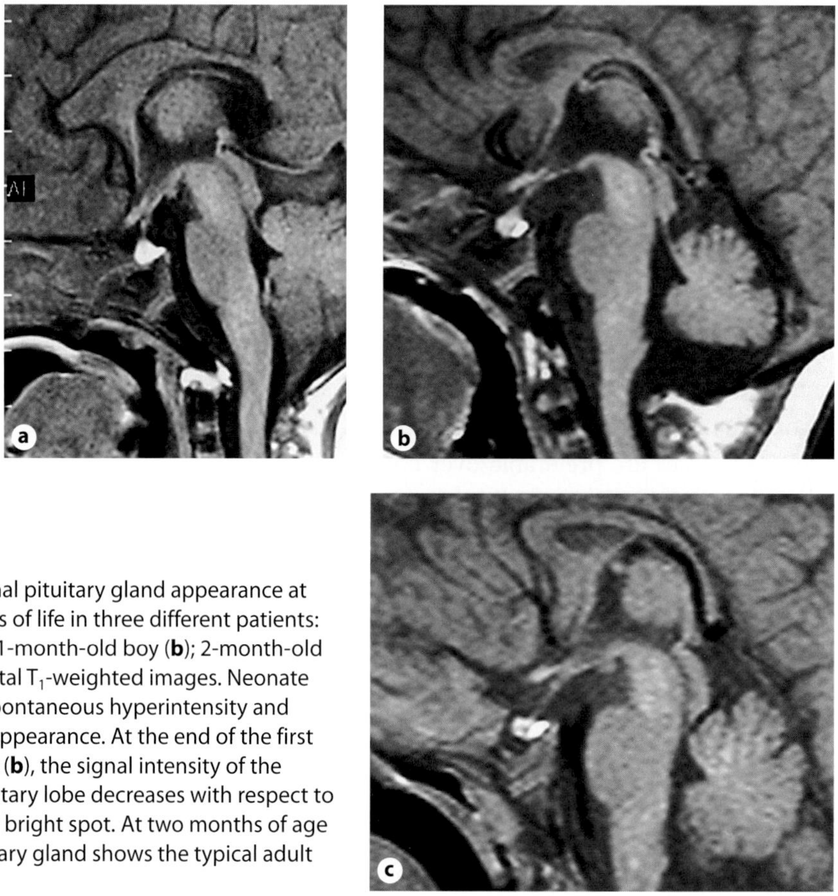

Fig. 1. Normal pituitary gland appearance at different ages of life in three different patients: neonate (**a**); 1-month-old boy (**b**); 2-month-old boy (**c**). Sagittal T_1-weighted images. Neonate (**a**): typical spontaneous hyperintensity and pear-shape appearance. At the end of the first month of life (**b**), the signal intensity of the anterior pituitary lobe decreases with respect to the posterior bright spot. At two months of age (**c**), the pituitary gland shows the typical adult pattern.

specifically result from the storage of vasopressin, a hormone synthesized by the hypothalamus [6, 7]. The vasopressin associated carrier protein, neurophysin, is a very high molecular weight glycoprotein that complexes with vasopressin to form insoluble crystal aggregates and typically shortens the T_1 signal [6]. Regardless of its chemical origin, the bright spot serves as an important marker of neurohypophyseal function and, when present, documents integrity of the hypothalamic-neurohypophyseal tract.

Following gadolinium administration, marked enhancement of the adenohypophysis, due to its high capillary density, and of the infundibulo-tuberal region is well evident [8]. Dynamic studies after i.v. contrast medium administration have shown that initial enhancement of the posterior pituitary lobe occurs simultaneously with that of the straight sinus in normal subjects; enhancement of the entire anterior pituitary lobe occurs within 30 s [9]. The normal pituitary stalk usually tapers smoothly along its course. It is approximately 3 mm in diameter near the optic chiasm and 2 mm where it inserts into the gland [10].

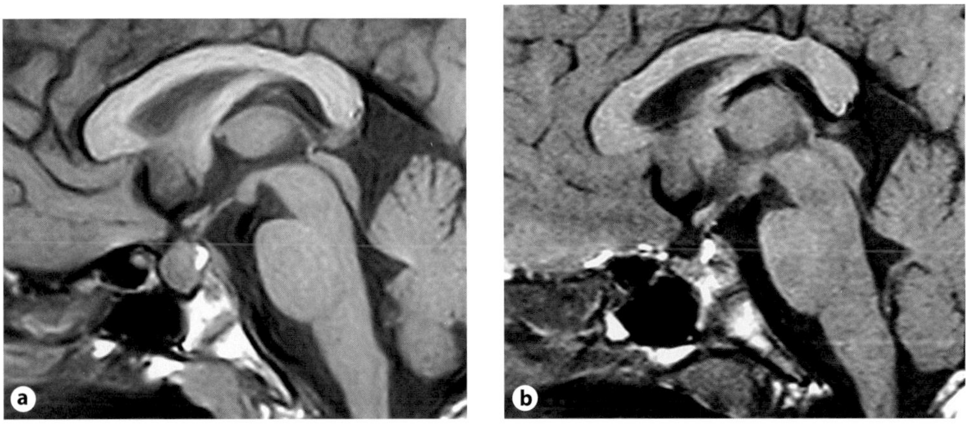

Fig. 2. Pituitary hyperplasia in a child affected with hypothiroidism. Sagittal T_1-weighted images. There is marked enlargement of the adenohypophysis at presentation (**a**). Note dramatic reduction of size following treatment of hypothiroidism (**b**).

Pituitary Hyperplasia

Physiological hyperplasia of the pituitary gland occurs during puberty. In girls, the gland may swell symmetrically to a height of 10 mm, appearing nearly spherical, whereas in pubertal boys it may reach 7–8 mm. On MRI, the anterior pituitary lobe is homogeneously enlarged and shows normal, homogeneous enhancement [11].

Pathological pituitary hyperplasia may occur in several circumstances, including central precocious puberty, ectopic production of hypothalamic-releasing hormones from hypothalamic and non pituitary tumors, and administration of exogenous estrogens. In primary hypothyroidism, insufficient amount of circulating thyroxine causes increased levels of thyrotropin-releasing hormones, with consequent pituitary gland enlargement resulting from lack of the normal negative feedback on the hypothalamus. Because benign pituitary hyperplasia can mimic macroadenomas, primary hypothyroidism should be excluded in any patient with pituitary enlargement [12]; follow-up studies after restoration of normal hormone levels will usually clear the view (fig. 2).

Pituitary Adenomas

Pituitary adenomas are relatively uncommon in children and account for less than 3% of all supratentorial tumors [13]. They are more frequent in adolescents than in younger age groups [14, 15]. Hormone secreting tumors predominate, while hormonally inactive adenomas are rare. Prepubertal children more frequently have ACTH-releasing adenomas, while pubertal and postpubertal patients are most likely to have prolactinomas [16]. The clinical presentation of prolactinoma varies with patient age and gender. Prepubertal children present with headache, visual disturbance, and growth failure; pubertal females present with symptoms of pubertal arrest and hypogonadism, possibly associated with galactorrhea; pubertal males may present with headache and visual impairment as well as delayed puberty or growth failure.

Growth failure with associated weight gain is one of the most reliable indicators of hypercortisolemia in pediatric Cushing disease. ACTH-releasing adenomas responsible of Cushing disease represents a diagnostic challenge because of their small (usually less than 5 mm) size, which is why MRI often fails to detect the lesion [17]; in a large series, only 50% of microadenomas were visible on pituitary MRI [18]. Bilateral inferior petrosal sinus sampling (BIPSS) in selected centers is reserved for patients who have ACTH-dependent Cushing syndrome and negative MRI [19]. In children, because of the extreme rarity of ectopic ACTH syndrome, the aim of BIPSS is primarily to demonstrate possible lateralization of ACTH secretion to one or the other side of the pituitary gland, thus guiding the surgeon during trans-sphenoidal surgery. Sensitivity for lateralization by BIPSS has been reported to be up to 60–90% before and after corticotrophin-releasing hormone stimulation [19–21]. BIPSS should be performed only in experienced medical centers to avoid potentially serious complications as well as improper procedures and data misinterpretation.

Hormonally inactive adenomas represent only 4–6% of cases in the pediatric literature and typically present with delayed puberty, short stature, or primary amenorrhea (in girls) [22]. Pituitary apoplexy, characterized by sudden enlargement of a pituitary adenoma secondary to extensive tumor infarction or hemorrhage, seldom occurs in children and adolescents. Clinically, acute headache and visual loss are the main manifestations [23, 24].

Depending on size, pituitary adenomas are classified into microadenomas and macroadenomas. Microadenomas are smaller than 10 mm in diameter and lie entirely within the pituitary gland. They appear as small, hypointense lesions on T_1-weighted images. Some may only become apparent as nonenhancing spots within the gland on post-contrast images (fig. 3). Their appearance on T_2-weighted images is variable. The pituitary stalk may or may not be displaced contralaterally, and the gland may show an upward convexity or a focal inferior bulging of the sellar floor. Thin coronal and sagittal sections both before and after half-dose gadolinium injection must be obtained in order to minimize the risk of small lesions remaining undetected because of partial volume averaging. Macroadenomas are larger than 10 mm in diameter (fig. 4). They expand the gland and may extend into the suprasellar cistern with a dumbbell shape on both sagittal and coronal sections. They may extend superiorly and stretch or compress the optic chiasm, compress the infundibulum, or extend laterally into the cavernous sinus. Macroadenomas show intermediate signal in unenhanced T_1-weighted images and enhance after contrast medium administration. Sometimes, adenomas can be hemorrhagic, in which case they show high T_1 signal intensity and variable T_2 signal intensity due to the presence of hemoglobin degradation products

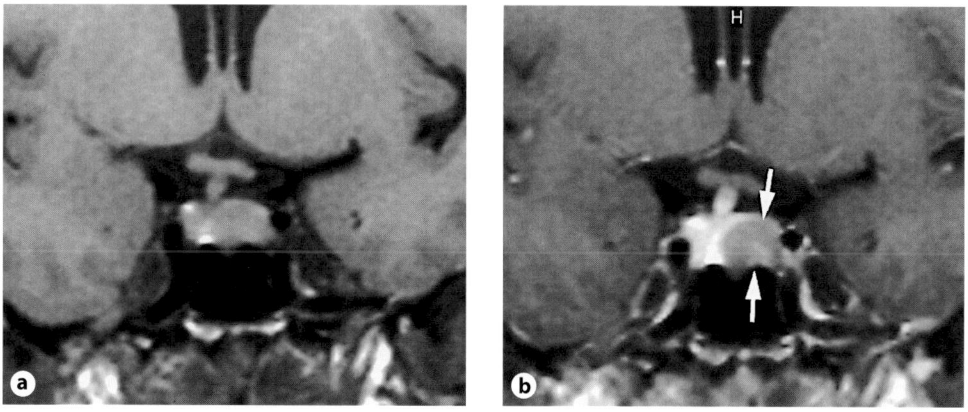

Fig. 3. PRL-releasing microadenoma in an 18-year-old girl. **a** Coronal T_1-weighted image. **b** Gd-enhanced coronal T_1-weighted image. The unenhanced coronal T_1-weighted image shows indirect signs of microadenoma: rising of the pituitary diaphragm on the left and contralateral shift of the pituitary stalk; however, the lesion itself is isointense with the normal pituitary gland parenchyma, and is therefore not immediately visible. Following gadolinium, the microadenoma is recognizable as a round hypointense area (arrows, **b**).

in various proportions [8]; sometimes, intralesional dependent fluid-fluid levels can be detected.

Diffusion-weighted MR imaging may assist in the early detection of acute pituitary infarction in clinically acute pituitary apoplexy showing areas of restricted diffusion [25]. Diffusion-weighted MR images with ADC maps can also provide information about the consistency of macroadenomas [26]. Proton MR spectroscopy may show marked reduction of N-acetylaspartate (NAA) peak, absence or presence of only residual creatine peak, moderate elevation of choline, and infrequent presence of small lipid and lactate peaks [27, 28].

Main Differential Diagnosis

Macroadenomas may be mistaken for other relatively frequent lesions in childhood, such as craniopharyngiomas, Rathke's cleft cysts, and suprasellar germinomas. Here, we describe these entities in order to propose an appropriate and accurate differential diagnosis.

Craniopharyngiomas

Craniopharyngiomas are benign epithelial tumors accounting for 5–13% of all intracranial neoplasms in the pediatric age group. Although may arise at any time in life,

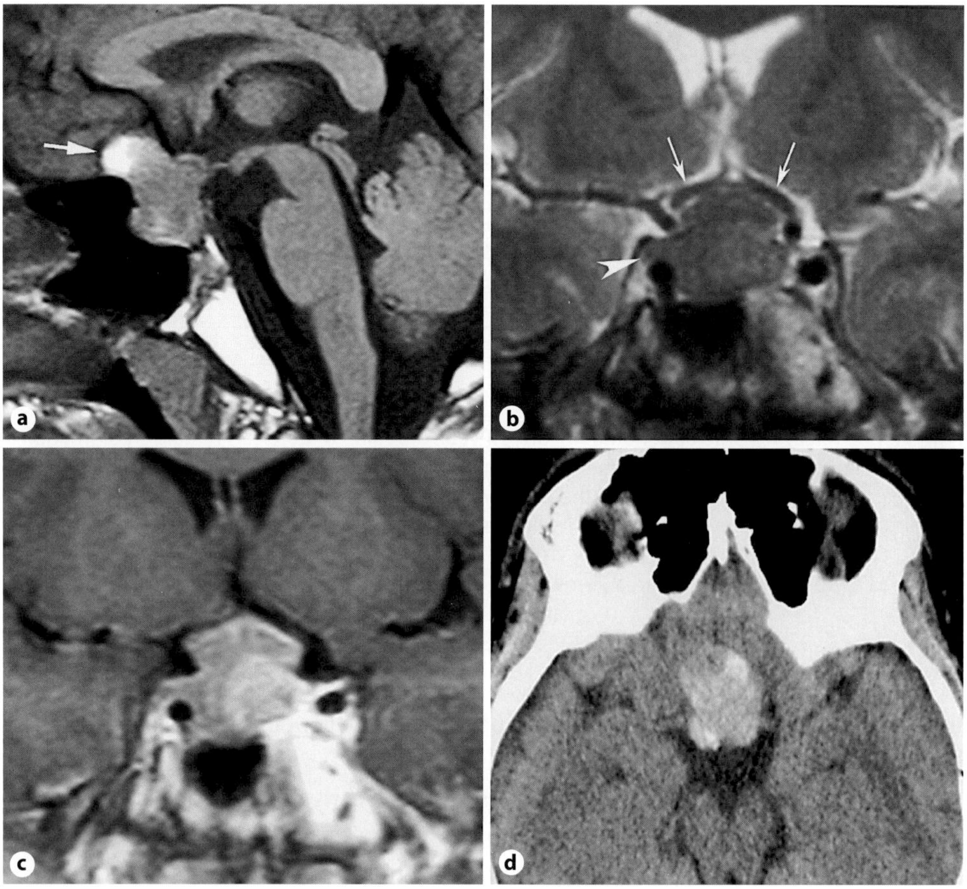

Fig. 4. GH-releasing macroadenoma in a 187-cm tall 11-year-old boy with McCune-Albright syndrome. **a** Sagittal T_1-weighted image. **b** Coronal T_2-weighted image. **c** Gd-enhanced coronal T_1-weighted image. **d** Axial CT scan. Huge lesion of the pituitary fossa extending cranially, with an anterior hemorrhagic portion (arrow, **a**). The lesion causes deformation of the chiasm and elevation of the A1 segments of the anterior cerebral arteries (arrows, **b**) in addition to the invasion of the right cavernous sinus (arrowhead, **b**). Following gadolinium administration, enhancement is moderate and diffuse (**c**). On CT scan (**d**), the lesion is spontaneously hyperdense, probably due to intralesional bleeding.

there is a bimodal incidence peak, at 5–14 years of age and in the 4th to 6th decade of life, respectively. Males are more commonly affected than females [8, 29, 30]. The clinical picture at the time of diagnosis is often characterized by non-endocrine manifestations, such as headache visual disturbances. However, up to 80% have evidence of endocrine dysfunction at diagnosis [31]. These tumors arise from remnants of the craniopharyngeal duct, connecting the stomodeal ectoderm with the evaginated Rathke's pouch. They may be intrasellar (25% of cases), suprasellar, or a combination of both. When the pituitary fossa is involved, the tumor has a hourglass shape and erodes the tuberculum and dorsum sellae. Pathologically, there are two separate types (adamantinous and squamous-papillary) with different histological, clinical, and radiological patterns [32]. Adamantinous craniopharyngiomas are cystic or predominantly cystic lobulated tumors, typical of childhood and only occasionally found in adults. Squamous-papillary craniopharyngiomas are typical of adults, and are believed to arise from squamous epithelial cells in the pars tuberalis of the adenohypophysis. They usually appear as predominantly solid or mixed solid-cystic spherical suprasellar masses [33].

Castillo and Mukherji [34] defined the «rule of the 90s» that characterizes craniopharyngiomas: 90% are cystic, 90% have calcifications, 90% enhance, and over 90% are suprasellar in location. On MRI (fig. 5), craniopahryngiomas show the most heterogeneous spectrum of signal behavior of all sellar/suprasellar masses. The most common pattern is represented by a cystic lesion that is hyperintense on both T_1-weighted and T_2-weighted images due to high protein concentration and/or to the presence of methemoglobin [35], with enhancing walls and subtle peripheral calcifications. Solid tumor components, often located in the intra- or parasellar region, are often heavily calcified and appear iso-hypointense in T_1-weighted images with variable, often low signal intensity on T_2-weighted images; these components typically enhance following gadolinium administration. CT is superior to MRI in the identification of calcifications that represent a hallmark of craniopharyngiomas; therefore, CT scans should always be obtained in case of suprasellar tumors. Morphologically, calcifications may appear as shell-like deposits along the cyst walls, or may form fine punctuations or lumps within the substance of the lesion.

Craniopharyngiomas may produce an elevation and deformation of the optic chiasm. The pituitary stalk and the posterior pituitary 'bright spot', albeit compressed and distorted, are usually preserved, even with large craniopharyngiomas; this sign can be useful in the differential diagnosis with other neoplastic and non-neoplastic conditions occurring in this region. Encasement of adjacent vessels, especially of the circle of Willis, is another recognized feature of craniopharyngiomas and represents an obstacle to radical surgery.

Proton MR spectroscopy may show a prominent lipid peak (fig. 6), with only small quantities of other metabolites or absence of any detectable metabolite peak [27, 28].

Rathke's Cleft Cysts

Rathke's cleft cysts (RCC) are intrasellar and/or suprasellar benign cysts containing mucoid material, accounting for fewer than 1% of all intracranial masses [8]. These congenital lesions arise from remnants of the Rathke's pouch; thus, they are embryologically related to craniopharyngiomas. Although usually stable, they may rarely enlarge, causing visual disturbances or pituitary dysfunction.

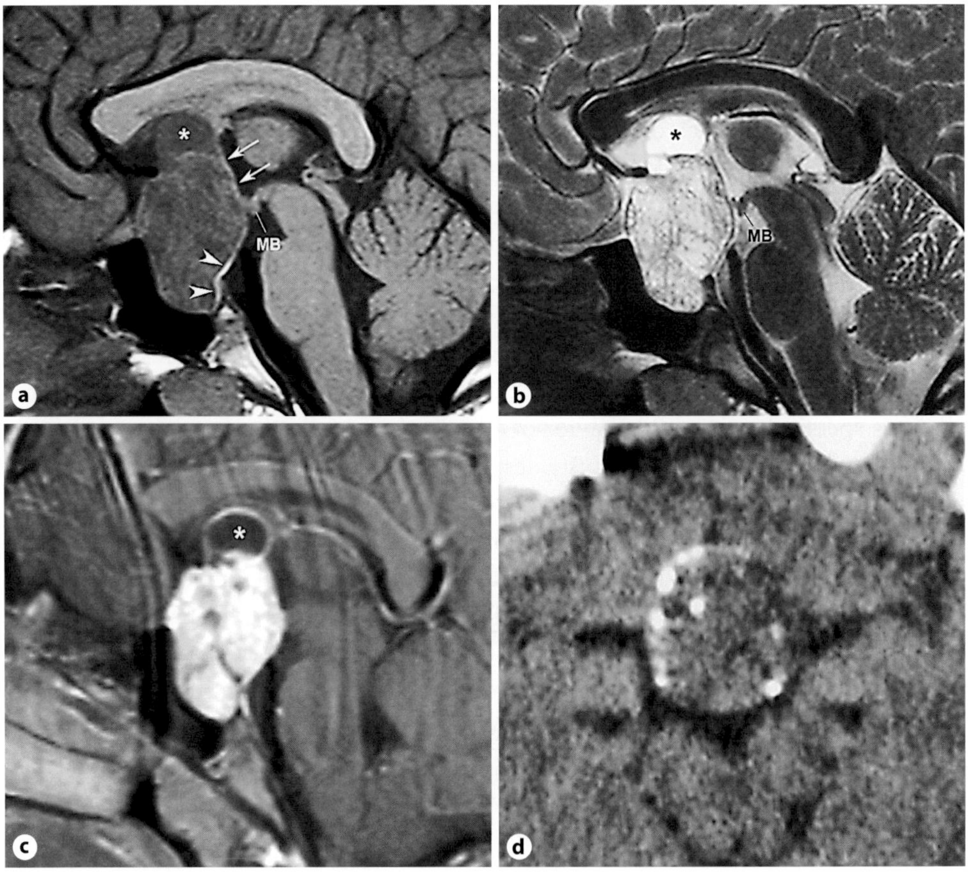

Fig. 5. Adamantinous craniopharyngioma in a 13-year-old girl presenting with visual disturbances. **a** Sagittal T_1-weighted image. **b** Sagittal T_2-weighted image. **c** Gd-enhanced sagittal T_1-weighted image. **d** Axial CT scan. Huge mass extending from the sellar floor up to the foramen of Monro. The lesion is markedly hypointense on T_1-weighted (**a**) and hyperintense on T_2-weighted images (**b**), and shows marginal cysts at the superior pole (asterisk, **a–c**). Following gadolinium administration, the whole solid lesion and the walls of the cyst enhance markedly and slightly inhomogeneously. The anterior third ventricle is amputated (arrows, **a**) and the mammillary bodies ('MB', **a**, **b**) are displaced. Note that the posterior pituitary lobe, albeit deformed and stretched, is still visible as a thin, spontaneously hyperintense stripe along the posterior margin of the tumor (arrowhead, **a**). CT scan (**d**) shows multiple small nodular calcifications prevailingly along the right antero-lateral surface of the mass.

On MRI (fig. 7) they appear as rounded cysts with variable signal behavior both on T_1- and T_2-weighted images. On T_1-weighted images, about two thirds are hyperintense to brain and one third shows low signal intensity, similar to CSF. On T_2-weighted images, about 50% are hyperintense, 25% isointense, and 25% hypointense; presence of a hypointense spot within a hyperintense cyst is said to be a characteristic finding. Contrast enhancement is absent. CT density varies with cyst content, with most cysts appearing hypodense to brain [8, 36].

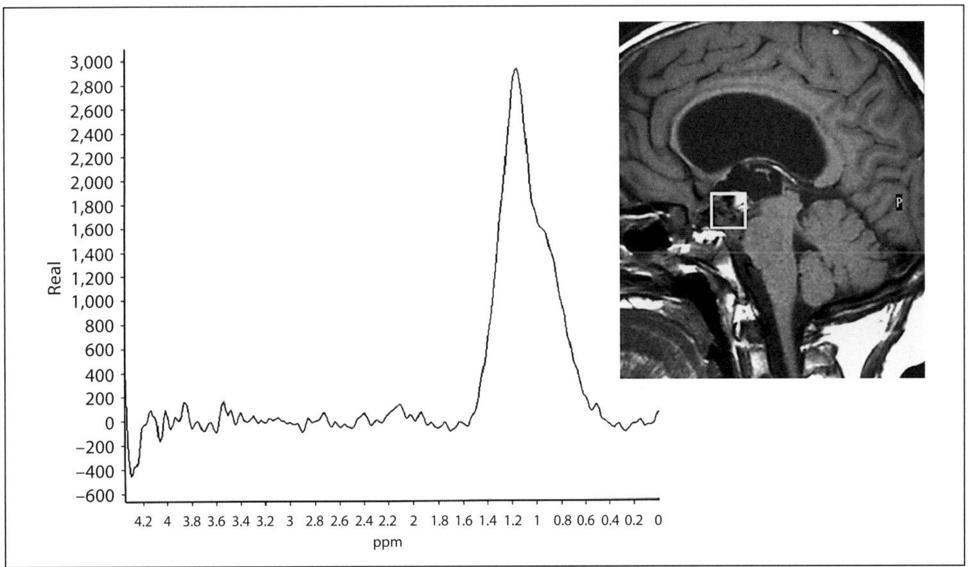

Fig. 6. MR spectroscopy in a case of craniopharyngioma. This single-voxel MR spectrum obtained with a PRESS technique at TE 144 ms shows prominent lipid peak with absence of other metabolites.

RCC are often difficult to differentiate from other sellar cystic lesions using conventional MR imaging. Differentiation from craniopharyngiomas is based on several factors, including location (prevailingly suprasellar in craniopharyngiomas and intrasellar in RCC) and presence of wall enhancement, calcification, and solid components (all features of craniopharyngiomas but not of RCC) [8, 37]. Regarding differentiation from pituitary adenomas, location is an important factor in that RCC typically lie centrally in the pars intermedia, i.e. between the anterior and posterior pituitary lobes, whereas pituitary adenomas are often eccentric and typically located within the adenohypophysis, whose tissue partially or completely surrounds the adenoma [37]. These features are particularly relevant in case of hemorrhagic adenomas, whose signal behavior may be indistinguishable from that of RCC.

On diffusion-weighted imaging, RCC are hypointense relative to normal brain parenchyma. It has recently been demonstrated that ADC values of RCC are significantly higher than those of the cystic components of craniopharyngiomas and hemorrhagic components of pituitary adenomas in the subacute phase, thus providing useful information in the differential diagnosis of RCC from other sellar cystic lesions [38]. Proton MR spectroscopy may show absence of all metabolites except lactate and lipid peaks [28].

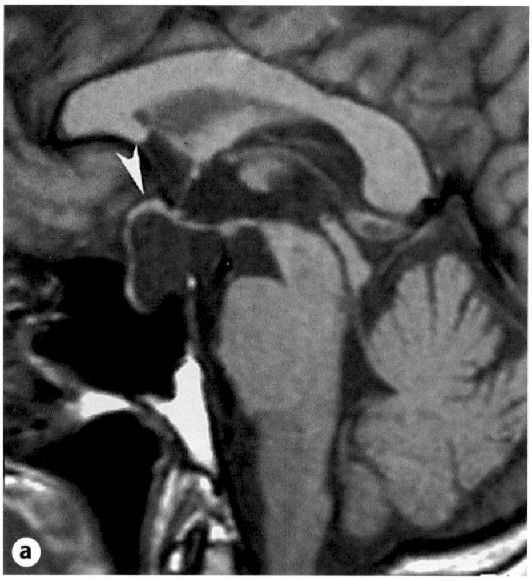

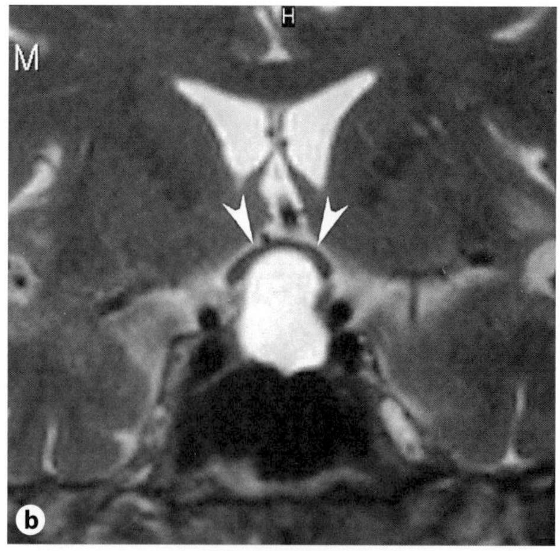

Fig. 7. Rathke's cleft cyst. **a** Sagittal T_1-weighted image. **b** Coronal T_2-weighted image. **c** Gd-enhanced coronal T_1-weighted image. A huge cystic intrasellar lesion developing in the suprasellar region is shown. Signal intensity of is slightly higher than that of CSF both on T_1-weighted (**a**) and T_2-weighted images (**b**). Following gadolinium, enhancement along the lateral aspect of the cyst is due to displaced adenohypophyseal tissue (arrows, **c**). Note stretched, elevated chiasm and anterior third ventricle (arrowhead, **a–c**).

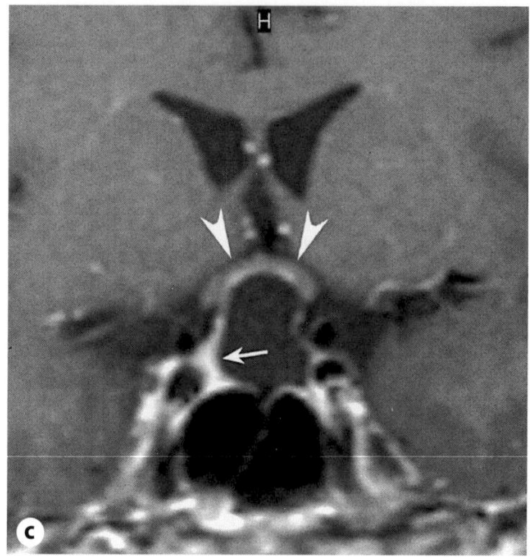

Suprasellar Germinomas

Suprasellar germinomas are rare intracranial neoplasms mainly occurring in children and adolescents with an incidence peak at 10–12 years. The suprasellar region is the second most common location of intracranial germinomas after the pineal region. Synchronous lesions in the hypothalamic and pineal regions account for 10% of all intracranial germ cell tumors. [8]. Affected children present with endocrine symptoms such as diabetes insipidus, delayed sexual development, growth hormone deficiency, and precocious puberty. Patients may also present with ophthalmic abnormalities such as bilateral temporal hemianopsia. Confirmation of the diagnosis requires measurement of serum and CSF tumor markers (α-fetoprotein and/or β-human chorionic gonadotropin) and/or biopsy [39].

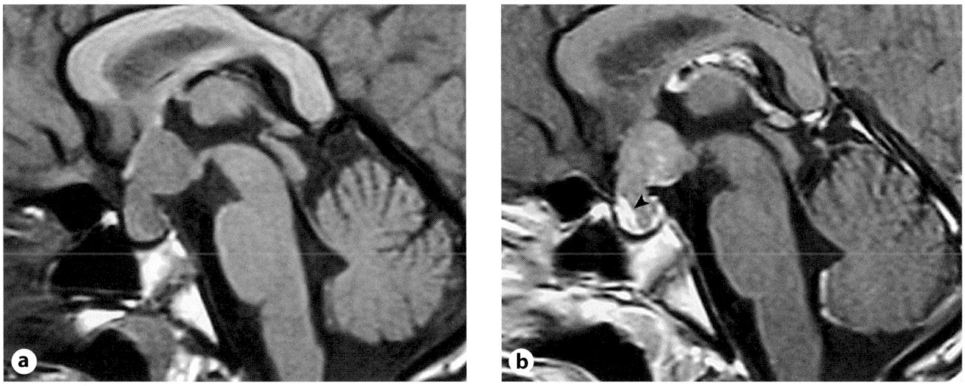

Fig. 8. Suprasellar germinoma in an 11-year-old girl. **a** Sagittal T_1-weighted image. **b** Gd-enhanced sagittal T_1-weighted image. Mass of the hypothalamic-hypophyseal region. The posterior bright spot is not recognizable (**a**), whereas the anterior pituitary lobe is seen following gadolinium (arrowhead, **b**) as a deformed and compressed structure.

Small tumors are characterized only by thickening of the infundibulum with dense homogeneous enhancement and no cystic components. With tumor growth, the normal pituitary gland may be compressed by the mass extending into the sella turcica. The tumor may also manifest as a giant sellar mass, without identification of the normal pituitary gland parenchyma [40].

On MRI (fig. 8), germinomas are generally isointense to gray matter on T_1-weighted images and isointense on T_2-weighted images [8]. The short T_2 relaxation time presumably reflects the diminished free water content of these tumors. Contrast enhancement is usually moderate to marked. Calcification and cystic-necrotic changes are rare.

Diffusion-weighted MR imaging shows restricted diffusion (DWI hyperintensity and ADC hypointensity) [41], while proton MR spectroscopy is characterized by predominance of choline peak, residual creatine peak, absence or marked reduction of NAA, and possible lactate and lipid peaks [28, 41].

It is important to recognize that, in children suffering from diabetes insipidus showing absence of visualization of the posterior 'bright spot', a small germinoma could not yet be visible on the initial MR images. A close follow-up with repeated imaging studies should therefore be carried out in these patients [8, 41]. A thickened infundibulum or pituitary stalk may also suggest lymphocytic hypophysitis, Langerhans cell histiocytosis, lymphoma, and granulomatous diseases (such as tuberculosis and sarcoidosis). However, it may also be present in idiopathic cases with central diabetes insipidus. MRI evidence of an increase in the size of the anterior pituitary with thickening of the stalk is strongly associated with the presence of a germinoma, whereas a decrease of normal gland parenchyma can suggest an inflammatory or autoimmune process such as lymphocytic infundibulohypophysitis [42].

Incidentalomas

Incidentalomas of the pituitary gland are defined as intrasellar mass lesions that are discovered incidentally on CT or MRI studies performed to evaluate unrelated problems. The increased availability and the advances in diagnostic imaging modalities have led to an increased identification of these lesions, which might therefore be termed 'modern technology diseases' [43, 44]. Very little is known about the exact incidence and prevalence of asymptomatic incidentalomas in childhood. An evaluation of nonselected autopsy pituitary specimens [45] revealed no incidental lesions in subjects aged 0–9 years, while the frequency of pituitary lesions in autopsy specimens from subjects aged 10–29 years was 1.7%; these lesions were represented by Rathke's cleft cysts, whereas pituitary adenomas were not found. Another study evaluating MR imaging studies in a group of 341 patients aged less than 15 years revealed only 4 pituitary cystic lesions (frequency 1.2%) [37]. In our routine work with children, pituitary cysts on MR imaging of asymptomatic (with respect to the hypothalamic-pituitary axis) patients are not rare, while incidental pituitary adenomas have been exceptional. In fact, small slow-growing hormonally inactive lesions that could be identified incidentally are very rare, accounting for only 4–6% of pituitary adenomas in the pediatric literature [22].

Although rare, incidentalomas may create management difficulties. Any incidental adenoma or cyst confined to the sella, discovered in an asymptomatic patient with normal pituitary function, should be managed by watchful waiting. Hormonally active prolactin-secreting tumors can be treated with dopamine agonists. Other hormonally active tumors and those that are causing a mass effect should be surgically removed [46].

References

1 Batista D, Courkoutsakis NA, Oldfield EH, Griffin KJ, Keil M, Patronas NJ, Stratakis CA: Detection of adrenocorticotropin-secreting pituitary adenomas by magnetic resonance imaging in children and adolescents with Cushing disease. J Clin Endocrinol Metab 2005;90:5134–5140.

2 Bartynski WS, Lin L: Dynamic and conventional spin-echo MR of pituitary microlesions. Am J Neuororadiol 1997;18:965–972.

3 Cox TD, Elster AD: Normal pituitary gland: changes in shape, size, and signal intensity during the 1st year of life at MR imaging. Radiology 1991;179:721–724.

4 Dietrich RB, Lis LE, Greensite FS, Duane P: Normal MR appearance of the pituitary gland in the first 2 years of life. Am J Neuroradiol 1995;16:1413–1419.

5 Asa SL, Kovacs K, Laszlo FA, Damokos I, Ezrin C: Human fetal adenohypophysis: histologic and immunocytochemical analysis. Neuroendocrinology 1986; 43:308–316.

6 Bonneville F, Cattin F, Marsot-Dupuch K, Dormonnt D, Bonneville JF, Chiras J: T_1 signal hyperintensity in the sellar region: spectrum of findings. Radiographics 2006;26:93–113.

7 Kurokawa H, Fujisawa I, Nakano Y, Kimura H, Akagi K, Ikeda K, Uokawa K, Tanaka Y: Posterior lobe of the pituitary gland: correlation between signal intensity on T_1-weighted MR images and vasopressin concentration. Radiology 1998;207:79–83.

8 Tortori-Donati P: Pediatric Neuroradiology. Heidelberg, Springer, 2005.

9 Maghnie M, Genovese E, Aricò M, Villa A, Beluffi G, Campani R, Severi F: Evolving pituitary hormone deficiency is associated with pituitary vasculopathy: dynamic MR study in children with hypopituitarism, diabetes insipidus, and Langerhans cell histiocytosis. Radiology 1994;193:493–499.

10 Simmons GE, Suchnicki JE, Rak KM, Damiano TR: MR imaging of the pituitary stalk: size, shape, and enhancement pattern. Am J Roentgenol 1992;159: 375–377.

11 Elster AD, Chen MTM, Williams DW III, Key LL: Pituitary gland: MR imaging of physiologic hypertrophy in adolescence. Radiology 1990;174:681–685.

12 Young M, Kattner K, Gupta K: Pituitary hyperplasia resulting from primary hypothyroidism mimicking macroadenomas. Br J Neurosurg 1999;13:138–142.

13 Gold FB: Epidemiology of pituitary adenomas. Epidemiol Rev 1981;3:163–183.

14 Haddad SF, Van Gilder JC, Menezes AH: Pediatric pituitary tumors. Neurosurgery 1991;29:509–514.

15 Laws ER, Sheithauer BW, Groover RV: Pituitary adenomas in childhood and adolescence. Prog Exp Tumor Res 1987;30:359–361.

16 Mindermann T, Wilson CB: Pediatric pituitary adenomas. Neurosurgery 1995;36:259–269.

17 Magiakou MA, Chrousos GP: Cushing's syndrome in children and adolescents: current diagnostic and therapeutic strategies. J Endocrinol Invest 2002;25: 181–194.

18 Magiakou MA, Mastorakos G, Oldfield EH, Gomez MT, Doppman JL, Cutler GB Jr, Nieman LK, Chrousos GP: Cushing's syndrome in children and adolescents. Presentation, diagnosis and therapy. N Engl J Med 1994;331:629–636.

19 Batista D, Gennari M, Riar J, Chang R, Keil MF, Oldfield EH, Stratakis CA: An assessment of petrosal sinus sampling for localization of pituitary microadenomas in children with Cushing disease. J Clin Endocrinol Metab 2006;91:221–224.

20 Storr HL, Chan Li F, Grossman AB, Savage MO: Paediatric Cushing's syndrome: epidemiology, investigation and therapeutic advances. Trends Endocrinol Metab 2007;18:167–174.

21 Savage MO, Chan Li F, Farhad Afshar P, Plowman N, Grossman AB, Storr HL: Advances in the management of paediatric Cushing's disease. Horm Res 2008;69:327–333.

22 Lafferty AR, Chrousos GP: Pituitary tumors in children and adolescents. J Clin Endocrinol Metab 1999;84:4317–4323.

23 Bills DC, Meyer FB: A retrospective analysis of pituitary apoplexy. Neurosurgery 1993;33:602–609.

24 Shah S, Pereira J, Becker C, Aronin P: Pituitary apoplexy in adolescence: case report. Pediatr Radiol 1995;25:26–27.

25 Rogg JM, Tung GA, Anderson G, Cortez S: Pituitary apoplexy: early detection with diffusion-weighted MR imaging. Am J Neuroradiol 2002;23:1240–1245.

26 Pierallini A, Caramia F, Falcone C, Tinelli E, Paonessa A, Ciddio AB, Fiorelli M, Bianco F, Natalizi S, Ferrante L, Bozzao L: Pituitary macroadenomas: preoperative evaluation of consistency with diffusion-weighted MR imaging: initial experience. Radiology 2006;239:223–231.

27 Sutton LN, Wang ZJ, Wehrli SL, Marwaha S, Molloy P, Phillips PC, Zimmerman RA: Proton spectroscopy of suprasellar tumors in pediatric patients. Neurosurgery 1997;41:388–395.

28 Chernov MF, Kawamata T, Amano K, Ono Y, Suzuki T, Nakamura R, Muragaki Y, Iseki H, Kubo O, Hori T, Takakura K: Possible role of single-voxel (1) H-MRS in differential diagnosis of suprasellar tumors. J Neurooncol 2009;91:191–198.

29 Bunin GR, Surawicz TS, Witman PA, Preston-Martin S, Davis F, Bruner JM: The descriptive epidemiology of craniopharyngioma. J Neurosurg 1998;89:547–551.

30 Rossi A, Cama A, Consales A, Gandolfo C, Garrè ML, Milanaccio C, Pavanello M, Piattelli G, Ravegnani M, Tortori-Donati P: Neuroimaging of pediatric craniopharyngiomas: a pictorial essay. J Pediatr Endocrinol Metab 2006;19(suppl 1):299–319.

31 Sklar CA: Craniopharyngioma: endocrine abnormalities at presentation. Pediatr Neurosurg 1994; 21(suppl 1):18–20.

32 Sartoretti-Schefer S, Wichmann W, Aguzzi A, Valavanis A: MR differentiation of adamantinous and squamous-papillary craniopharyngiomas. Am J Neuroradiol 1997;18:77–87.

33 Eldevik OP, Blaivas M, Gabrielsen TO, Hald JK, Chandler WF: Craniopharyngioma: radiologic and histologic findings and recurrence. Am J Neuroradiol 1996;17:1427–1439.

34 Castillo M, Mukherji SK: Imaging of the Pediatric Head, Neck, and Spine. Philadelphia, Lippincott-Raven, 1996.

35 Ahmadi J, Destian S, Apuzzo ML, Segall HD, Zee CS: Cystic fluid in craniopharyngiomas: MR imaging and quantitative analysis. Radiology 1992;182: 783–785.

36 Naylor MF, Scheithauer BW, Forbes GS, Tomlinson FH, Young WF: Rathke cleft cyst: CT, MR, and pathology of 23 cases. J Comput Assist Tomogr 1995;19:853–859.

37 Takanashi J, Tada H, Barkovich AJ, Saeki N, Kohno Y: Pituitary cysts in childhood evaluated by MR imaging. Am J Neuroradiol 2005;26:2144–2147.

38 Kunii N, Abe T, Kawamo M, Tanioka D, Izumiyama H, Moritani T: Rathke's cleft cysts: differentiation from other cystic lesions in the pituitary fossa by use of single-shot fast spin-echo diffusion-weighted MR imaging. Acta Neurochir 2007;149:759–769.
39 Echevarría ME, Fangusaro J, Goldman S: Pediatric central nervous system germ cell tumors: a review. Oncologist 2008;13:690–699.
40 Liang L, Korogi Y, Sugahara T, Ikushima I, Shigematsu Y, Okuda T, Takahashi M, Kochi M, Ushio Y: MRI of intracranial germ-cell tumours. Neuroradiology 2002;44:382–388.
41 Barkovich AJ: Diagnostic Imaging: Pediatric Neuroradiology. Salt Lake City, Amirsys Inc, 2007.
42 Maghnie M, Cosi G, Genovese E, Manca-Bitti ML, Cohen A, Zecca S, Tinelli C, Gallucci M, Bernasconi S, Boscherini B, Severi F, Aricò M: Central diabetes insipidus in children and young adults. N Engl J Med 2000;343:998–1007.
43 Krikorian A, Aron D: Evaluation and management of pituitary incidentalomas: revisiting an acquaintance. Nat Clin Pract Endocrinol Metab 2006;2:138–145.
44 Chidiac RM, Aron DC: Incidentalomas: a disease of modern technology. Endocrinol Metab Clin North Am 1997;26:233–253.
45 Teramoto A, Hirakawa K, Sanno N, Osamura Y: Incidental pituitary lesions in 1,000 unselected autopsy specimens. Radiology 1994;193:161–164.
46 Serhal D, Weil RJ, Hamrahian AH: Evaluation and management of pituitary incidentalomas. Cleve Clin J Med 2008;75:793–801.

Giovanni Morana, MD
Department of Pediatric Neuroradiology, IRCCS 'G. Gaslini'
Largo G. Gaslini 5, IT–16147 Genoa (Italy)
Tel. +39 0105636516, Fax +39 0103779798
E-Mail giovannimorana@ospedale-gaslini.ge.it, giomorana@yahoo.it

Loche S, Cappa M, Ghizzoni L, Maghnie M, Savage MO (eds): Pediatric Neuroendocrinology.
Endocr Dev. Basel, Karger, 2010, vol 17, pp 175–184

Resistin: Regulation of Food Intake, Glucose Homeostasis and Lipid Metabolism

Ruben Nogueiras · Marta G. Novelle · María Jesús Vazquez · Miguel Lopez · Carlos Dieguez

Department of Physiology, School of Medicine, University of Santiago de Compostela, Instituto de Investigación Sanitaria, and CIBER Fisiopatología de la Obesidad y Nutrición (CIBERobn), Santiago de Compostela, Spain

Abstract

Resistin has been identified as a hormone secreted by adipocytes that is under hormonal and nutritional control. This hormone has been suggested to be the link between obesity and type 2 diabetes. In rodents, resistin is mainly located and secreted from adipocytes, even though its expression was also found in several other tissues. However, in humans resistin is expressed primarily by macrophages and seems to be involved in the recruitment of other immune cells and the secretion of pro-inflammatory factors, although its role in insulin resistance cannot be ruled out. In addition to its role in glucose metabolism, resistin has been also involved in the control of hypothalamic and peripheral lipid metabolism and in the regulation of food intake. In this short review, we will summarize the most relevant findings of this hormone in rodents.

The primary role of adipocytes is to store triacylglycerol during periods of caloric excess and to mobilize this reserve when expenditure exceeds intake. However, there is now compelling evidence that adipocytes act as endocrine secretory cells, since it has been shown that several hormones, growth factors, and cytokines are actually expressed in white adipose tissue (WAT). A growing number of adipocyte-derived factors have been described and their contribution to the pathophysiology of the metabolic syndrome, characterized by central adiposity, insulin resistance, dyslipidemia, hypertension, chronic inflammation and a prothrombotic state, is being investigated. These adipocyte-specific or enriched proteins, termed adipokines, have been shown to have a variety of local, peripheral, and central effects. Adipose tissue is therefore able to integrate signals from other organs and respond by regulating secretion of multiple proteins, and is an active participant in whole body energy homeostasis regulation.

Since an excess of adipose tissue is associated with dyslipidemia, obesity and the insulin resistance of type 2 diabetes, it was accepted that overloading the capacity for fat storage, combined with excessive lipolysis and release of free fatty acid, caused defects in glucose homeostasis. However, the severe loss of fat tissue, as characterized by lipodystrophy, also leads to numerous metabolic abnormalities such as insulin resistance and type 2 diabetes. During the last years, many efforts have been made to understand the role of adipokines on the regulation of energy homeostasis. In this review, we will focus on some novel aspects of resistin.

The Discovery of Resistin

Resistin was discovered independently by three different groups, thus it received three different names (FIZZ3, resistin and ADSF). Holcomb et al. [1] described three murine genes and two human homologs, which together composed a novel gene family. Each encoded protein had an N-terminal signal peptide, a processed N-terminal domain of 28–44 residues having only limited homology among the family and a well-conserved cysteine-rich C-terminal domain of 57–60 residues with little primary amino acid homology to any known proteins [1]. Independently, another group [2] identified a serine/cysteine-rich adipocyte-specific secretory factor (ADSF). The cDNA sequence of rat ADSF revealed a 1,174-bp cDNA [2] specifically expressed in adipose tissue [2]. Finally, the laboratory of Dr. Lazar discovered the same peptide and called it resistin [3], because it caused insulin resistance.

Regulation of Resistin by Obesity and Insulin/Glucose Alterations

The quantification of resistin has been quite controversial since its discovery. Serum levels of resistin were found to be increased in several rodent models of obesity and diabetes such as leptin- and leptin receptor-deficient mice [3]. On the contrary, it was also reported that resistin gene and protein levels were markedly decreased in adipose and serum of several obese models when compared to lean controls [4, 5]. Another group reported no changes in resistin gene expression in WAT from leptin-deficient mice [6]. The discrepancies were also observed in models of insulin resistance such as the fructose-fed rats [7] or in a transgenic mouse model fed a high-fat diet (HFD) [8], which showed lower levels of resistin but the opposite result was found in rats with alcohol-induced insulin resistance [9] or Fischer 344 rats [10], where resistin levels were increased.

In addition to studies in which resistin regulation was assessed in obesity and diabetes, its expression was also measured in response to insulin and glucose. An in vivo report has shown that insulin itself stimulate resistin expression and secretion in WAT [2]. However, an intro study showed a marked suppressive effect of insulin on resistin mRNA levels in 3T3-L1 adipocytes [11]. Consistent with this in vitro observation, a population of wild-type mice on a HFD showed that hyperinsulinemia reduced resistin mRNA and protein levels [8]. The findings with glucose were more consistent since resistin levels were increased in response to hyperglycemia in mice [4] and in 3T-L1 adipocytes [12].

The controversial results on resistin expression were also found after treatment with antidiabetic agents. Thiazolidinediones (TZDs) are antidiabetic drugs including rosiglitazone, which reduced serum resistin levels and WAT gene and protein expression in lean and obese/diabetic mice compared to the lean controls [3, 13]. Surprisingly, another study showed that treatment with TZDs increased WAT resistin expression in ob/ob mice and Zucker diabetic fatty rats [5]. Metformin, which is widely used as an oral glucose-lowering drug to treat type 2 diabetic patients, increased resistin protein expression in adipose tissue of mice lacking the leptin receptor, even though an improvement in hyperinsulinemia and hyperglycemia was found [14].

The regulation of resistin by factors inducing insulin resistance was also studied. Dexamethasone, a synthetic glucocorticoid, which is well known to impair insulin sensitivity, increased resistin expression in both 3T3-L1 adipocytes and white adipose tissue [12]. On the contrary, tumor necrosis factor-α (TNFα) which potently induces insulin resistance inhibited resistin gene expression and protein secretion resistin gene expression [15]. Increased serum levels of thyroid hormones can also impair glucose tolerance and it was found that resistin was downregulated in hyperthyroid rats [16].

In humans, the primary site of expression of resistin is circulating mononuclear cells [17]. Some studies were unable to detect resistin in human adipocytes [17], but others detected resistin in adipose tissue and found that resistin levels were increased in the serum and adipose tissue of obese subjects compared with lean control subjects [17–19], which positively correlated with body mass index and visceral fat content [17, 20, 21]. On the contrary, other laboratories did not find any correlation between resistin gene expression in human adipocytes and insulin resistance [22]. Although the role of resistin in humans is largely unknown, one report has demonstrated that resistin slightly but significantly reduced glucose uptake in human adipocytes [19]. The reasons for these discrepancies are unclear but may well be related to the limited reliability of some of the immunoassays used for resistin measurements and that the mRNA levels assessed in WAT may well be dependent on the degree of infiltration by mononuclear cells.

Effects of Resistin on Glucose Metabolism

Resistin has been postulated to participate in the regulation of glucose metabolism because its administration to rodents increased blood glucose levels [3] whereas immunoneutralization of this protein improved insulin action [3]. Consistent with the increased glucose levels, the hepatic glucose production increased by the upregulation of the enzyme glucose-6-phosphatase [23]. As a matter of fact, resistin induced all the pathways involved in the formation of liver glucose-6-phosphatase: gluconeogenesis, glycogenolysis and glucose cycling [23]. In vitro studies have also detected a decrease in glucose uptake that is independent of insulin signaling and glucose transporter 4 (GLUT4) translocation [24]. Resistin has been also detected in human and murine pancreatic islets [25]. In vitro studies have shown that resistin decreases the expression of the insulin receptor but not insulin secretion in rodent pancreatic beta cells [26]. Consistent with that report, transiently resistin-expressing mice showed an impaired insulin secretory response to glucose, leading to insulin resistance [27].

The role of chronic hyperresistinemia was also studied in different reports. The administration of an adenovirus encoding resistin, which induced insulin resistance in skeletal muscle, liver and adipose tissue, resulted in glucose intolerance, hyperinsulinemia, and hypertriglyceridemia [28]. The mechanism whereby resistin decreased insulin sensitivity involved a reduction in AMP-activated protein kinase (AMPK) activity in skeletal muscle, adipose tissue and liver and of insulin receptor substrate-1 (IRS-1) in adipose tissue and skeletal muscle [28]. Consistent with that report, transgenic mice that have high circulating levels of resistin showed higher fasting blood glucose levels, glucose intolerance and elevated hepatic glucose production [29]. In this report, the increase in glucose production was partially explained by the increased expression of hepatic phosphoenolpyruvate carboxykinase (PEPCK), but no changes were found in glucose-6-phosphatase levels [29].

Another study aimed to determine if the elevation in circulating levels of resistin associated with HFD played an important role in the onset of insulin resistance. To test that hypothesis, a sequence-specific antisense oligonucleotide directed against resistin mRNA was administered during 1 week in rodents fed on HFD [30]. This treatment normalized the plasma resistin levels and completely reversed the hepatic insulin resistance [30]. The molecular mechanism mediating those actions seems to be AMPK, since the decrease of plasma resistin concentration by the antisense oligonucleotide increased AMPK phosphorylation, whereas the infusion of resistin decreased AMPK phosphorylation [30].

The administration of resistin in the central nervous system also impaired glucose homeostasis. Resistin injection into the cerebral ventricle in rat blunted insulin action in the liver [30]. Central infusion of resistin was associated with neuronal activation in the arcuate, paraventricular and dorsomedial nuclei, and increased neuropeptide Y (NPY) expression [31]. The ability of resistin to increase hepatic insulin resistance and modulate the levels of various mediators in the liver was mediated by NPY [31]. For instance, the capacity of resistin to increase hepatic insulin resistance in the liver was blunted in mice lacking NPY as well as mice pretreated with a central NPY Y1 receptor antagonist [31].

Finally, mice lacking endogenous resistin have been also generated. These mice did not show any difference in body weight or food intake, but they exhibited low blood glucose levels after fasting, due to reduced hepatic glucose production [32]. Consistent with the pharmacological data stated above, the beneficial effects of the lack of resistin were partially mediated by the activation of AMPK and the decreased expression of gluconeogenic enzymes in the liver such as glucose-6-phosphatase and PEPCK [32]. Another study determined the role of resistin in the obese and insulin-resistant ob/ob mice, which do not have leptin [33]. Surprisingly, the loss of resistin increased obesity in ob/ob mice without affecting food intake [33]. The increased body weight and fat mass in the double knockout mice was explained by a decrease in the energy expenditure and the expression of uncoupling protein-1 (UCP-1) and peroxisome proliferator-activated receptor-coactivator-1α in brown adipose tissue [33]. Nevertheless, resistin deficiency improved glucose tolerance and insulin sensitivity. Although the hepatic glucose production was unmodified, the double knockouts showed an enhanced insulin-mediated glucose disposal in muscle and white and brown adipose tissues [33]. The molecular pathway involved in the improvement of glucose metabolism in the double knockout mice seems to be related with AKT and suppressor of cytokine signaling 3 (SOCS-3), since phosphorylation of AKT (protein kinase B; PKB) was increased while the expression of SOCS-3 was decreased when compared to ob/ob mice [33]. Interestingly, the molecular mechanisms by which the lack of resistin improves glucose metabolism were different in double knockout mice and in diet-induced (DIO) obese mice, since the lack of resistin in DIO mice reduced hepatic glucose production and increased peripheral glucose uptake [33].

Resistin and Lipid Metabolism

Adipocytes play an essential role in storing triglycerides which provide energy in the form of free fatty acids (FFA), and the released FFA may contribute to insulin resistance in peripheral tissues. Therefore, it was plausible to hypothesize that resistin might represent a link between increased FFA plasma levels and insulin resistance. However, the results obtained by different laboratories are controversial and this hypothesis has been not clearly proven. In one of the first studies, FFA levels were found to suppress the expression of resistin [7]. These results were in agreement with a prior observation that resistin mRNA expression was inhibited by starvation, a condition accompanied by increased lipolysis and elevated concentrations of intracellular FFA. Another work assessed the effect of specific dietary FFAs on resistin mRNA expression and found that stearic acid promoted a small increase in resistin expression, whereas arachidonic acid and eicosapentaenoic acid reduced resistin mRNA levels [34]. On the contrary, another report found that FFA increased the release of resistin, hypothesizing that the FFA-induced release of resistin may contribute to the development of FFA-induced insulin resistance in rats [35]. Consistent with that report, obese Zucker rats fed a conjugated linoleic acids (CLA) mixture showed higher adipose resistin expression than control obese Zucker rats [36].

Although several reports have studied the regulation of resistin by fatty acids, little is known about the effect of resistin on lipid metabolism. An in vitro study has found that treating rat skeletal muscle cells with resistin decreased the uptake of palmitate

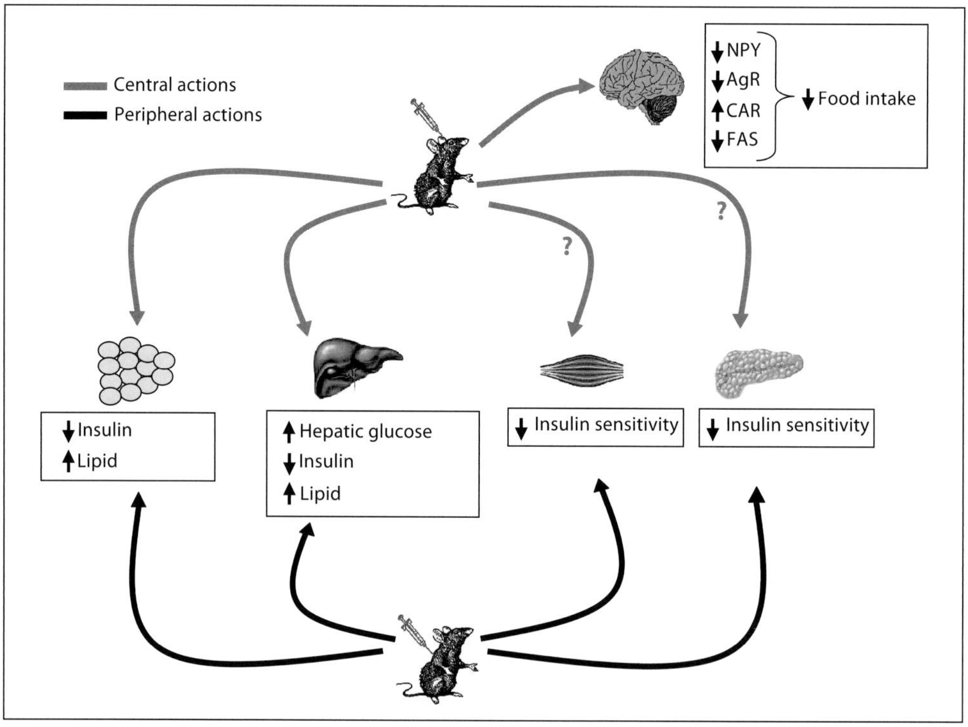

Fig. 1. Effects of central vs. peripheral resistin on food intake, lipid metabolism and insulin sensitivity in different tissues.

and fatty acid oxidation, while it increased intracellular lipid accumulation [37]. Those effects seem to be mediated by the reduced cell surface cluster of differentiation 36 (CD36) content, lower expression of fatty acid transport protein 1 (FATP1) and a decrease in phosphorylation of AMPK and acetyl CoA carboxilase (ACC) [37]. Another study differentiated the effects of human vs. mouse resistin, which only has 53% homology. That report found that chronic treatment of cultured human adipocytes with human resistin resulted in hypotrophic cells with smaller lipid droplets [38]. Recombinant human resistin stimulated adipocyte triglyceride lipolysis, whereas recombinant mouse resistin had no detectable effects on lipolysis [38]. Interestingly, insulin-stimulated glucose uptake and AKT phosphorylation were not altered in human resistin-treated adipocytes, indicating an intact insulin response. In mouse adipose explants, human resistin simultaneously accelerated triglyceride lipolysis and fatty acid reesterification. Consistent with the in vitro findings, the acute administration of recombinant human resistin into normal mice caused a significant increase in serum glycerol concentration with no elevation in FFAs [38].

The central administration of resistin has been also demonstrated to exert a relevant effect on hypothalamic and peripheral lipid metabolism in a nutritional-dependent fashion [39]. Central acute resistin administration stimulated the phosphorylation of AMPK and ACC in fed but not fasted states and decreased the expression of fatty acid synthase specifically in the ventromedial nucleus of the hypothalamus [39], suggesting that resistin may decrease de novo fatty acid synthesis in the hypothalamus in periods of nutritional restriction. Contrary to its central actions, the acute administration of resistin in the brain did not modify peripheral lipid metabolism [39]. However, when the animals were infused with resistin during 1 week, an increase in the hepatic fatty acid synthesis of fed rats and in the WAT of fasted rats was found [39]. This increase in fat deposition might at least partially explain the central resistin-induced insulin resistance.

Resistin and Food Intake

Resistin mRNA and protein was localized in the ARC of the hypothalamus [40]. The ARC plays a major role by connecting afferent signals with central circuitries orchestrating efferent commands to govern food intake, motor activity and peripheral cell metabolism. Neurons in the hypothalamic ARC are expressing specific neuropeptides with orexigenic or anorexigenic effects. Small amounts of resistin were also found in the ventromedial and periventricular areas of the hypothalamus [40]. Interestingly, resistin was found to decrease food intake in rats [41, 42].

Central administration of resistin promotes short-term satiety in rats [42]. The effect is transient since it could only be observed during the first 90 min after challenge but not at later time points [42]. Importantly, resistin's anorectic effects were not the result of an unpleasant/toxic side effect of the resistin treatment [42]. The anorectic effect of resistin is associated with marked changes in the level of neuropeptide gene expression, namely agouti-related protein (AgRP), NPY, and cocaine and amphetamine-regulated transcript (CART) [39], as well as changes in the hypothalamic expression of enzymes involved in fatty acid metabolism as stated above. More specifically, resistin decreased NPY and AgRP expression, while it increased CART gene levels in the ARC [39]. Since resistin is expressed in the hypothalamus, this raises the question of whether some of its central effects are exerted by peripherally- or central-synthesized resistin.

Concluding Remarks

It is clear that the metabolic syndrome is a multifactorial process affected by several adipokines. Although the role of resistin on obesity and insulin resistance has been clearly demonstrated in preclinical models (fig. 1), its role in humans is still far from being elucidated. The low homology between human and mouse resistin and its different location (adipocytes in rodents and macrophages in humans) are likely the main difficulties in the research of this hormone. A great step for the understanding of the physiological actions of human resistin has been the generation of mice lacking adipocyte-derived mouse resistin but producing human resistin specifically in macrophages [43]. When those mice were fed on HFD, they showed an increase in WAT inflammation, which led to a higher accumulation of lipids in the muscle and thereby insulin resistance [43]. Those findings suggested that even though human resistin is not located in adipocytes, it contributed to inflammation and insulin resistance. However, further studies will be necessary to confirm those results. Indeed, the discovery of the receptor(s) will be a crucial step for the understanding of the biology of resistin, and given the low homology of this hormone between humans and rodents, it will be necessary to assess if the receptor is similar in both species. The identification of the receptor(s) will allow researchers to design resistin receptor antagonists, which would be supposed to exert some beneficial actions. Another gap in the investigation of resistin is that resistin or an antibody blocking resistin's actions has not been administered to human patients. So far, there are a number of reports with some degree of controversy, indicating the correlation between resistin circulating levels with obesity, body mass index, inflammatory factors and cardiovascular disease. However, the physiological or pharmacological role of resistin (i.e. its effects on glucose tolerance, serum glucose, insulin, inflammatory markers, etc.) is still to be found. Similarly, the physiological role of resistin in other tissues such as the pituitary and the gonads remains to be elucidated. Nevertheless, we are in the early stages of resistin research, it is only 8 years old, and every year new studies are shedding more light on its intriguing biology, and those new findings are encouraging the potential use of resistin as a pharmacological target for the treatment of the metabolic syndrome in the future. The resistin story will be continued.

Acknowledgements

This work was supported by grants from Xunta de Galicia (C.D.: PGIDIT06PXIB208063PR and M.L.: GRC2006/66), Fondo Investigationes Sanitarias (M.L.: PI061700), Ministerio de Educacion y Ciencia (C.D.: BFU2008, M.L.: RYC-2007-00211, and R.N.: RYC-2008-02219), European Union (C.D.: Health-F2-2008-223713), and Mútua Madrileña (C.D. and M.L.). CIBER de Fisiopatología de la Obesidad y Nutrición is an initiative of ISCIII, Spain.

References

1 Holcomb IN, Kabakoff RC, Chan B, Baker TW, Gurney A, Henzel W, Nelson C, Lowman HB, Wright BD, Skelton NJ, Frantz GD, Tumas DB, Peale FV Jr, Shelton DL, Hebert CC: FIZZ1, a novel cysteine-rich secreted protein associated with pulmonary inflammation, defines a new gene family. EMBO J 2000;19:4046–4055.

2 Kim KH, Lee K, Moon YS, Sul HS: A cysteine-rich adipose tissue-specific secretory factor inhibits adipocyte differentiation. J Biol Chem 2001;276:11252–11256.

3 Steppan CM, Bailey ST, Bhat S, Brown EJ, Banerjee RR, Wright CM, Patel HR, Ahima RS, Lazar MA: The hormone resistin links obesity to diabetes. Nature 2001;409:307–312.

4 Rajala MW, Lin Y, Ranalletta M, Yang XM, Qian H, Gingerich R, Barzilai N, Scherer PE: Cell type-specific expression and coregulation of murine resistin and resistin-like molecule-alpha in adipose tissue. Mol Endocrinol 2002;16:1920–1930.
5 Way JM, Gorgun CZ, Tong Q, Uysal KT, Brown KK, Harrington WW, Oliver WR Jr, Willson TM, Kliewer SA, Hotamisligil GS: Adipose tissue resistin expression is severely suppressed in obesity and stimulated by peroxisome proliferator-activated receptor gamma agonists. J Biol Chem 2001;276: 25651–25653.
6 Makimura H, Mizuno TM, Bergen H, Mobbs CV: Adiponectin is stimulated by adrenalectomy in ob/ob mice and is highly correlated with resistin mRNA. Am J Physiol Endocrinol Metab 2002;283: E1266–E1271.
7 Juan CC, Au LC, Fang VS, Kang SF, Ko YH, Kuo SF, Hsu YP, Kwok CF, Ho LT: Suppressed gene expression of adipocyte resistin in an insulin-resistant rat model probably by elevated free fatty acids. Biochem Biophys Res Commun 2001;289:1328–1333.
8 Le Lay S, Boucher J, Rey A, Castan-Laurell I, Krief S, Ferre P, Valet P, Dugail I: Decreased resistin expression in mice with different sensitivities to a high-fat diet. Biochem Biophys Res Commun 2001;289:564–567.
9 Chen L, Nyomba BL: Glucose intolerance and resistin expression in rat offspring exposed to ethanol in utero: modulation by postnatal high-fat diet. Endocrinology 2003;144:500–508.
10 Levy JR, Davenport B, Clore JN, Stevens W: Lipid metabolism and resistin gene expression in insulin-resistant Fischer 344 rats. Am J Physiol Endocrinol Metab 2002;282:E626–E633.
11 Haugen F, Jorgensen A, Drevon CA, Trayhurn P: Inhibition by insulin of resistin gene expression in 3T3-L1 adipocytes. FEBS Lett 2001;507:105–108.
12 Shojima N, Sakoda H, Ogihara T, Fujishiro M, Katagiri H, Anai M, Onishi Y, Ono H, Inukai K, Abe M, Fukushima Y, Kikuchi M, Oka Y, Asano T: Humoral regulation of resistin expression in 3T3-L1 and mouse adipose cells. Diabetes 2002;51:1737–1744.
13 Moore GB, Chapman H, Holder JC, Lister CA, Piercy V, Smith SA, Clapham JC: Differential regulation of adipocytokine mRNAs by rosiglitazone in db/db mice. Biochem Biophys Res Commun 2001;286:735–741.
14 Fujita H, Fujishima H, Morii T, Koshimura J, Narita T, Kakei M, Ito S: Effect of metformin on adipose tissue resistin expression in db/db mice. Biochem Biophys Res Commun 2002;298:345–349.
15 Fasshauer M, Klein J, Neumann S, Eszlinger M, Paschke R: Tumor necrosis factor alpha is a negative regulator of resistin gene expression and secretion in 3T3-L1 adipocytes. Biochem Biophys Res Commun 2001;288:1027–1031.
16 Nogueiras R, Gualillo O, Caminos JE, Casanueva FF, Dieguez C: Regulation of resistin by gonadal, thyroid hormone, and nutritional status. Obes Res 2003;11:408–414.
17 Savage DB, Sewter CP, Klenk ES, Segal DG, Vidal-Puig A, Considine RV, O'Rahilly S: Resistin/Fizz3 expression in relation to obesity and peroxisome proliferator-activated receptor-gamma action in humans. Diabetes 2001;50:2199–2202.
18 McTernan CL, McTernan PG, Harte AL, Levick PL, Barnett AH, Kumar S: Resistin, central obesity, and type 2 diabetes. Lancet 2002;359:46–47.
19 McTernan PG, Fisher FM, Valsamakis G, Chetty R, Harte A, McTernan CL, Clark PM, Smith SA, Barnett AH, Kumar S: Resistin and type 2 diabetes: regulation of resistin expression by insulin and rosiglitazone and the effects of recombinant resistin on lipid and glucose metabolism in human differentiated adipocytes. J Clin Endocrinol Metab 2003;88: 6098–6106.
20 Azuma K, Katsukawa F, Oguchi S, Murata M, Yamazaki H, Shimada A, Saruta T: Correlation between serum resistin level and adiposity in obese individuals. Obes Res 2003;11:997–1001.
21 Degawa-Yamauchi M, Bovenkerk JE, Juliar BE, Watson W, Kerr K, Jones R, Zhu Q, Considine RV: Serum resistin (FIZZ3) protein is increased in obese humans. J Clin Endocrinol Metab 2003;88:5452–5455.
22 Janke J, Engeli S, Gorzelniak K, Luft FC, Sharma AM: Resistin gene expression in human adipocytes is not related to insulin resistance. Obes Res 2002; 10:1–5.
23 Rajala MW, Obici S, Scherer PE, Rossetti L: Adipose-derived resistin and gut-derived resistin-like molecule-beta selectively impair insulin action on glucose production. J Clin Invest 2003;111:225–230.
24 Moon B, Kwan JJ, Duddy N, Sweeney G, Begum N: Resistin inhibits glucose uptake in L6 cells independently of changes in insulin signaling and GLUT4 translocation. Am J Physiol Endocrinol Metab 2003; 285:E106–E115.
25 Minn AH, Patterson NB, Pack S, Hoffmann SC, Gavrilova O, Vinson C, Harlan DM, Shalev A: Resistin is expressed in pancreatic islets. Biochem Biophys Res Commun 2003;310:641–645.
26 Brown JE, Onyango DJ, Dunmore SJ: Resistin down-regulates insulin receptor expression, and modulates cell viability in rodent pancreatic beta-cells. FEBS Lett 2007;581:3273–3276.

27 Nakata M, Okada T, Ozawa K, Yada T: Resistin induces insulin resistance in pancreatic islets to impair glucose-induced insulin release. Biochem Biophys Res Commun 2007;353:1046–1051.
28 Satoh H, Nguyen MT, Miles PD, Imamura T, Usui I, Olefsky JM: Adenovirus-mediated chronic 'hyper-resistinemia' leads to in vivo insulin resistance in normal rats. J Clin Invest 2004;114:224–231.
29 Rangwala SM, Rich AS, Rhoades B, Shapiro JS, Obici S, Rossetti L, Lazar MA: Abnormal glucose homeostasis due to chronic hyperresistinemia. Diabetes 2004;53:1937–1941.
30 Muse ED, Obici S, Bhanot S, Monia BP, McKay RA, Rajala MW, Scherer PE, Rossetti L: Role of resistin in diet-induced hepatic insulin resistance. J Clin Invest 2004;114:232–239.
31 Singhal NS, Lazar MA, Ahima RS: Central resistin induces hepatic insulin resistance via neuropeptide Y. J Neurosci 2007;27:12924–12932.
32 Banerjee RR, Rangwala SM, Shapiro JS, Rich AS, Rhoades B, Qi Y, Wang J, Rajala MW, Pocai A, Scherer PE, Steppan CM, Ahima RS, Obici S, Rossetti L, Lazar MA: Regulation of fasted blood glucose by resistin. Science 2004;303:1195–1198.
33 Qi Y, Nie Z, Lee YS, Singhal NS, Scherer PE, Lazar MA, Ahima RS: Loss of resistin improves glucose homeostasis in leptin deficiency. Diabetes 2006;55: 3083–3090.
34 Haugen F, Zahid N, Dalen KT, Hollung K, Nebb HI, Drevon CA: Resistin expression in 3T3-L1 adipocytes is reduced by arachidonic acid. J Lipid Res 2005;46:143–153.
35 Yang G, Li L, Fang C, Zhang L, Li Q, Tang Y, Boden G: Effects of free fatty acids on plasma resistin and insulin resistance in awake rats. Metabolism 2005; 54:1142–1146.
36 Noto A, Zahradka P, Ryz NR, Yurkova N, Xie X, Taylor CG: Dietary conjugated linoleic acid preserves pancreatic function and reduces inflammatory markers in obese, insulin-resistant rats. Metabolism 2007;56:142–151.
37 Palanivel R, Sweeney G: Regulation of fatty acid uptake and metabolism in L6 skeletal muscle cells by resistin. FEBS Lett 2005;579:5049–5054.
38 Ort T, Arjona AA, MacDougall JR, Nelson PJ, Rothenberg ME, Wu F, Eisen A, Halvorsen YD: Recombinant human FIZZ3/resistin stimulates lipolysis in cultured human adipocytes, mouse adipose explants, and normal mice. Endocrinology 2005;146:2200–2209.
39 Vazquez MJ, Gonzalez CR, Varela L, Lage R, Tovar S, Sangiao-Alvarellos S, Williams LM, Vidal-Puig A, Nogueiras R, Lopez M, Dieguez C: Central resistin regulates hypothalamic and peripheral lipid metabolism in a nutritional-dependent fashion. Endocrinology 2008;149:4534–4543.
40 Morash BA, Willkinson D, Ur E, Wilkinson M: Resistin expression and regulation in mouse pituitary. FEBS Lett 2002;526:26–30.
41 Cifani C, Durocher Y, Pathak A, Penicaud L, Smih F, Massi M, Rouet P, Polidori C: Possible common central pathway for resistin and insulin in regulating food intake. Acta Physiol (Oxf) 2009;196:395–400.
42 Tovar S, Nogueiras R, Tung LY, Castaneda TR, Vazquez MJ, Morris A, Williams LM, Dickson SL, Dieguez C: Central administration of resistin promotes short-term satiety in rats. Eur J Endocrinol 2005;153:R1–R5.
43 Qatanani M, Szwergold NR, Greaves DR, Ahima RS, Lazar MA: Macrophage-derived human resistin exacerbates adipose tissue inflammation and insulin resistance in mice. J Clin Invest 2009;DOI: 10.1172/JCI37273.

Carlos Dieguez, PhD
Department of Physiology, School of Medicine, University of Santiago de Compostela
Instituto de Investigación Sanitaria, and CIBER Fisiopatología de la Obesidad y Nutrición (CIBERobn)
S. Francisco s/n
ES–15782 Santiago de Compostela (A Coruña) (Spain)
Tel. +34 981 582658, Fax +34 981 574145, E-Mail carlos.dieguez@usc.es

Loche S, Cappa M, Ghizzoni L, Maghnie M, Savage MO (eds): Pediatric Neuroendocrinology.
Endocr Dev. Basel, Karger, 2010, vol 17, pp 185–196

Hypothalamic Obesity

Irit Hochberg · Ze'ev Hochberg

Rambam Medical Center, Rappaport Family Faculty of Medicine and Research Institute, Technion, Israel Institute of Technology, Haifa, Israel

Abstract

Following extensive suprasellar operations for excision of hypothalamic tumors, some patients develop morbid obesity, the so-called hypothalamic obesity (HyOb). HyOb complicates disorders related to the hypothalamus, including those that cause structural damage to the hypothalamus, pituitary macroadenoma with suprasellar extension, glioma, meningioma, teratoma, germ cell tumors, radiotherapy, Prader–Willi syndrome, and mutations in leptin, leptin receptor, POMC, MC4R and CART genes. It is conceivable that a subgroup of patients with 'simple obesity' also have HyOb. The hypothalamus regulates body weight by precisely balancing the intake of food, energy expenditure and body fat tissue. Orexigenic and anorexigenic hypothalamic centers (hyperphagia when impaired) play a central role, connecting to adipose tissue by means of an intricate efferent and afferent signals circuit. Other mechanisms by which the brain regulates adipose tissue and beta cells of the pancreas include the sympathetic nervous system, vagally mediated hyperinsulinemia and the endocrine system, namely growth hormone, thyroid-stimulating hormone and the hypothalamo-pituitary-adrenal axis. Corticotropin-releasing hormone, adrenocorticotropic hormone glucocorticoids and the 11β-HSD-1 shuttle regulate lipolysis both directly and indirectly. All the above mechanisms may be impaired in HyOb. Management of HyOb targets the major manifestations: hyperphagia, autonomic dysfunction, hyperinsulinemia and impaired energy expenditure. Individual variation is considerable. Satisfactory therapy is currently unavailable.

The hypothalamus plays a key role in energy and weight homeostasis as evidenced by the fact that most monogenic syndromes of morbid obesity result from mutations in genes expressed in the hypothalamus. Following extensive suprasellar operations for excision of hypothalamic tumors, some patients develop morbid obesity, the so-called hypothalamic obesity (HyOb). HyOb complicates disorders that cause structural damage, tumors and genetic defects in the hypothalamus. A recent study detected apoptosis of hypothalamic neurons in rats in which obesity was induced by a high-fat diet [1]. This suggests a role for hypothalamic decompensation in obesity induced by nutritional changes.

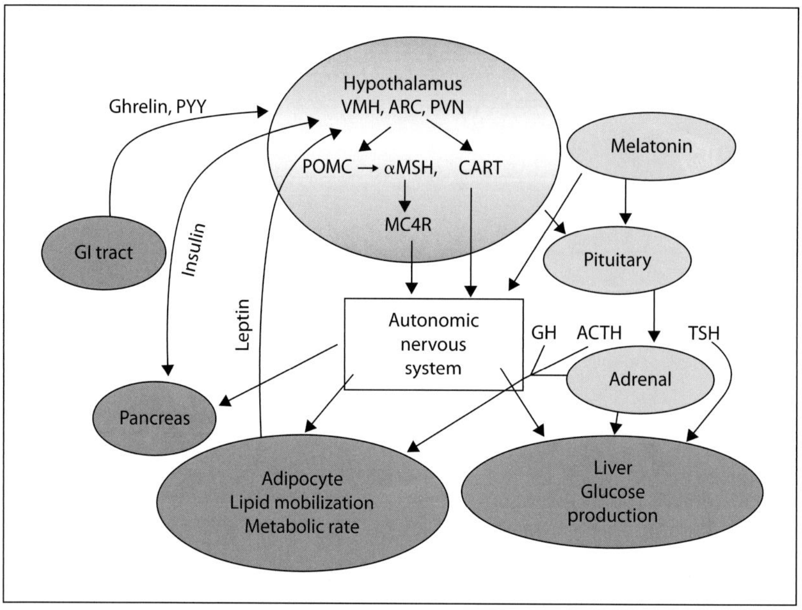

Fig. 1. Pathways involved in the pathogenesis of hypothalamic obesity. The main hypothalamic areas involved in energy regulation are the ventromedial nuclei (VMH), paraventricular nuclei (PVN) and arcuate nucleus (ARC). ARC generates the anorexigenic pro-opiomelanocortin (POMC) and cocaine- and amphetamine-related transcript (CART). The PVN expresses receptors for the POMC derived melanocyte-stimulating hormone (MC3R/MC4R), and secrete neuropeptides that have an anorexigenic and catabolic action, including CRH and oxytocin. Signals from the fat tissue mass, particularly leptin, the pancreas (insulin) and the gastrointestinal tract, including ghrelin and PYY, affect hypothalamic centers. These centers control tissues regulating energy homeostasis, primarily through the autonomic nervous system and pituitary hormone secretion. Melatonin also affects the metabolic rate through the sympathetic nervous system. Impediment of each of these pathways leads to dramatic weight gain (table 2), demonstrating the non-redundant nature of each factor.

It is conceivable that a substantial subgroup of patients with 'simple obesity' also have HyOb. This chapter will review the clinical characteristics and therapeutic approaches of HyOb, as well as its mechanisms: impaired energy regulation by the hypothalamus, nonredundant effects of hypothalamic proteins, and defective communication between the brain and periphery.

Hypothalamic Energy Regulation

The hypothalamus regulates body weight by precisely balancing the intake of food, energy expenditure and body fat tissue. To perform these tasks, the hypothalamus receives afferent messages from the periphery, and sends back efferent messages. The main hypothalamic areas involved in energy regulation are the ventromedial nuclei

Table 1. Structural damage leading to HyOb

Neoplastic – Craniopharyngioma, epithelioma, angiosarcoma, cholesteatoma, pinealoma, greminoma, endothelioma, hamartoma, chordoma, colloid cysts, epidermoid, ganglioneuroma, enpendymoma, glioma, meningioma, pituitary macroadenoma, teratoma, leukemia, Langerhans cell, metastasis
Inflammatory – sarcoidosis, tuberculosis, arachnioditis, histiocytosis X, encephalitis
Traumatic – head injury
Neurosurgery
Cranial radiotherapy
Cerebral aneurysm

(VMH), paraventricular nuclei (PVN), arcuate nucleus (ARC) and the lateral hypothalamic area (LH) (fig. 1). ARC contains two sets of neurons. One generates the orexigenic agouti-related protein (AGRP) and neuropeptide Y (NPY), and the other generates the anorexigenic proopiomelanocortin (POMC) and cocaine- and amphetamine-related transcript (CART). The PVN express both melanocortin receptors 3 and 4 (MC3R/MC4R) and NPY receptors, and secrete neuropeptides, such as corticotropin-releasing hormone (CRH) and oxytocin, that have an anorexigenic and catabolic action. These centers control tissues and the hormones that regulate energy homeostasis, primarily through the autonomic nervous system and pituitary hormone secretion (reviewed in [2]). The efferent signals CRH, GHRH, somatostatin and TRH regulate pituitary ACTH, GH and TSH, which in turn regulate the metabolic rate and adipose tissue metabolism. Afferent signals from fat tissue mass, particularly leptin, and from the pancreas (insulin) and the gastrointestinal tract (ghrelin and PYY), affect hypothalamic centers.

Etiologies of Hypothalamic Obesity

Anatomic Hypothalamic Damage

Severe obesity as a consequence of hypothalamic damage has been described in several hundreds of individuals during the last century (reviewed in [3]). While many mechanisms of acquired hypothalamic damage can lead to obesity (table 1), the paradigm of HyOb remains the morbid obesity that develops after aggressive surgery of hypothalamic tumors, particularly craniopharyngioma.

Genetic Syndromes

The majority of currently recognized monogenic obesity syndromes involve regulatory hypothalamic pathways (table 2), and can be considered a subtype of HyOb.

Table 2. Genetic obesity disorders of hypothalamic origin

Gene/protein	Function	Phenotype when mutated	Correlation with 'simple' obesity
Leptin	secreted by adipocytes, regulation of food intake and energy expenditure	hyperphagia, severe obesity, hypogonadotrophic hypogonadism [14]	
Leptin receptor	leptin signaling	early-onset morbid obesity, severe hyperphagia, hypogonadotrophic hypogonadism, reduced secretion of GH and IGF-1, hypothalamic hypothyroidism, hyperleptinemia; normal glucose, insulin and lipid profile	
CART	ARC peptide, modulated by leptin, signaling in the SNS [55]	heterozygote missense mutation associated with childhood and adult obesity, reduced basal metabolic rate and normal leptin levels [56]	
POMC	precursor of αMSH and ACTH, anorexigenic, decrease of food intake and increases energy expenditure	early-onset obesity, hyperphagia, red hair pigmentation and adrenal insufficiency	polymorphisms associated with hyperinsulinemia and high leptin
Prohormone convertase-1	conversion of POMC to αMSH and ACTH	severe obesity, 2nd hypocortisolism; impaired glucose tolerance; postprandial hypoglycemia; hypogonadotrophic hypogonadism; elevated POMC and proinsulin, with very low insulin levels; elevated progastrin and proglucagon levels, normal leptin levels	
MC4R	αMSH and ACTH signaling	early-onset severe obesity in homozygotes, less severe early- or late-onset obesity in heterozygotes Increased linear growth, higher bone mineral density, hyperphagia, normal resting metabolic rate, hyperinsulinemia, normal leptin	nearby SNPs associated with obesity
BDNF, TrkB	TrkB is the receptor for BDNF. Together, regulation of short-term synaptic functions and long-term potentiation of brain synapses, involvement in MC4R signaling [66]	a single case of TrkB mutation: hyperphagia, morbid obesity and mental retardation TrkB and BDNF are reduced in mice with high-fat induced obesity	

Table 2. Continued

Gene/protein	Function	Phenotype when mutated	Correlation with 'simple' obesity
Prader-Willi syndrome Loss of paternally imprinted genes on chromosome 15q11-q13	unknown	severe hyperphagia and obesity beginning in childhood, other endocrine deficiencies; elevated fasting and postprandial ghrelin [71, 72], hyperleptinemia normal insulin small PVN and few oxytocin neurons	
Bardel-Biedl syndrome	defects in several proteins involved in cilia function and intracellular protein/ vesicle trafficking; defective hypothalamic leptin receptor signaling and reduced POMC expression [79, 80]	obesity reduced physical activity with no difference in BMR	BBS gene variants associated with obesity
Single-minded 1 (Sim-1)	a transcription factor essential for formation of the supraoptic and PVN nuclei in the hypothalamus	haploinsufficiency – profound obesity and hyperphagia [85–87]; animal model – decreased PVN volume, reduced hypothalamic oxytocin, obesity with increased linear growth, hyperleptinemia, hyperinsulinemia	polymorphisms associated with a slight but significant increase in BMI in males

Table 3. Psychotropic drugs causing obesity (adapted from [4])

Antidepressants – amitriptyline, doxepin, imipramine, clomipramine, maprotiline, nortriptyline, trimipramine, paroxetine, mirtazapine, deipramine, isocarboxazide
Mood stabilizers – lithium, valproate, carbamazepine
Antipsychotic – clozapine, olanzepine, zotepine, quetiapine, chlorpromazine, thioridazine, perphenazine, trifluoperazine, risperidone, clopenthioxol, sulpiride

Even more common are obesity-associated polymorphisms in the genes involved in these pathways. Thus, the pathophysiology of 'essential' or 'simple' obesity is related to inter-individual variability in hypothalamic weight-regulating mechanisms.

Obesity Induced by Psychotropic Drugs

Many psychotropic drugs, including antidepressants, mood stabilizers, and antipsychotic and antiepileptic drugs, induce weight gain (table 3). The mechanism of weight gain is likely related to the agonist and antagonist effects on neurotransmitter signaling in pathways involved in weight regulation (reviewed in [4]). Indeed, recent studies have confirmed the specific role of neurotransmitters including GABA [5], dopamine [6], serotonin [7] and histamine [8, 9] in hypothalamic weight regulation.

Clinical Characteristics of HyOb

Hyperphagia

Voracious hyperphagia appears within a day or two and is hard to contain. Patients consume in excess of their caloric need, and display unusual food-seeking behaviors, including foraging for food, stealing food and stealing money for food [3, 10].

Reduced Physical Activity

Craniopharyngioma patients with hypothalamic involvement were significantly less physically active than those without [11]. Similarly, the intensity of physical activity was less in children with hypothalamic obesity than in those with simple obesity [12].

Associated Hypothalamic Malfunction

Hypothalamic damage in patients with HyOb compromises many additional functions of the hypothalamus, and results in somnolence, behavioral changes, hypopituitarism with growth hormone deficiency, hypogonadotrophic hypogonadism, secondary hypocortisolism, central hypothyroidism and diabetes insipidus [3].

Hormonal and Metabolic Characteristics of HyOb

Hyperleptinemia

Leptin is secreted by adipocytes and regulates body weight by decreasing food intake and energy expenditure (reviewed recently in [13]). Patients with leptin deficiency or leptin receptor mutations display the clinical features of HyOb: hyperphagia, severe obesity and hypogonadotropic hypogonadism [14].

Interestingly, patients with post- surgical HyOb usually have higher serum leptin levels than expected for their BMI, possibly the result of damaged leptin sensitivity [12, 15–17]. Leptin insensitivity may be involved in other aspects of HyOb, including hypogonadotropic hypogonadism and central hypothyroidism.

Hyperinsulinemia

Patients with anatomic HyOb are hyperinsulinemic more than would be predicted by their excess weight, and display higher than expected fasting insulin, severe insulin resistance and loss of diurnal insulin variation [3, 16, 18]. Hyperinsulinemia is thought to contribute to the normal or even accelerated growth in HyOb children with growth hormone deficiency, the so-called 'growth without growth hormone' [19].

In HyOb rat models hyperinsulinemia appeared instantaneously after VMH damage, and persisted even when food intake was restricted and weight gain prevented, suggesting a direct hypothalamic regulation of insulin release by beta cells [20–22]. The significant reduction in hyperinsulinemia subsequent to denervation of pancreatic tissue by pancreatectomy with ectopic pancreas transplantation indicates a neuronal link [23]. Hyperinsulinemia in HyOb may be due to loss of hypothalamic insulin regulation by POMC, α-MSH and insulin itself, regulation that is transmitted through signals of the sympathetic system [24–26]. Vagal hyperactivity contributes to hyperinsulinemia and reduced gastric acidity in HyOb. Both vagotomy and atropine prevent obesity, proliferation of pancreatic beta cells and hyperinsulinemia in rats with VMH lesions [27–30].

Impaired Activity of the Sympathetic Nervous System

The sympathetic nervous system (SNS) regulates the metabolic rate of adipose tissue, controlling fat mobilization and thermogenesis (reviewed in [31]). Several clinical studies have shown defective SNS activity and reduction of basal metabolic rate (BMR) in human subjects with HyOb (reviewed in [3, 11]). Animal models of HyOb displayed reduced turnover of norepinephrine in various tissues, most significantly in abdominal adipocytes [32, 33], reduced urinary epinephrine excretion, reduced thermogenic capacity of brown adipose tissue, reduced oxygen consumption [34, 35] and a reduction in adrenal catecholamine content and secretion in response to stress [36]. Disruption of ARCs CART, and αMSH activity, which act as regulators of the SNS downstream to leptin (reviewed in [37–40]), may explain the defective sympathetic activity and reduction in BMR in HyOb.

Enhanced 11β-Hydroxysteroid Dehydrogenase 1 (11β-HSD1) Activity

Similarity of the HyOb and Cushing's syndrome phenotypes prompted investigation of prereceptor modification of glucocorticoids. A study in patients with HyOb and ACTH deficiency after surgical removal of craniopharyngioma demonstrated a striking increase in the 11-OH/11-oxo ratio in HyOb patients. This suggests enhanced activity of 11β-HSD1, probably through damage to the hypothalamic message that modulates peripheral 11β-HSD1. This enzyme catalyzes conversion of inactive cortisone to active cortisol. Enhanced11β-HSD1 activity is associated with obesity in animal models [41]. Inter-individual variability in its activity has been proposed as a molecular etiology for both human visceral obesity and the metabolic syndrome [42–45]. In vitro, 11β-HSD1 activity in preadipocytes was downregulated by CRH, ACTH and α2 adrenergic activation; and upregulated by β_2-adrenergic activation and TNFα [46], all of which may be hypothalamic elements affected by HyOb.

Detected hypercorticosteronemia in leptin-deficient and leptin receptor-deficient mice suggests that loss of leptin signaling may also have a role in 11β-HSD1 dysregulation.

Table 4. Pharmacologic treatment of anatomic HyOb

Drug	n	Results	Reference
Dextroamphetamine	5	weight stabilization	[90]
	11	weight stabilization or reduction	[91]
Ephedrine and caffeine	3	weight stabilization in 2 patients	[92]
Octreotide	8	weight loss in 5 patients and weight stabilization in 3	[18]
	10	weight stabilization	[93]
Triiodothyronine	3	weight reduction	[94]
Sibutramine	19	weight reduction	[95]

Leptin suppressed secretion of ACTH and corticosterone in response to stressful events, and decreased mRNA expression and release of CRH in the hypothalamus [47].

Melatonin Dysregulation

Melatonin affects energy metabolism in seasonal animals [48], as well as in other species, through upregulation of the SNS. Recently, a polymorphism of melatonin receptor 2 was identified as a marker for insulin resistance and diabetes [49]. Disruption of normal circadian melatonin signaling may play a role in the development of hyperinsulinemia and obesity in HyOb. In children with HyOb secondary to tumors, morning and nighttime (but not midday and evening) salivary melatonin was increased as compared to controls. Morning and nighttime melatonin correlated positively with BMI and daytime sleepiness [50].

Treatment

Treatment of HyOb is palliative and requires comprehensive command of the affected mechanisms in the damaged hypothalamus. While diet is the first-line approach for hyperphagia, it often fails. Trials of dietary treatment alone have not been documented. Exercise, the logical approach to reduced activity, has failed as well. While physical activity is shown to promote weight reduction in experimental HyOb [51–54] and in MC4R knockout mice [54], there are no data on the affect of exercise in human HyOb.

Drugs affecting the damaged pathways in HyOb include sympathomimetics, triiodothyronine and somatostatin analogues (table 4). 11β-HSD-1 inhibitors, when available for clinical use, may prove effective. Sibutramine and bariatric surgery have benefited patients with HyOb.

The few human studies conducted with these drugs are small-scale, short- term and only showed limited effectiveness.

Conclusions

The clinical findings in patients with HyOb, including hypersecretion of insulin and leptin, enhanced 11βHSD1 activity, and decreased SNS activity and basal metabolic rate, can all be explained by damage to hypothalamic nuclei regulating these functions. We expect the increasing understanding of cerebral regulation of appetite and weight to reveal additional pathways, mutations and polymorphisms characteristic of HyOb. Similarities in the characteristics and affected pathways between HyOb induced by anatomic damage and HyOb resulting from monogenic syndromes may promote treatment options in the future.

References

1 Moraes JC, et al: High-fat diet induces apoptosis of hypothalamic neurons. PLoS ONE 2009;4:e5045.

2 Woods SC, D'Alessio DA: Central control of body weight and appetite. J Clin Endocrinol Metab 2008; 93(11 suppl 1):S37–S50.

3 Bray GA, Gallagher TF Jr: Manifestations of hypothalamic obesity in man: a comprehensive investigation of eight patients and a reveiw of the literature. Medicine (Baltimore) 1975;54:301–330.

4 Zimmermann U, et al: Epidemiology, implications and mechanisms underlying drug-induced weight gain in psychiatric patients. J Psychiatr Res 2003;37: 193–220.

5 Tong Q, et al: Synaptic release of GABA by AgRP neurons is required for normal regulation of energy balance. Nat Neurosci 2008;11:998–1000.

6 Abizaid A, et al: Ghrelin modulates the activity and synaptic input organization of midbrain dopamine neurons while promoting appetite. J Clin Invest 2006;116:3229–3239.

7 Heisler LK, et al: Serotonin reciprocally regulates melanocortin neurons to modulate food intake. Neuron 2006;51:239–249.

8 Masaki T, et al: Involvement of hypothalamic histamine H1 receptor in the regulation of feeding rhythm and obesity. Diabetes 2004;53:2250–2260.

9 Kim SF, et al: From the Cover: Antipsychotic drug-induced weight gain mediated by histamine H1 receptor-linked activation of hypothalamic AMP-kinase. Proc Natl Acad Sci USA 2007;104:3456–3459.

10 Skorzewska A, et al: Abnormal food-seeking behavior after surgery for craniopharyngioma. Neuropsychobiology 1989;21:17–20.

11 Roth CL, et al: Reduced sympathetic metabolites in urine of obese patients with craniopharyngioma. Pediatr Res 2007;61:496–501.

12 Shaikh MG, Grundy RG, Kirk JM: Hyperleptinaemia rather than fasting hyperinsulinaemia is associated with obesity following hypothalamic damage in children. Eur J Endocrinol 2008;159:791–797.

13 Farooqi IS, O'Rahilly S: Leptin: a pivotal regulator of human energy homeostasis. Am J Clin Nutr 2009;89:980S–984S.

14 Clement K, et al: A mutation in the human leptin receptor gene causes obesity and pituitary dysfunction. Nature 1998;392:398–401.

15 Roth C, et al: Hyperphagia in children with craniopharyngioma is associated with hyperleptinaemia and a failure in the downregulation of appetite. Eur J Endocrinol 1998;138:89–91.

16 Guran T, et al: The role of leptin, soluble leptin receptor, resistin, and insulin secretory dynamics in the pathogenesis of hypothalamic obesity in children. Eur J Pediatr 2008.

17 Brabant G, et al: Serum leptin levels following hypothalamic surgery. Horm Metab Res 1996;28:728–731.

18 Lustig RH, et al: Hypothalamic obesity caused by cranial insult in children: altered glucose and insulin dynamics and reversal by a somatostatin agonist. J Pediatr 1999;135:162–168.

19 Bucher H, et al: Insulin-like growth factors I and II, prolactin, and insulin in 19 growth hormone-deficient children with excessive, normal, or decreased longitudinal growth after operation for craniopharyngioma. N Engl J Med 1983;309:1142–1146.
20 Frohman LA, Bernardis LL: Growth hormone and insulin levels in weanling rats with ventromedial hypothalamic lesions. Endocrinology 1968;82:1125–1132.
21 Rohner F, et al: Immediate effect of lesion of the ventromedial hypothalamic area upon glucose-induced insulin secretion in anaesthetized rats. Diabetologia 1977;13:239–242.
22 Slaunwhite WR 3rd, Goldman JK, Bernardis LL: Sequential changes in glucose metabolism by adipose tissue and liver of rats after destruction of the ventromedial hypothalamic nuclei: effect of three dietary regimens. Metabolism 1972;21:619–631.
23 Bray GA, Inoue S, Nishizawa Y: Hypothalamic obesity. The autonomic hypothesis and the lateral hypothalamus. Diabetologia 1981(20 suppl):366–377.
24 Fan W, et al: The central melanocortin system can directly regulate serum insulin levels. Endocrinology 2000;141:3072–3079.
25 Obici S, et al: Central melanocortin receptors regulate insulin action. J Clin Invest 2001;108:1079–1085.
26 Bruning JC, et al: Role of brain insulin receptor in control of body weight and reproduction. Science 2000;289:2122–2125.
27 Inoue S, Bray GA: The effects of subdiaphragmatic vagotomy in rats with ventromedial hypothalamic obesity. Endocrinology 1977;100:108–114.
28 Berthoud HR, Jeanrenaud B: Acute hyperinsulinemia and its reversal by vagotomy after lesions of the ventromedial hypothalamus in anesthetized rats. Endocrinology 1979;105:146–151.
29 Cox JE, Powley TL: Prior vagotomy blocks VMH obesity in pair-fed rats. Am J Physiol 1981;240: E573–E583.
30 Kiba T, et al: Ventromedial hypothalamic lesion-induced vagal hyperactivity stimulates rat pancreatic cell proliferation. Gastroenterology 1996;110: 885–893.
31 Penicaud L, et al: The autonomic nervous system, adipose tissue plasticity, and energy balance. Nutrition 2000;16:903–908.
32 Vander Tuig JG, Knehans AW, Romsos DR: Reduced sympathetic nervous system activity in rats with ventromedial hypothalamic lesions. Life Sci 1982; 30:913–920.
33 Balkan B, et al: Altered sympathetic control of nutrient mobilization during physical exercise after lesions in the VMH. Am J Physiol 1991;260: R368–R372.
34 Vander Tuig JG, Kerner J, Romsos DR: Hypothalamic obesity, brown adipose tissue, and sympathoadrenal activity in rats. Am J Physiol 1985;248:E607–E617.
35 Monda M, Sullo A, De Luca B: Lesions of the ventromedial hypothalamus reduce postingestional thermogenesis. Physiol Behav 1997;61:687–691.
36 Martins AC, et al: Adrenal medullary function and expression of catecholamine-synthesizing enzymes in mice with hypothalamic obesity. Life Sci 2004; 74:3211–3222.
37 Dun SL, et al: Cocaine- and amphetamine-regulated transcript peptide and sympatho-adrenal axis. Peptides 2006;27:1949–1955.
38 Wang C, et al: Effect of CART in the hypothalamic paraventricular nucleus on feeding and uncoupling protein gene expression. Neuroreport 2000;11:3251–3255.
39 Gullicksen PS, et al: Energy metabolism and expression of uncoupling proteins 1, 2, and 3 after 21 days of recovery from intracerebroventricular mouse leptin in rats. Physiol Behav 2002;75:473–482.
40 Haynes WG, et al: Interactions between the melanocortin system and leptin in control of sympathetic nerve traffic. Hypertension 1999;33(1 Pt 2):542–547.
41 Masuzaki H, et al: A transgenic model of visceral obesity and the metabolic syndrome. Science 2001; 294:2166–2170.
42 Stewart PM, et al: Cortisol metabolism in human obesity: impaired cortisone->cortisol conversion in subjects with central adiposity. J Clin Endocrinol Metab 1999;84:1022–1027.
43 Rask E, et al: Tissue-specific dysregulation of cortisol metabolism in human obesity. J Clin Endocrinol Metab 2001;86:1418–1421.
44 Draper N, et al: Association studies between microsatellite markers within the gene encoding human 11beta-hydroxysteroid dehydrogenase type 1 and body mass index, waist to hip ratio, and glucocorticoid metabolism. J Clin Endocrinol Metab 2002;87: 4984–4990.
45 Gelernter-Yaniv L, et al: Associations between a polymorphism in the 11 beta hydroxysteroid dehydrogenase type I gene and body composition. Int J Obes Relat Metab Disord 2003;27:983–986.
46 Friedberg M, et al: Modulation of 11 beta-hydroxysteroid dehydrogenase type 1 in mature human subcutaneous adipocytes by hypothalamic messengers. J Clin Endocrinol Metab 2003;88:385–393.
47 Lu XY: The leptin hypothesis of depression: a potential link between mood disorders and obesity? Curr Opin Pharmacol 2007;7:648–652.
48 Le Gouic S, et al: Effects of both a melatonin agonist and antagonist on seasonal changes in body mass and energy intake in the garden dormouse. Int J Obes Relat Metab Disord 1996;20:661–667.

49 Staiger H, et al: Polymorphisms within the novel type 2 diabetes risk locus MTNR1B determine beta-cell function. PLoS ONE 2008;3:e3962.
50 Muller HL, et al: Melatonin secretion and increased daytime sleepiness in childhood craniopharyngioma patients. J Clin Endocrinol Metab 2002;87: 3993–3996.
51 Gobatto CA, et al: The monosodium glutamate (MSG) obese rat as a model for the study of exercise in obesity. Res Commun Mol Pathol Pharmacol 2002;111:89–101.
52 de Mello MA, et al: Glucose tolerance and insulin action in monosodium glutamate (MSG) obese exercise-trained rats. Physiol Chem Phys Med NMR 2001;33:63–71.
53 Jenkins RR, Lamb DR: Effects of physical training on hypothalamic obesity in rats. Eur J Appl Physiol Occup Physiol 1982;48:355–359.
54 Haskell-Luevano C, et al: Voluntary exercise prevents the obese and diabetic metabolic syndrome of the melanocortin-4 receptor knockout mouse. Faseb J 2009;23:642–655.
55 Elias CF, et al: Leptin activates hypothalamic CART neurons projecting to the spinal cord. Neuron 1998;21:1375–1385.
56 del Giudice EM, et al: Mutational screening of the CART gene in obese children: identifying a mutation (Leu34Phe) associated with reduced resting energy expenditure and cosegregating with obesity phenotype in a large family. Diabetes 2001;50:2157–2160.
57 Coll AP, et al: Proopiomelanocortin and energy balance: insights from human and murine genetics. J Clin Endocrinol Metab 2004;89:2557–2562.
58 Krude H, et al: Severe early-onset obesity, adrenal insufficiency and red hair pigmentation caused by POMC mutations in humans. Nat Genet 1998;19: 155–157.
59 Krude H, et al: Obesity due to proopiomelanocortin deficiency: three new cases and treatment trials with thyroid hormone and ACTH4–10. J Clin Endocrinol Metab 2003;88:4633–4640.
60 Santoro N, et al: An insertional polymorphism of the proopiomelanocortin gene is associated with fasting insulin levels in childhood obesity. J Clin Endocrinol Metab 2004;89:4846–4849.
61 Comuzzie AG, et al: A major quantitative trait locus determining serum leptin levels and fat mass is located on human chromosome 2. Nat Genet 1997; 15:273–276.
62 Jackson RS, et al: Obesity and impaired prohormone processing associated with mutations in the human prohormone convertase 1 gene. Nat Genet 1997;16: 303–306.
63 Farooqi IS, et al: Clinical spectrum of obesity and mutations in the melanocortin 4 receptor gene. N Engl J Med 2003;348:1085–1095.
64 Lubrano-Berthelier C, et al: Melanocortin 4 receptor mutations in a large cohort of severely obese adults: prevalence, functional classification, genotype-phenotype relationship, and lack of association with binge eating. J Clin Endocrinol Metab 2006; 91:1811–1818.
65 Loos RJ, et al: Common variants near MC4R are associated with fat mass, weight and risk of obesity. Nat Genet 2008;40:768–775.
66 Xu B, et al: Brain-derived neurotrophic factor regulates energy balance downstream of melanocortin-4 receptor. Nat Neurosci 2003;6:736–742.
67 Yeo GS, et al: A de novo mutation affecting human TrkB associated with severe obesity and developmental delay. Nat Neurosci 2004;7:1187–1189.
68 Yu Y, Wang Q, Huang XF: Energy-restricted pair-feeding normalizes low levels of brain-derived neurotrophic factor/tyrosine kinase B mRNA expression in the hippocampus, but not ventromedial hypothalamic nucleus, in diet-induced obese mice. Neuroscience 2009.
69 Goldstone AP, et al: Recommendations for the diagnosis and management of Prader-Willi syndrome. J Clin Endocrinol Metab 2008;93:4183–4197.
70 Cummings DE, et al: Elevated plasma ghrelin levels in Prader Willi syndrome. Nat Med 2002;8:643–644.
71 DelParigi A, et al: High circulating ghrelin: a potential cause for hyperphagia and obesity in prader-willi syndrome. J Clin Endocrinol Metab 2002;87: 5461–5464.
72 Haqq AM, et al: Serum ghrelin levels are inversely correlated with body mass index, age, and insulin concentrations in normal children and are markedly increased in Prader-Willi syndrome. J Clin Endocrinol Metab 2003;88:174–178.
73 Eiholzer U, Blum WF, Molinari L: Body fat determined by skinfold measurements is elevated despite underweight in infants with Prader-Labhart-Willi syndrome. J Pediatr 1999;134:222–225.
74 Hoybye C, et al: Peptides associated with hyperphagia in adults with Prader-Willi syndrome before and during GH treatment. Growth Horm IGF Res 2003;13:322–327.
75 Schuster DP, Osei K, Zipf WB: Characterization of alterations in glucose and insulin metabolism in Prader-Willi subjects. Metabolism 1996;45:1514–1520.

76 Goldstone AP, et al: Fasting and postprandial hyperghrelinemia in Prader-Willi syndrome is partially explained by hypoinsulinemia, and is not due to peptide YY3–36 deficiency or seen in hypothalamic obesity due to craniopharyngioma. J Clin Endocrinol Metab 2005;90:2681–2690.
77 Swaab DF, Purba JS, Hofman MA: Alterations in the hypothalamic paraventricular nucleus and its oxytocin neurons (putative satiety cells) in Prader-Willi syndrome: a study of five cases. J Clin Endocrinol Metab 1995;80:573–579.
78 Moore SJ, et al: Clinical and genetic epidemiology of Bardet-Biedl syndrome in Newfoundland: a 22-year prospective, population-based, cohort study. Am J Med Genet A 2005;132:352–360.
79 Rahmouni K, et al: Leptin resistance contributes to obesity and hypertension in mouse models of Bardet-Biedl syndrome. J Clin Invest 2008;118:1458–1467.
80 Seo S, et al: Requirement of Bardet-Biedl syndrome proteins for leptin receptor signaling. Hum Mol Genet 2009;18:1323–1331.
81 Beales PL, et al: New criteria for improved diagnosis of Bardet-Biedl syndrome: results of a population survey. J Med Genet 1999;36:437–446.
82 Grace C, et al: Energy metabolism in Bardet-Biedl syndrome. Int J Obes Relat Metab Disord 2003; 27:1319–1324.
83 Benzinou M, et al: Bardet-Biedl syndrome gene variants are associated with both childhood and adult common obesity in French Caucasians. Diabetes 2006;55:2876–2882.
84 Holder JL Jr, Butte NF, Zinn AR: Profound obesity associated with a balanced translocation that disrupts the SIM1 gene. Hum Mol Genet 2000;9:101–108.
85 Faivre L, et al: Deletion of the SIM1 gene (6q16.2) in a patient with a Prader-Willi-like phenotype. J Med Genet 2002;39:594–596.
86 Wang JC, et al: A 5-Mb microdeletion at 6q16.--q16.3 with SIM gene deletion and obesity. Am J Med Genet [A] 2008;146A:2975–2978.
87 Bonaglia MC, et al: Detailed phenotype-genotype study in five patients with chromosome 6q16 deletion: narrowing the critical region for Prader-Willi-like phenotype. Eur J Hum Genet 2008;16: 1443–1449.
88 Michaud JL, et al: Sim1 haploinsufficiency causes hyperphagia, obesity and reduction of the paraventricular nucleus of the hypothalamus. Hum Mol Genet 2001;10:1465–1473.
89 Hung CC, et al: Studies of the SIM1 gene in relation to human obesity and obesity-related traits. Int J Obes (Lond) 2007;31:429–434.
90 Mason PW, Krawiecki N, Meacham LR: The use of dextroamphetamine to treat obesity and hyperphagia in children treated for craniopharyngioma. Arch Pediatr Adolesc Med 2002;156:887–892.
91 Ismail D, O'Connell MA, Zacharin MR: Dexamphetamine use for management of obesity and hypersomnolence following hypothalamic injury. J Pediatr Endocrinol Metab 2006;19:129–134.
92 Greenway FL, Bray GA: Treatment of hypothalamic obesity with caffeine and ephedrine. Endocr Pract 2008;14:697–703.
93 Lustig RH, et al: Octreotide therapy of pediatric hypothalamic obesity: a double-blind, placebo-controlled trial. J Clin Endocrinol Metab 2003;88:2586–2592.
94 Fernandes JK, et al: Triiodothyronine supplementation for hypothalamic obesity. Metabolism 2002;51: 1381–1383.
95 Danielsson P, et al: Impact sibutramine therapy in children with hypothalamic obesity or obesity with aggravating syndromes. J Clin Endocrinol Metab 2007;92:4101–4106.

Ze'ev Hochberg
Meyer Children's Hospital, Rambam Medical Center
Faculty of Medicine, Technion, Israel Institute of Technology
POB 9602, IL–31096 Haifa (Israel)
Tel. +972 4 854 2157, Fax +972 4 854 21 57, E-Mail z_hochberg@rambam.health.gov.il

Loche S, Cappa M, Ghizzoni L, Maghnie M, Savage MO (eds): Pediatric Neuroendocrinology.
Endocr Dev. Basel, Karger, 2010, vol 17, pp 197–214

Neuroendocrine Consequences of Anorexia Nervosa in Adolescents

Madhusmita Misra · Anne Klibanski

Neuroendocrine and Pediatric Endocrine Units, Massachusetts General Hospital and Harvard Medical School, Boston, Mass., USA

Abstract

Anorexia nervosa (AN) is a condition of severe undernutrition characterized by alterations in multiple neuroendocrine axes and peptides that signal or regulate energy intake. These alterations include a state of hypogonadotropic hypogonadism, a nutritionally acquired resistance to growth hormone (GH) with low IGF-1 levels, relative hypercortisolemia, low total T3 despite normal TSH, low levels of leptin and insulin, and elevated levels of ghrelin, peptide YY (PYY) and possibly adiponectin. Although many of these changes are adaptive to low weight, they can impact bone metabolism, body composition, reproductive function and statural growth. Low bone mass is characteristic of AN in both adolescent boys and girls. In girls, sites of trabecular bone are more likely to be affected than sites of cortical bone, whereas in boys with AN, sites of cortical bone are more commonly affected. Bone microarchitecture is also affected in adolescent girls with AN, with a decrease in trabecular thickness and bone trabecular volume, and an increase in trabecular separation. Important predictors of low bone density include nutritional factors, body composition, hypogonadism, low IGF-1, elevated cortisol and PYY levels, with possible contributions of low insulin. Weight gain is associated with a stabilization of bone density, although residual deficits persist in the short term, and in some cases, long term.

Anorexia nervosa (AN) is primarily a psychiatric disorder characterized by severe self-imposed nutritional deprivation and reduction in caloric intake associated with (1) weight loss, a failure to gain weight or to maintain weight leading to body weight that is less than 85% of what is considered ideal for age and for height, (2) BMI less than 17.5 kg/m^2 in older adolescents, (3) an intense fear of gaining weight, (4) an impaired body image, and (5) in postmenarchal girls, amenorrhea for at least three consecutive cycles [1]. 0.2–4.0% of adolescent girls and college aged young women suffer from this eating disorder, and this has been reported to be the third most

The author has consulted for Ipsen within the past year and has previously received grant support from Tercica.

common chronic illness in teenage girls [2]. In the restrictive form of AN, which is more common in adolescents, reduction in caloric intake is primarily a consequence of marked decreases in absolute fat intake, whereas protein and carbohydrate intake do not significantly differ from normal-weight healthy adolescents [3]. This nutritional deprivation is associated with significant alterations in various endocrine axes, and these are typically adaptive responses to a state of reduced energy availability. In addition, AN is associated with significant impairment of normal bone metabolism, a consequence of both the low energy state and of adaptive changes in various endocrine axes. This review describes alterations that occur in these endocrine axes in AN and reviews the pathophysiology underlying low bone density in adolescents with AN. Electrolyte abnormalities such as hypokalemia and hypophosphatemia can occur in patients with eating disorders, as well as hematologic abnormalities, but will not be reviewed here.

Hypothalamo-Pituitary-Gonadal Axis

AN is characterized by hypogonadotropic hypogonadism, and at this time, amenorrhea remains a necessary diagnostic criterion for AN according to the DSM-IV. The condition may present as primary or secondary amenorrhea, and in one study, 28% of adolescent girls 12–18 years old with AN were premenarchal compared to only 11% of healthy normal-weight adolescents of the same age range [4]. Studies by Boyar et al. [5] in adult women with AN have demonstrated that luteinizing hormone (LH) pulsatility reverts to either a prepubertal pattern of low amplitude LH pulses or an early pubertal pattern of nighttime entrainment of LH pulses. Of note, with recovery, the pattern of gonadotropin secretion recapitulates normal pubertal patterns. Estradiol levels in adolescent girls with AN are lower than in healthy adolescent girls, even when the latter are examined in the early follicular phase of their cycles when estradiol levels are at a nadir [4], and free testosterone levels trend lower in girls with AN than in controls [6]. Similarly, boys with AN have lower testosterone and estradiol levels than healthy adolescent boys [7].

Hypogonadotropic hypogonadism is likely the consequence of a marked reduction in energy availability associated with low fat mass, and resumption of menstrual function in girls with AN is associated with significant increases in fat mass [8] (fig. 1). In one study, all girls whose percent fat mass reached 24% resumed menstrual function, whereas none of the girls with percent fat mass of less than 18% resumed menses [8]. Research is ongoing to identify neuroendocrine factors that signal a state of low energy availability to hypothalamic neurons in, but possible signals include alterations in levels of hormones such as leptin, ghrelin, cortisol, insulin and IGF-1. Low leptin and high ghrelin levels have been demonstrated to predict lower levels of estradiol and gonadotropins in AN [9, 10]. Menstrual recovery is expected to occur within six months of weight gain (to 90% of ideal body weight) in girls with AN,

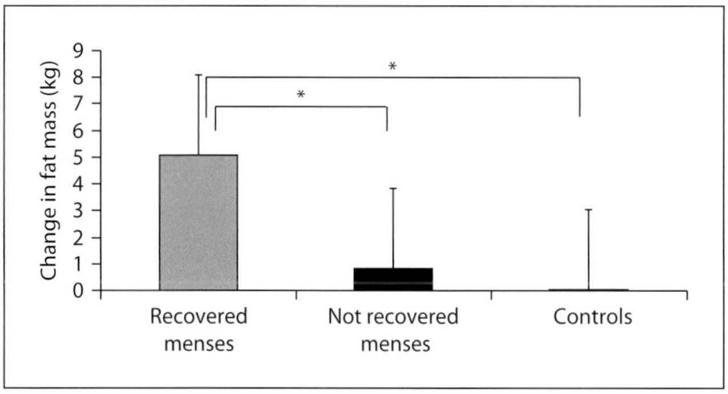

Fig. 1. Changes in fat mass in AN girls who recovered menses (n = 19) (gray bar), AN girls who did not recover menses (n = 14) (black bar) and controls (n = 33) (white). ANOVA demonstrated a significant difference between the groups ($p < 0.0001$). AN girls who recovered menses had greater increases in fat mass than AN girls who did not resume menses and controls ($p < 0.05$ for both). Reprinted with permission from Misra et al. [8].

however, this is not universal. A corresponding increase in fat mass is necessary, and persistent alterations in hormones such as ghrelin, leptin and cortisol may prevent resumption of menses in some instances even after adequate weight gain. In addition, some girls with AN who do not resume menses with weight gain have features of the lean form of polycystic ovary syndrome (PCOS), and examination for clinical and biochemical correlates of PCOS may become necessary in such instances. It is unknown whether such girls revert to a pre-morbid phenotype, or, whether weight gain in a subset of girls alters hypothalamic- pituitary-ovarian sensitivity.

Growth Hormone-Insulin-Like Growth Factor Axis

In adolescents with AN, levels of insulin-like growth factor-1 (IGF-1) are low despite high concentrations of growth hormone (GH), indicating a state of hepatic GH resistance that is nutritionally acquired [11, 12]. Low levels of GH-binding protein in adults with this disorder suggest that reduced expression of the GH receptor may account for resistance to GH effects [13]. IGF-1 levels are a direct marker of nutritional status and correlate inversely with GH concentrations [11]. Elevated GH concentrations appear to be a consequence of (1) reduced negative feedback from low IGF-1 levels resulting from inadequate liver production of IGF-1, (2) an increase in ghrelin, which is a GH secretatgogue [14], with the possible contribution of (3) low leptin levels [9–11, 15]. Deconvolution analyses indicate that increased GH concentrations in AN are consequent to increases in both basal and pulsatile GH secretion [11, 15], and the latter results from increased secretory burst frequency [11, 15] and burst mass [15] (fig. 2). Studies have proposed both a decrease in hypothalamic somatostatinergic tone

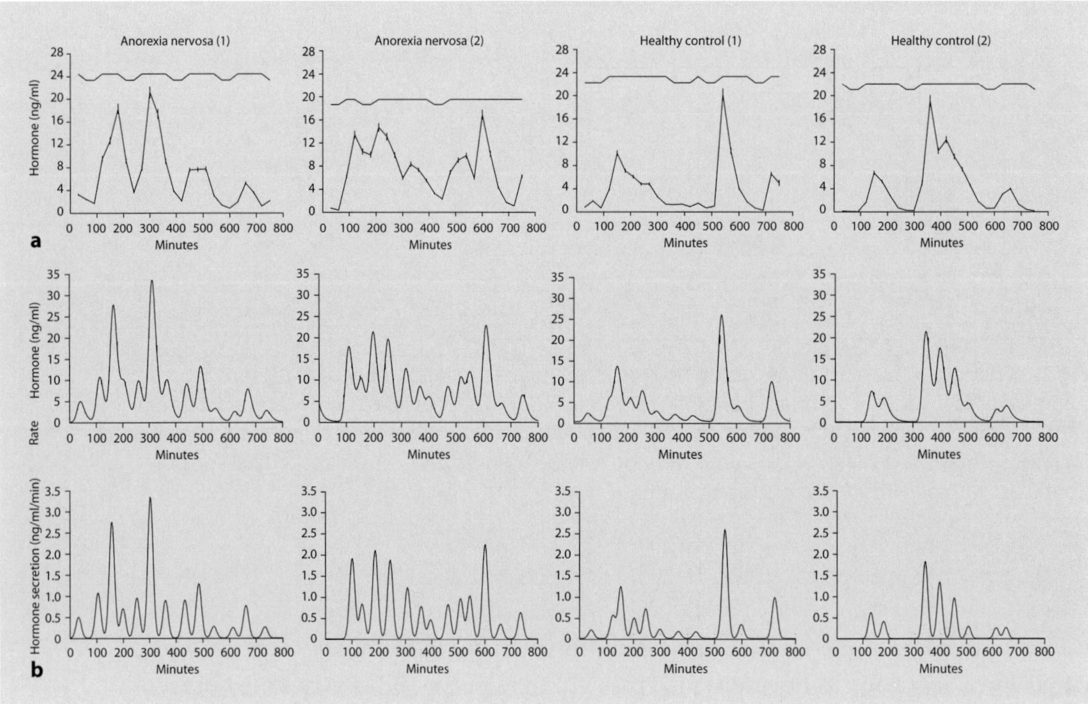

Fig. 2. Cluster and deconvolutional analyses in AN patients and controls. **a** Cluster analysis in 2 girls with AN (two left panels) and 2 healthy adolescent girls (two right panels). The mean and nadir GH concentrations and the total AUC were greater in girls with AN than in controls. **b** Deconvolutional analysis in the 2 girls with AN and the 2 healthy controls analyzed by cluster in **a**. The upper panels show GH concentrations over the sampling period; the lower panels show the individual secretory bursts. Girls with AN had higher basal GH secretion and a greater number of secretory episodes than healthy adolescents of comparable chronological and bone ages. Reprinted with permission from Misra et al. [11].

and an increase in gonadotropin hormone-releasing hormone pulses in AN, although definitive data are lacking [16]. Increased approximate entropy scores in AN in both adults and adolescents also indicate an increased disorderliness of GH secretion [11, 15]. Although absolute suppression of GH following an oral glucose load does not differ from controls, because baseline GH concentrations are higher in AN, nadir GH concentrations are also higher [17]. Weight gain is associated with an increase in IGF-1 levels and a lowering of GH concentrations. Because GH is a counter-regulatory hormone, an increase in GH concentrations in this state of severe undernutrition should help maintain euglycemia, and likely represents an adaptive response to an undernourished state.

IGF-binding proteins have been studied in AN, and the results are variable. IGFBP-1 and IGFBP-2 levels are typically high in AN and decrease with weight gain

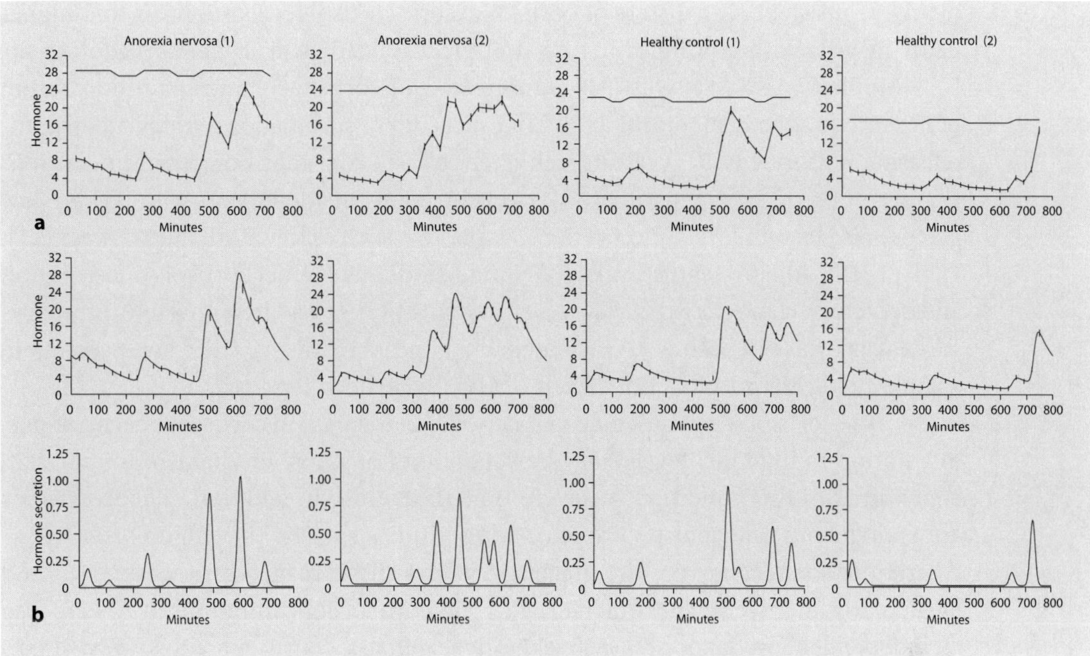

Fig. 3. Cluster analysis of cortisol concentration and deconvolutional analysis of cortisol secretion AN and healthy adolescents. **a** Cluster analysis in 2 girls with AN (two left panels) and 2 healthy adolescent girls (two right panels). Mean, nadir, valley mean, peak mass, peak amplitude of cortisol concentration, and total AUC were greater in girls with AN than in controls. **b** Deconvolutional analysis in the 2 girls with AN and the 2 healthy controls analyzed by cluster in **a**. The upper panels show cortisol concentrations over the sampling period, whereas the lower panels show the individual secretory bursts. Girls with AN had a greater number of secretory episodes than healthy adolescents of comparable CA and BA and higher pulsatile and total cortisol secretion. Reprinted with permission from Misra et al. [11].

[12, 13]. IGFBP-3 levels, however, have been variably reported to be low [12, 13] or normal in AN [6, 18], and unlike other catabolic states, AN is not associated with increased proteolysis of IGFBP-3 [19]. IGFBP-4 and IGFBP-5 have important effects on bone and are both very low in AN [20].

Hypothalamo-Pituitary-Adrenal Axis

Both 24-hour urinary cortisol concentrations and serum cortisol measured by frequent sampling overnight are higher in adolescent girls with AN compared with controls, associated with an increased frequency of secretory bursts and longer half-life [21] (fig. 3). The frequency of secretory bursts decreases following weight gain, with or without menstrual recovery. Diurnal rhythmicity of cortisol secretion is preserved in AN. Consistent with a state of cortisol excess, cortisol levels suppress to a higher nadir in girls with AN following an oral glucose load than in healthy adolescents [21]. Similarly, in adults with AN, suppression of cortisol following administration of dexamethasone is suboptimal [22] and subsequent stimulation with corticotropin-releasing hormone (CRH) results in higher cortisol concentrations than in controls. Important predictors of high cortisol concentrations in adolescents with AN are low glucose and insulin levels and nutritional markers such as low BMI and fat mass [21]. High ghrelin and low leptin levels in AN independently predict cortisol concentration and secretory characteristics. The level of activation of the hypothalamo-pituitary-adrenal axis has not been well elucidated, but appears to involve CRH hypersecretion, and elevated cerebrospinal fluid levels of CRH have been reported.

Because cortisol stimulates gluconeogenesis, an increase in cortisol concentrations, in addition to high GH levels, may be yet another adaptive mechanism to maintain euglycemia in this condition of severe undernutrition. In addition, glucocorticoids are endogenous antagonists of leptin. Some studies suggest that high cortisol concentrations in AN may predict greater increases in fat mass with recovery [8] and particularly an increase in trunk fat [23]. High cortisol concentrations in AN are also an independent predictor of lower extremity lean mass, consistent with known effects of cortisol on muscle [24].

Hypothalamo-Pituitary-Thyroid Axis

Changes in the hypothalamo-pituitary-thyroid axis in adolescents with AN are reminiscent of the sick euthyroid syndrome. TSH levels are usually normal, total T3 levels are low, and free T4 levels are normal or low normal [21]. The low T3 levels are consequent to increased peripheral deiodination of T4 to reverse T3 rather than T3. Total T3 levels correlate directly with measures of nutritional status in AN including BMI, fat mass, insulin, glucose, IGF-1 and leptin. A decrease in thyroid hormone levels could contribute to the low resting energy expenditure observed in AN, and preservation of consumed energy for vital functions. A blunted response of TSH to exogenously administered TRH has been previously reported in up to 50% of adults with AN [25]. Changes in thyroid hormones normalize with weight gain.

Peptides and Cytokines that Signal Energy Availability

Various peptides and cytokines are affected by the state of energy availability and may impact other endocrine axes and also bone metabolism. AN is associated with marked reductions in BMI and fat mass, and adolescents with AN have as much as a 50% reduction in fat mass and 40% reduction in percent body fat compared with normal-weight adolescents [4]. Consistent with reductions in fat mass, there is a marked reduction in the adipokine, leptin [10]. In addition, peptides regulating appetite, food intake and satiety are markedly altered in this state of nutritional deprivation, usually as adaptive phenomena [9, 10, 26]. In addition to leptin, data are available regarding levels of insulin, adiponectin, ghrelin and PYY in AN.

Insulin and Adiponectin

Low body weight and low fat mass in AN are associated with lower levels of fasting insulin and glucose compared with normal-weight adolescent girls [21, 27]. Measures of insulin resistance, such as HOMA-IR, are also markedly reduced in AN [27]. CT and MRI measures of regional body composition are limited in AN, however, reports using dual-energy X-ray absorptiometry indicate marked reductions in trunk fat, consistent with increased insulin sensitivity in AN [23, 28]. Adiponectin is an adipokine that mediates insulin sensitivity and resistance through effects on PPAR-γ, and levels of adiponectin have been variably reported to be elevated, unchanged or low in AN and may reflect difficulties assessing this adipokine in extreme states of reduced fat mass [27, 29–31]. Although adiponectin levels are typically high in conditions of increased insulin sensitivity, as observed in some studies of AN, it is also possible that high levels of adiponectin may not be evident if fat mass is markedly reduced given that adiponectin is secreted by adipocytes. In fact, in at least one study in which absolute adiponectin levels were reported to be unchanged compared with controls, levels were higher per unit fat mass in AN than in normal-weight controls [27].

Leptin

Leptin is an adipokine that correlates strongly with fat mass [10]. Adolescent girls with AN have almost 72% lower levels of leptin than normal-weight girls, associated with increases in the soluble leptin receptor, which is the binding protein for circulating leptin. The free leptin index, which is the ratio of leptin and the soluble leptin receptor is 84 % lower in AN than in controls [32]. Lower leptin levels in girls with AN are a consequence of reduced leptin burst mass and basal secretion, and are predicted strongly by fat mass [10]. Because leptin inhibits the orexigenic neuropeptide Y (NPY) and AgRP neurons and stimulates the anorexigenic POMC and CART neurons in the hypothalamus, low leptin levels in AN may represent an adaptive response to nutritional deprivation, and an attempt to suppress anorexigenic and facilitate orexigenic stimuli and thereby stimulate caloric intake. Leptin also has a potentiating effect on gonadotropin-releasing hormone neurons, and resumption of menstrual function in AN is associated with and may in part be mediated by an increase in leptin levels [8, 10]. Leptin concentrations increase with weight gain and an increase in fat mass, although this increase may not be evident with only partial weight recuperation. Interestingly, in contrast to girls with AN, boys with AN do not have lower leptin levels than normal-weight boys, despite lower fat mass [7]. Larger studies in boys are necessary to confirm these findings.

Ghrelin

Ghrelin is an orexigenic peptide that is secreted by the oxyntic cells of the stomach [33], and levels of ghrelin typically peak right before a meal and reach a nadir between 30 and 60 min following a meal. Ghrelin stimulates the NPY and AgRP neurons in the arcuate nucleus of the hypothalamus, and girls with AN have significantly higher ghrelin levels than normal-weight controls [9, 34]. Nadir ghrelin levels following an oral glucose load are higher in AN than in controls [9,17]. High ghrelin levels are a consequence of increased ghrelin secretory burst mass [9], and decrease with weight gain. Low insulin levels and lower HOMA-IR are important predictors of high ghrelin levels in AN, with other predictors being lower BMI, fat mass, IGF-1 and leptin. High ghrelin levels in AN are an indicator of low energy availability, and the increase in ghrelin is likely an adaptive response to stimulate hunger and food intake. In addition, ghrelin is a GH and ACTH secretagogue, and also has inhibitory effects on gonadotropin pulsatility as demonstrated in animal and human studies [35, 36]. In our studies, higher ghrelin levels in AN were an independent predictor of higher GH and cortisol and lower LH and estradiol levels [9]. Stimulation of ACTH and subsequently cortisol may also be an adaptive response to stimulate hunger. Importantly, in contrast to high ghrelin levels in girls with AN, levels in boys with AN are not significantly higher than in controls [7]. A recent study reports high levels of obestatin, a ghrelin gene product that inhibits appetite and gastric motility, in adults with AN [37] with positive associations with acyl- and desacyl-ghrelin, and inverse associations with BMI, glucose, insulin and leptin. Further studies are necessary to better understanding the implication of high levels of this hormone in AN.

Peptide YY

PYY is an anorexigenic peptide secreted by the L or endocrine cells of the distal gut in response to food intake. Levels rise within 15–30 min of food intake, and induce satiety through the binding of PYY to the Y2 receptor of NPY, which causes a reduction in NPY secretion. Typically, PYY levels would be expected to be low in AN as an adaptive response to a low energy state in order to reduce satiety, and would be expected to be high in obesity. However, contrary to expectations, adolescent girls with AN have high levels of PYY [26] whereas obese individuals have low levels of PYY [38]. PYY levels are predicted inversely by body weight and BMI, and the reason behind this paradox remains unclear at this time. Whether elevated PYY levels represent a more primary disease mechanism rather than an adaptation to starvation is unknown. Similar to girls with AN, PYY levels are high in boys with AN [7].

Other Hormones

There are limited data regarding other gut and hypothalamic peptides in AN. Activation of NPY neurons stimulates feeding behavior, and leptin, ghrelin and PYY all impact NPY secretion with consequent effects on appetite. It is unclear whether peripheral NPY levels in any way reflect central expression of NPY, and data regarding NPY levels in AN are conflicting. The serotoninergic system has been strongly implicated in eating disorders, and specific polymorphisms in the promoter of the 5-HT 2A receptor gene have been associated with restrictive AN and with reduced caloric intake. Similar to NPY, the importance of peripheral serotonin levels, which are gut rather than brain derived remains unknown in AN. Gut hormones such as GLP-1 and GLP-2, amylin, cholecystokinin, bombesin and gastrin inhibitory peptide are altered in states of energy deficit and excess; however, there are limited data regarding these hormones in AN.

Bone Metabolism

An important consequence of impaired nutrition and alterations in various neuroendocrine axes in AN is low bone density. This disorder can result in suboptimal bone mass accrual and marked reduction in bone mass at multiple skeletal sites. AN is characterized by impaired bone metabolism in both adults [39] and adolescents [4, 40] (fig. 4, 5). In adults, more than 90% of ambulatory nonhospitalized women with AN are osteopenic and almost 40% are osteoporotic by WHO criteria based on bone density assessment by dual-energy X-ray absorptiometry (DXA) [39]. In adolescents with AN, about half have Z-scores of < -1 at one or more skeletal site, and 11% have Z-scores of < -2 [4]. Both trabecular and cortical bone are affected in this condition, although trabecular bone appears to be affected more than cortical based on lower Z-scores (for adolescents) and T-scores (for adults) for the spine, than for the hip or femoral neck [4, 39]. In adolescents, low spine bone density is a consequence of decreased spine bone mineral content for bone area, with sparing of bone area for height. In contrast, low whole body bone density is a consequence of low bone area for height, with a sparing of bone mineral content for bone area [41]. Lower bone density as assessed by DXA is corroborated by reports of impaired bone microarchitecture as assessed by ultra-high resolution CT of the radius. Adults with AN have a decrease in trabecular number and bone trabecular volume and an increase in trabecular separation, as well as a decrease in cortical thickness [42]. In addition, in adults with AN, lower bone density at the spine is associated with greater marrow

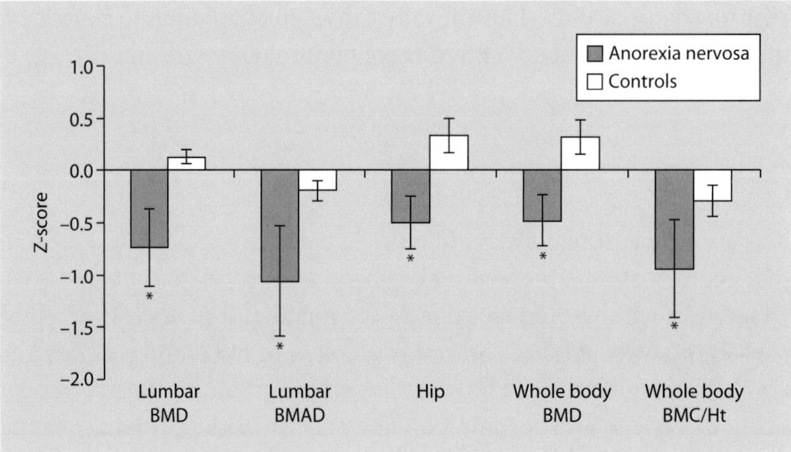

Fig. 4. Bone density Z-scores in adolescent girls with AN and controls. Z-scores for lumbar spine bone mineral density (BMD), lumbar spine bone mineral apparent density (BMAD), hip bone density, whole body bone density and whole body bone mineral content/height (BMC/Ht) were lower in girls with AN (black bars) than in healthy controls (white bars). * $p < 0.05$.

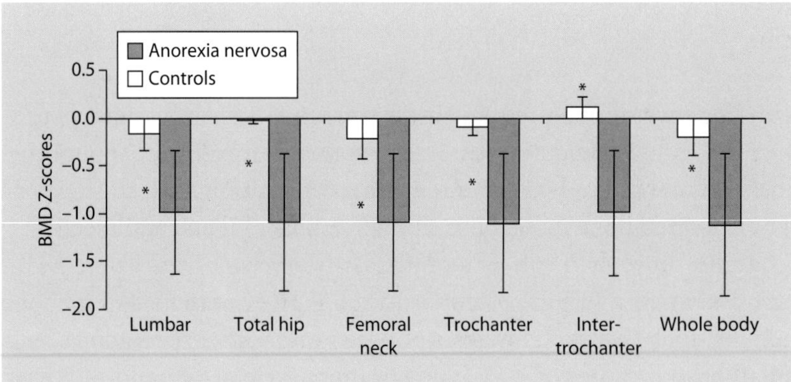

Fig. 5. Bone density Z-scores in adolescent boys with anorexia nervosa and controls. Z-scores of the lumbar spine, total hip and its sub-regions (femoral neck, trochanter, intertrochanteric region) and the whole body were significantly lower in boys with anorexia nervosa than in controls. * $p < 0.05$. Reprinted with permission from Misra et al. [7].

fat corroborating the bone-fat connection [43]. In adolescents with AN, trabecular thickness and bone trabecular volume are lower than in controls, whereas trabecular separation is increased [44].

Similar to females with AN, males with AN are also at high risk for low bone density. Adolescent boys and young men with AN have significantly lower bone density than normal-weight controls at all sites [7, 45]. However, unlike females, males with AN have greater involvement of the hip and femoral neck than of the spine [7, 45].

Bone turnover is uncoupled in adults with AN with a decrease in surrogate markers of bone formation and an increase in surrogate markers of bone resorption [46]. In male and female adolescents with AN, both bone formation and bone resorption markers are lower than in healthy adolescents, indicating a coupled decrease in bone turnover [6, 7, 47]. This is in contrast to normal adolescence, typically a high bone turnover state. With weight recovery, markers of bone formation and resorption both increase, and are predicted by the corresponding increase in lean mass and IGF-1 [48].

Nutritional markers such as BMI and lean mass are important determinants of low bone density in AN in both males and females [4, 6, 7], consistent with the known beneficial effects of weight loading and muscle pull on bone. In the absence of weight gain, girls with AN have a decrease in bone density and corresponding Z-scores over time [41, 48]. This is in contrast to healthy girls, who have the expected pubertal increase in bone mass and areal density, and maintain their Z-scores over the follow-up period. In one study, areal bone density at the spine decreased at an annual rate of 0.3% in girls not recovering weight or menses, and increased at the rate of 2.8% per year in normal-weight girls (fig. 6). Similar trends were observed with bone mineral content. Because the adolescent years are a critical time during which to optimize bone mass accrual towards attainment of peak bone mass, this decreased rate of bone mass accrual in AN is of significant concern. In fact, data indicate that individuals who develop AN during the adolescent years have lower subsequent bone density than those who develop this disorder in adult life, despite a similar duration of amenorrhea [49]. Of note, in girls with AN who gain weight and resumed menses, spine areal bone density increases at an intermediate rate of 1.4% per year, and bone mineral content for bone area at the spine, and bone area for height for the whole body also increase [41]. Although this rate of bone mass accrual falls short of complete catch-up, the trend is positive, emphasizing the importance of early and sustained weight gain and menstrual recovery in AN. Associated increases in lean mass with weight gain are an important predictor of increases in levels of bone turnover markers and bone density in girls with AN [48].

In adults with AN, in the absence of weight or menstrual recovery, women lose bone density at an annual rate of 2.6% at the spine and 2.4% at the hip [50]. Weight gain favors an increase in bone density at the hip, whereas menstrual recovery is associated with an increase in bone density at the spine, consistent with known effects of estrogen deficiency on trabecular bone density.

Although an optimal nutritional status is essential for optimizing bone mass accrual and calcium and vitamin D are nutrients essential for bone mineralization, multiple studies have demonstrated that adults and adolescents are not calcium or vitamin D deficient. Intake of calcium and vitamin D in this population is typically better than in controls, subsequent to increased use and patient acceptance of non-caloric supplements. Importantly, supplementation with calcium and vitamin D is not effective in increasing bone density in AN [6, 51].

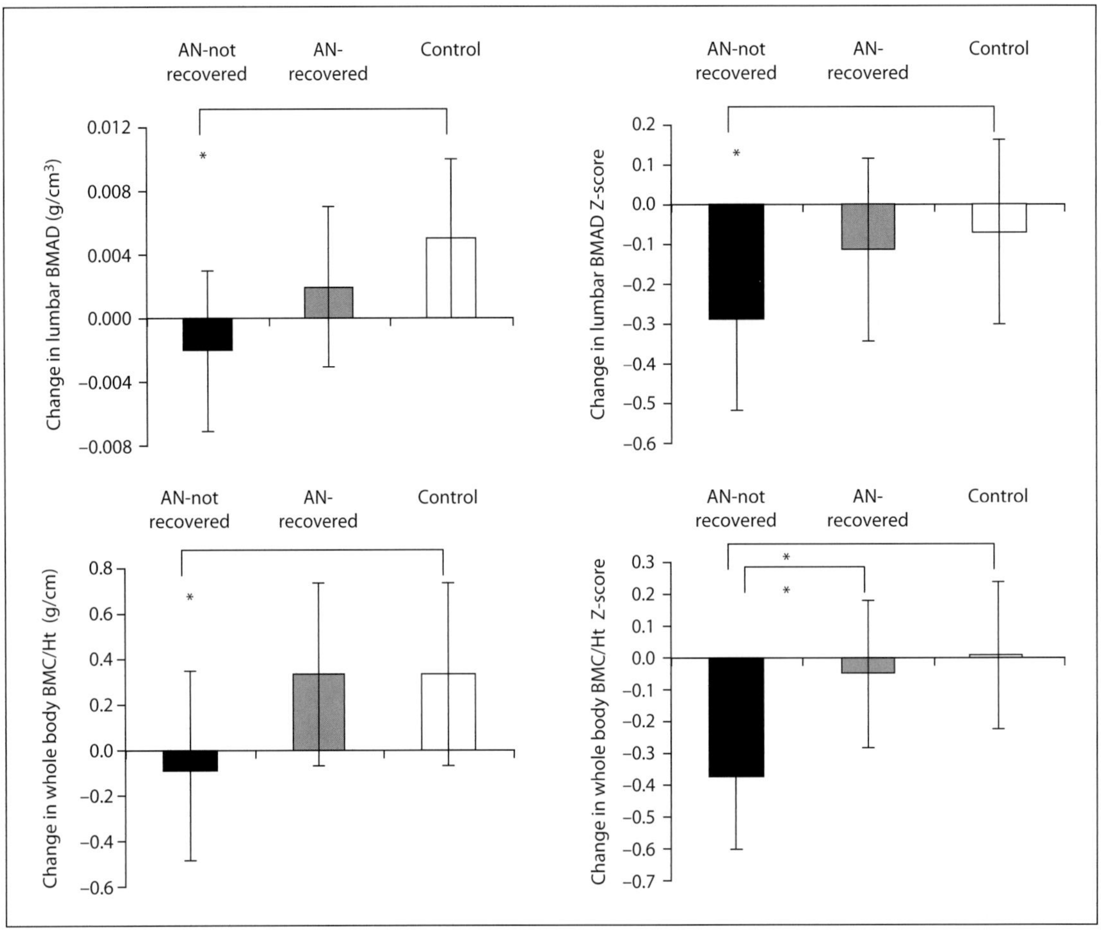

Fig. 6. Change in lumbar BMAD and WB BMC/Ht measures in AN-not recovered (black bar), AN-recovered (gray bar), and healthy adolescents (white bar). AN-not recovered continued to lose bone mass over the 1-year follow-up period, and change in bone density measures was significantly lower in this group, compared with controls (Tukey-Kramer test for multiple comparisons). AN-recovered did not differ from controls for change in bone density parameters and differed significantly from AN-not recovered for change in whole body bone density Z-scores. * $p < 0.05$. Reprinted with permission from Misra et al. [41].

Hormonal Determinants of Low Bone Density in Anorexia Nervosa

Hypogonadism

Hypogonadism is an important contributor to low bone density in AN. The duration of amenorrhea predicts the extent of bone loss in females with AN [40], and low testosterone levels are an independent predictor of low bone density in both boys and girls with AN [7, 48]. Estrogen is primarily antiresorptive and decreases osteoclast differentiation and activity through its effect on pro-inflammatory cytokines and the

RANK-RANKL-osteoprotegerin (OPG) pathway [52]. It inhibits secretion of the pro-inflammatory cytokines and increases OPG, with a consequent reduction in osteoclast differentiation and activation and an increase in osteoclast apoptosis. A state of hypogonadism would thus be expected to result in an increase in pro-inflammatory cytokines and a decrease in OPG. Levels of cytokines such as IL-6 are elevated in AN [27]; however, OPG levels are also high [53]. OPG levels correlate inversely with bone density measures suggesting that high OPG levels in AN may be an adaptive response to preserve bone mass. Testosterone has direct anabolic effects on bone but a major impact of its effect on bone metabolism is through its aromatization to estrogen [54].

Importantly, contrary to expectations, bone density does not increase with administration of oral estrogen in both adults and adolescent females with AN [51, 55, 56]. This has been attributed to IGF-1 and androgen suppressive effect of oral estrogens, although it is also possible that weight normalization is necessary for beneficial effects of estrogen replacement on bone. In addition, oral contraceptives may further decrease IGF-1 levels, and in adolescents, the doses of estrogen in such preparations may not be physiological. The effect of testosterone replacement on bone density in hypogonadal males with AN has not been reported. Data regarding levels of adrenal androgens in AN are conflicting with studies indicating either normal or low levels of DHEAS in adolescents and young adults with AN [48, 57]. Long-term DHEA administration does not increase bone density in AN after controlling for effects of weight gain [57].

GH Resistance and Low IGF-1

Another important cause of low bone density in AN is the state of GH resistance, with low levels of IGF-1, a hormone known to be anabolic to bone [11]. GH has direct and IGF-1 mediated effects on osteoblast and osteoclast differentiation and activity, and low IGF-1 levels in AN predict both lower bone density and lower levels of bone formation markers [6]. In addition, whereas GH concentrations are positive predictors of bone turnover markers in healthy adolescent girls, this association is absent in girls with AN, suggesting that the resistance to GH effects seen at the liver, may also occur in bone [11]. Increases in IGF-1 levels seen with weight gain are associated with increases in markers of bone formation and in bone density [6]. Short-term administration of rhIGF-1 at a dose of 30 mcg/kg twice daily selectively increases bone formation markers in adults with AN within days [58]. A higher dose of 100 μg/kg twice daily increases markers of both bone formation and bone resorption. Chronic administration of rhIGF-1 (30 μg/kg s.c. doses twice daily) with daily estrogen given as an oral contraceptive for nine months (an anabolic and an antiresorptive agent, respectively) caused a significant increase in spine bone density in adult women with AN [58]. This effect was not seen with estrogen alone, highlighting the importance of an anabolic agent in the treatment of this low formation state. This combination was associated with an increase in surrogate markers of bone formation and a decrease in surrogate markers of bone resorption, consistent with known effects of IGF-1 and estrogen on bone. It is important to emphasize that IGF-1 is locally produced by bone and the impact of circulating versus locally produced IGF-1 is unknown.

Other Hormones

Hypercortisolemia has multiple deleterious effects on bone. Cortisol excess inhibits osteoblasts and stimulates osteoclasts, impairs calcium absorption from the gut and the renal handling of calcium, and impacts negatively on the GH-IGF-1 axis. Cortisol levels are higher in both adults and adolescents with AN than in controls, and are an important and inverse predictor of bone density [21, 49]. In girls with AN, elevated cortisol concentrations independently predicted low levels of bone formation markers [21], again emphasizing the importance of weight gain and weight maintenance in AN.

Other possible determinants of low bone density include high levels of adiponectin (in relation to fat mass) [27], ghrelin [59] and PYY [26, 60] and low levels of insulin and leptin [27]. Adiponectin has been demonstrated to increase osteoclast activity through effects on RANKL and OPG, and ghrelin increases osteoblast activity in in vitro models. In addition, PYY, which acts through the Y2 receptor of NPY, may impact osteoblast activity based on data from the Y2 receptor knockout mouse, which demonstrates increased osteoblastic activity and high bone mass [61]. Thyroid hormones stimulate local IGF-1 secretion at the level of bone, and low total T3 levels may contribute to lower bone density by reducing local IGF-1 secretion. In adolescents with AN, high PYY and low levels of insulin are important predictors of lower levels of bone turnover markers [26, 27]. High PYY predicts lower bone density in adults with AN [60], and adiponectin is an inverse predictor of bone density measures in adolescents with AN [27]. Ghrelin was an independent predictor of bone density in controls, but not in an AN population, and one may postulate a resistance to ghrelin effects in AN given that effects of ghrelin on bone in controls seem to be mediated through increases in GH and cortisol by ghrelin [59].

Body Composition

Both fat and lean mass are lower in adults and adolescents with AN as compared to normal-weight controls. Regional fat distribution is also affected with a decrease in percent trunk fat and a decrease in the trunk/extremity fat ratio in adult and adolescent females with AN [23, 28]. With weight gain, percent trunk fat and trunk/extremity fat increase in girls with AN to approximate that in healthy adolescent girls [28]. In contrast, weight gain in adults with AN is associated with an increase in percent trunk fat during recovery such that this may exceed percent trunk fat in healthy adults [23].

Reassuringly, MRI measures of body composition indicate that although there is an acute increase in visceral fat with weight gain in adult women with AN to exceed that seen in controls, this normalizes over time with sustained weight gain. In adolescent girls with AN, high GH concentrations predict lower trunk fat, whereas high cortisol levels predict lower extremity lean mass [24]. Boys with AN have a sparing of trunk fat unlike females with AN, which appears to be related to their low testosterone levels [62].

Statural Growth

Reports have indicated lower than expected, normal and even higher than expected stature in girls with AN compared with genetic potential or controls [63–65]. Similarly, both height deficits and height within range of genetic potential have been reported in boys with AN [7, 66]. Whether or not height is affected may depend on the age of onset, severity and duration of the disease, and the pubertal stage of the specific individual. Greater severity and longer duration of the disorder, and onset of AN before puberty or in early puberty (when significant growth potential exists) may cause statural deficits. In contrast, later onset of AN (when growth is almost complete) would not be expected to cause significant statural deficits. Studies that have reported no change in height potential or height SDS in AN suggest that a delay in bone age associated with high GH concentrations (and direct GH effects on the growth plate) may cause a sparing of height deficits in adolescents with AN, particularly when the disease is not very severe [63].

Conclusion

AN is associated with adaptive changes in multiple endocrine systems leading to hypogonadotropic hypogonadism, a nutritionally acquired resistance to GH with low IGF-1 levels, relative hypercortisolemia, low levels of insulin and leptin, and high levels of ghrelin and adiponectin. In addition, PYY levels are high in AN. The adaptive changes, however, can cause significant pathology, particularly in the context of bone metabolism. Low bone density and impaired bone microarchitecture are important consequences of nutritional, body composition and hormonal changes in AN and in some patients bone deficits can persist throughout adult life.

Grant Support

This work was supported in part by NIH grant K23 RR018851.

References

1 Diagnostic and Statistical Manual of Mental Disorders, ed 3. Washington, American Psychiatric Association, 1987.

2 Lucas AR, Beard CM, O'Fallon WM, Kurland LT: 50-year trends in the incidence of anorexia nervosa in Rochester, Minn.: a population-based study. Am J Psychiatry 1991;148:917–922.

3 Misra M, Tsai P, Anderson EJ, et al: Nutrient intake in community-dwelling adolescent girls with anorexia nervosa and in healthy adolescents. Am J Clin Nutr 2006;84:698–706.

4 Misra M, Aggarwal A, Miller KK, et al: Effects of anorexia nervosa on clinical, hematologic, biochemical, and bone density parameters in community-dwelling adolescent girls. Pediatrics 2004;114:1574–1583.

5 Boyar RM, Katz J, Finkelstein JW, et al: Anorexia nervosa. Immaturity of the 24-hour luteinizing hormone secretory pattern. N Engl J Med 1974;291:861–865.

6 Soyka LA, Misra M, Frenchman A, et al: Abnormal bone mineral accrual in adolescent girls with anorexia nervosa. J Clin Endocrinol Metab 2002;87:4177–4185.

7 Misra M, Katzman DK, Cord J, et al: Bone metabolism in adolescent boys with anorexia nervosa. J Clin Endocrinol Metab 2008;93:3029–3036.

8 Misra M, Prabhakaran R, Miller KK, et al: Role of cortisol in menstrual recovery in adolescent girls with anorexia nervosa. Pediatr Res 2006;59:598–603.

9 Misra M, Miller K, Kuo K, et al: Secretory dynamics of ghrelin in adolescent girls with anorexia nervosa and healthy adolescents. Am J Physiol Endocrinol Metab 2005;289:E347–E356.

10 Misra M, Miller KK, Kuo K, et al: Secretory dynamics of leptin in adolescent girls with anorexia nervosa and healthy adolescents. Am J Physiol Endocrinol Metab 2005;289:E373–E381.

11 Misra M, Miller K, Bjornson J, et al: Alterations in growth hormone secretory dynamics in adolescent girls with anorexia nervosa and effects on bone metabolism. J Clin Endocrinol Metab 2003;88:5615–5623.

12 Scacchi M, Pincelli A, Caumo A, et al: Spontaneous nocturnal growth hormone secretion in anorexia nervosa. J Clin Endocrinol Metab 1997;82:3225–3229.

13 Counts D, Gwirtsman H, Carlsson L, Lesem M, Cutler G: The effect of anorexia nervosa and refeeding on growth hormone-binding protein, the insulin-like growth factors (IGFs), and the IGF-binding proteins. J Clin Endocrinol Metab 1992;75:762–767.

14 Takaya K, Ariyasu H, Kanamoto N, et al: Ghrelin strongly stimulates growth hormone release in humans. J Clin Endocrinol Metab 2000;85:4908–4911.

15 Stoving R, Veldhuis J, Flyvbjerg A, et al: Jointly amplified basal and pulsatile growth hormone secretion and increased process irregularity in women with anorexia nervosa: indirect eveidence for disruption of feedback regulatin within the growth hormone-insulin like growth factor-I axis. J Clin Endocrinol Metab 1999;84:2056–2063.

16 Stoving RK, Andersen M, Flyvbjerg A, et al: Indirect evidence for decreased hypothalamic somatostatinergic tone in anorexia nervosa. Clin Endocrinol (Oxf) 2002;56:391–396.

17 Misra M, Miller KK, Herzog DB, et al: Growth hormone and ghrelin responses to an oral glucose load in adolescent girls with anorexia nervosa and controls. J Clin Endocrinol Metab 2004;89:1605–1612.

18 Grinspoon S, Miller K, Herzog D, Clemmons D, Klibanski A: Effects of recombinant human insulin-like growth factor (IGF)-I and estrogen administration on IGF-I, IGF binding protein (IGFBP)-2, and IGFBP-3 in anorexia nervosa: a randomized-controlled study. J Clin Endocrinol Metab 2003;88:1142–1149.

19 Stoving RK, Flyvbjerg A, Frystyk J, et al: Low serum levels of free and total insulin-like growth factor I (IGF-I) in patients with anorexia nervosa are not associated with increased IGF-binding protein-3 proteolysis. J Clin Endocrinol Metab 1999;84:1346–1350.

20 Munoz MT, Argente J: Anorexia nervosa in female adolescents: endocrine and bone mineral density disturbances. Eur J Endocrinol 2002;147:275–286.

21 Misra M, Miller KK, Almazan C, et al: Alterations in cortisol secretory dynamics in adolescent girls with anorexia nervosa and effects on bone metabolism. J Clin Endocrinol Metab 2004;89:4972–4980.

22 Lawson EA, Misra M, Meenaghan E, et al: Adrenal glucocorticoid and androgen precursor dissociation in anorexia nervosa. J Clin Endocrinol Metab 2009;94:1367–1371.

23 Grinspoon S, Thomas L, Miller K, et al: Changes in regional fat redistribution and the effects of estrogen during spontaneous weight gain in women with anorexia nervosa. Am J Clin Nutr 2001;73:865–869.

24 Misra M, Miller KK, Almazan C, et al: Hormonal determinants of regional body composition in adolescent girls with anorexia nervosa and controls. J Clin Endocrinol Metab 2005;90:2580–2587.

25 Leslie RD, Isaacs AJ, Gomez J, Raggatt PR, Bayliss R: Hypothalamo-pituitary-thyroid function in anorexia nervosa: influence of weight gain. Br Med J 1978;ii:526–528.
26 Misra M, Miller KK, Tsai P, et al: Elevated peptide YY levels in adolescent girls with anorexia nervosa. J Clin Endocrinol Metab 2006;91:1027–1033.
27 Misra M, Miller KK, Cord J, et al: Relationships between serum adipokines, insulin levels, and bone density in girls with anorexia nervosa. J Clin Endocrinol Metab 2007;92:2046–2052.
28 Misra M, Soyka L, Miller K, et al: Regional body composition in adolescents with anorexia nervosa and changes with weight recovery. Am J Clin Nutr 2003;77:1361–1367.
29 Housova J, Anderlova K, Krizova J, et al: Serum adiponectin and resistin concentrations in patients with restrictive and binge/purge form of anorexia nervosa and bulimia nervosa. J Clin Endocrinol Metab 2005;90:1366–1370.
30 Pannacciulli N, Bunt JC, Ortega E, et al: Lower total fasting plasma adiponectin concentrations are associated with higher metabolic rates. J Clin Endocrinol Metab 2006;91:1600–1603.
31 Tagami T, Satoh N, Usui T, et al: Adiponectin in anorexia nervosa and bulimia nervosa. J Clin Endocrinol Metab 2004;89:1833–1837.
32 Misra M, Miller KK, Almazan C, et al: Hormonal and body composition predictors of soluble leptin receptor, leptin, and free leptin index in adolescent girls with anorexia nervosa and controls and relation to insulin sensitivity. J Clin Endocrinol Metab 2004;89:3486–3495.
33 Nakazato M, Murakami N, Date Y, et al: A role for ghrelin in the central regulation of feeding. Nature 2001;409:194–198.
34 Soriano-Guillen L, Barrios V, Campos-Barros A, Argente J: Ghrelin levels in obesity and anorexia nervosa: effect of weight reduction or recuperation. J Pediatr 2004;144:36–42.
35 Kluge M, Schussler P, Uhr M, Yassouridis A, Steiger A: Ghrelin suppresses secretion of luteinizing hormone in humans. J Clin Endocrinol Metab 2007;92:3202–3205.
36 Vulliemoz NR, Xiao E, Xia-Zhang L, et al: Decrease in luteinizing hormone pulse frequency during a five-hour peripheral ghrelin infusion in the ovariectomized rhesus monkey. J Clin Endocrinol Metab 2004;89:5718–5723.
37 Nakahara T, Harada T, Yasuhara D, et al: Plasma obestatin concentrations are negatively correlated with body mass index, insulin resistance index, and plasma leptin concentrations in obesity and anorexia nervosa. Biol Psychiatry 2008;64:252–255.
38 Batterham RL, Cohen MA, Ellis SM, et al: Inhibition of food intake in obese subjects by peptide YY3–36. N Engl J Med 2003;349:941–948.
39 Grinspoon S, Thomas E, Pitts S, et al: Prevalence and predictive factors for regional osteopenia in women with anorexia nervosa. Ann Intern Med 2000;133:790–794.
40 Soyka LA, Grinspoon S, Levitsky LL, Herzog DB, Klibanski A: The effects of anorexia nervosa on bone metabolism in female adolescents. J Clin Endocrinol Metab 1999;84:4489–4496.
41 Misra M, Prabhakaran R, Miller KK, et al: Weight gain and restoration of menses as predictors of bone mineral density change in adolescent girls with anorexia nervosa-1. J Clin Endocrinol Metab 2008;93:1231–1237.
42 Milos G, Spindler A, Ruegsegger P, et al: Cortical and trabecular bone density and structure in anorexia nervosa. Osteoporos Int 2005;16:783–790.
43 Bredella MA, Fazeli PK, Miller KK, et al: Increased bone marrow fat in anorexia nervosa. J Clin Endocrinol Metab 2009;94:2129–2136.
44 Bredella MA, Misra M, Miller KK, et al: Distal radius in adolescent girls with anorexia nervosa: trabecular structure analysis with high-resolution flat-panel volume CT. Radiology 2008;249:938–946.
45 Castro J, Toro J, Lazaro L, Pons F, Halperin I: Bone mineral density in male adolescents with anorexia nervosa. J Am Acad Child Adolesc Psychiatry 2002;41:613–618.
46 Grinspoon S, Baum H, Lee K, et al: Effects of short-term recombinant human insulin-like growth factor I administration on bone turnover in osteopenic women with anorexia nervosa. J Clin Endocrinol Metab 1996;81:3864–3870.
47 Misra M, Prabhakaran R, Miller KK, et al: Prognostic indicators of changes in bone density measures in adolescent girls with anorexia nervosa-II. J Clin Endocrinol Metab 2008;93:1292–1297.
48 Soyka L, Misra M, Frenchman A, et al: Abnormal bone mineral accrual in adolescent girls with anroexia nervosa. J Clin Endocrinol Metab 2002;87:4177–4185.
49 Biller B, Saxe V, Herzog D, et al: Mechanisms of osteoporosis in adult and adolescent women with anorexia nervosa. J Clin Endocrinol Metab 1989;68:548–554.
50 Miller KK, Lee EE, Lawson EA, et al: Determinants of skeletal loss and recovery in anorexia nervosa. J Clin Endocrinol Metab 2006;91:2931–2937.
51 Klibanski A, Biller B, Schoenfeld D, Herzog D, Saxe V: The effects of estrogen administration on trabecular bone loss in young women with anorexia nervosa. J Clin Endocrinol Metab 1995;80:898–904.

52 Riggs B: The mechanisms of estrogen regulation of bone resorption. J Clin Invest 2000;106:1203–1204.
53 Misra M, Soyka LA, Miller KK, et al: Serum osteoprotegerin in adolescent girls with anorexia nervosa. J Clin Endocrinol Metab 2003;88:3816–3822.
54 Riggs BL, Khosla S, Melton LJ III: Sex steroids and the construction and conservation of the adult skeleton. Endocr Rev 2002;23:279–302.
55 Golden NH, Lanzkowsky L, Schebendach J, et al: The effect of estrogen-progestin treatment on bone mineral density in anorexia nervosa. J Pediatr Adolesc Gynecol 2002;15:135–143.
56 Strokosch GR, Friedman AJ, Wu SC, Kamin M: Effects of an oral contraceptive (norgestimate/ethinyl estradiol) on bone mineral density in adolescent females with anorexia nervosa: a double-blind, placebo-controlled study. J Adolesc Health 2006;39: 819–827.
57 Gordon CM, Grace E, Emans SJ, et al: Effects of oral dehydroepiandrosterone on bone density in young women with anorexia nervosa: a randomized trial. J Clin Endocrinol Metab 2002;87:4935–4941.
58 Grinspoon S, Thomas L, Miller K, Herzog D, Klibanski A: Effects of recombinant human IGF-I and oral contraceptive administration on bone density in anorexia nervosa. J Clin Endocrinol Metab 2002;87:2883–2891.
59 Misra M, Miller KK, Stewart V, et al: Ghrelin and bone metabolism in adolescent girls with anorexia nervosa and healthy adolescents. J Clin Endocrinol Metab 2005;90:5082–5087.
60 Utz AL, Lawson EA, Misra M, et al: Peptide YY (PYY) levels and bone mineral density (BMD) in women with anorexia nervosa. Bone 2008;43:135–139.
61 Baldock PA, Sainsbury A, Couzens M, et al: Hypothalamic Y2 receptors regulate bone formation. J Clin Invest 2002;109:915–921.
62 Misra M, Katzman DK, Cord J, et al: Percentage extremity fat, but not percentage trunk fat, is lower in adolescent boys with anorexia nervosa than in healthy adolescents. Am J Clin Nutr 2008;88:1478–1484.
63 Prabhakaran R, Misra M, Miller KK, et al: Determinants of height in adolescent girls with anorexia nervosa. Pediatrics 2008;121:e1517–e1523.
64 Roze C, Doyen C, Le Heuzey MF, et al: Predictors of late menarche and adult height in children with anorexia nervosa. Clin Endocrinol (Oxf) 2007;67: 462–467.
65 Nussbaum M, Baird D, Sonnenblick M, Cowan K, Shenker IR: Short stature in anorexia nervosa patients. J Adolesc Health Care 1985;6:453–455.
66 Modan-Moses D, Yaroslavsky A, Novikov I, et al: Stunting of growth as a major feature of anorexia nervosa in male adolescents. Pediatrics 2003;111: 270–276.

Madhusmita Misra, MD, MPH
BUL 457, Neuroendocrine Unit, Massachusetts General Hospital
55 Fruit Street
Boston, MA 02114 (USA)
Tel. +1 617 724 5602, Fax +1 617 726 8528, E-Mail mmisra@partners.org

Author Index

Subject Index